Rheumatology
and Orthopaedics

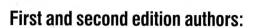

First and second edition authors:

Annabel Coote

Paul Haslam

Daniel Marsland

Sabrina Kapoor

Third edition authors:

Cameron Elias-Jones

Martin Perry

4th Edition
CRASH COURSE

SERIES EDITORS

Philip Xiu
MA, MB BChir, MRCP
GP Registrar
Yorkshire Deanery
Leeds, UK

Shreelata Datta
MD, MRCOG, LLM, BSc (Hons), MBBS
Honorary Senior Lecturer
Imperial College London;
Consultant Obstetrician and Gynaecologist
King's College Hospital
London, UK

FACULTY ADVISOR

Cameron Elias-Jones
FRCS (Tr + Orth)
Consultant Orthopaedic Surgeon
Glasgow Royal Infirmary
Glasgow, UK

Martin Perry
MBChB BSc (Hons), MRCP (UK), FHEA, MMEd
Consultant Rheumatologist and Physician
Honorary Senior Clinical Lecturer
Royal Alexandra Hospital, Paisley, UK;
University of Glasgow, Glasgow UK

Rheumatology and Orthopaedics

Marc Joseph Aitken
MBChB, MRCP (UK)
Rheumatology Specialist Trainee ST5
West of Scotland Deanery
University Hospital Wishaw
Wishaw UK

Anthony Gibson
BA Oxon(Hons), MBBS, MRCS
Speciality Registrar
Trauma and Orthopaedics
Royal Alexandra Hospital
Paisley, UK.

For additional online content visit StudentConsult.com

ELSEVIER

ELSEVIER

Content Strategist: Jeremy Bowes
Content Development Specialist: Alexandra Mortimer
Project Manager: Andrew Riley
Design: Christian Bilbow
Illustration Manager: Karen Giacomucci
Illustrator: MPS North America LLC
Marketing Manager: Deborah Watkins

First edition 1998
First edition 2004
Second edition 2008
Third edition 2013
Updated Third edition 2015
Fourth edition 2019

Notices

Practitioners and researchers must always rely on their own experience and knowledge in evaluating and using any information, methods, compounds or experiments described herein. Because of rapid advances in the medical sciences, in particular, independent verification of diagnoses and drug dosages should be made. To the fullest extent of the law, no responsibility is assumed by Elsevier, authors, editors or contributors for any injury and/or damage to persons or property as a matter of products liability, negligence or otherwise, or from any use or operation of any methods, products, instructions, or ideas contained in the material herein.

ISBN: 978-0-7020-7360-1
eISBN: 978-0-7020-7361-8

your source for books,
journals and multimedia
in the health sciences
www.elsevierhealth.com

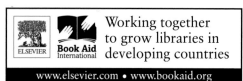
Working together
to grow libraries in
developing countries
www.elsevier.com • www.bookaid.org

The
publisher's
policy is to use
**paper manufactured
from sustainable forests**

Printed in Poland
Last digit is the print number: 9 8 7 6 5 4 3 2 1

Series Editors' foreword

The *Crash Course* series was conceived by Dr Dan Horton-Szar who as series editor presided over it for more than 15 years – from publication of the first edition in 1997, until publication of the fourth edition in 2011. His inspiration, knowledge and wisdom lives on in the pages of this book. As the new series editors, we are delighted to be able to continue developing each book for the twenty-first century undergraduate curriculum.

The flame of Medicine never stands still, and keeping this all-new fifth series relevant for today's students is an ongoing process. Each title within this new fifth edition has been re-written to integrate basic medical science and clinical ractice, after extensive deliberation and debate. We aim to build on the success of the previous titles by keeping the series up-to-date with current guidelines for best practice, and recent developments in medical research and pharmacology.

We always listen to feedback from our readers, through focus groups and student reviews of the *Crash Course* titles. For the fifth editions we have reviewed and re-written our self-assessment material to reflect today's 'single-best answer' and 'extended matching question' formats. The artwork and layout of the titles has also been largely re-worked and are now in colour, to make it easier on the eye during long sessions of revision. The new on-line materials supplement the learning process.

Despite fully revising the books with each edition, we hold fast to the principles on which we first developed the series. *Crash Course* will always bring you all the information you need to revise in compact, manageable volumes that still maintain the balance between clarity and conciseness, and provide sufficient depth for those aiming at distinction. The authors are junior doctors who have recent experience of the exams you are now facing, and the accuracy of the material is checked by a team of faculty editors from across the UK.

We wish you all the best for your future careers!

Philip Xiu and Shreelata Datta

Preface

Musculoskeletal problems represent an increasing problem in primary and secondary care as a result of an ageing population, the anticipated obesity epidemic and active sporting young adults. It is inevitable that all doctors will encounter patients with orthopaedic and rheumatological problems. Musculoskeletal medicine is a rapidly changing field, subject to much clinical and basic science research.

This *Crash Course* has been redesigned, rewritten and reformatted to help medical students develop a basic knowledge of diseases that affect the musculoskeletal system and the new understanding that underlies their pathologies and treatments.

We hope you enjoy reading and learning from this book and that it will help you pass your exams, and perhaps stimulate you toward a career in orthopaedics or rheumatology.

Marc Aitken, Anthony Gibson, Cameron Elias-Jones, Martin Perry

Acknowledgements

Thanks to my husband Paul and son William, for your endless support.

Marc Aitken

Thanks to Alison and Leon for their patience and help.

Anthony Gibson

To Audrey, my family and all those who supported me whilst working on this book.

Cameron Elias-Jones

Thanks to my retired Colleague Dr Max Field who helped me develop a love of medical education.

Martin Perry

FIGURE ACKNOWLEDGEMENTS

Dr Anna Ciechomska, Consultant, Rheumatology, University Hospital Wishaw, for supplying ultrasound images.

Dr Aziz Marzoug, Radiology Specialist Trainee ST2, Aberdeen Royal Infirmary, for supplying X-ray images.

Dr Stuart Gallacher, Core Medical Trainee CT1, University Hospital Wishaw, for participating in examination images.

Series Editors' acknowledgements

We would like to thank the support of our colleagues who have helped in the preparation of this edition, namely the junior doctor contributors who helped write the manuscript as well as the faculty editors who check the veracity of the information.

We are extremely grateful for the support of our publisher, Elsevier, whose staffs' insight and persistence has maintained the quality that Dr Horton-Szar has set-out since the first edition. Jeremy Bowes, our commissioning editor, has been a constant support. Alex Mortimer and Barbara Simmons our development editors have managed the day-to-day work on this edition with extreme patience and unflaggable determination to meet the ever looming deadlines, and we are ever grateful for Kim Benson's contribution to the online editions and additional online supplementary materials.

Contents

Contents

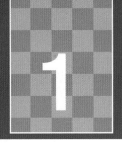

Taking a good history is vital in making a correct diagnosis. A clear history can often give many clues to diagnosis long before you have examined the patient or ordered any tests. It is important to establish a rapport and make the patient feel at ease: patients will find it easier to share information if they feel comfortable.

> **HINTS AND TIPS**
>
> Politely introduce yourself to the patient using your name and grade. Remember to ask for the patient's consent, particularly if you plan to take notes.
>
> The first points to document in your history are:
>
> - The patient's full name, date of birth, sex and hospital number.
> - The time, date and place of the consultation (e.g., Accident and Emergency Department).
> - The source of the referral, e.g., GP referral.

PRESENTING COMPLAINT

This is a short statement summarizing the patient's presenting symptoms, for example:

- Painful right knee.
- Stiffness and swelling in both hands.

HISTORY OF THE PRESENTING COMPLAINT

This should contain details of the patient's presenting symptoms from their onset to the current time. The following areas are important to discuss when taking a history:

> **COMMUNICATION**
>
> Begin your history taking with open questions, e.g., 'Tell me about your pain', then ask closed questions if necessary, e.g., 'Does your knee swell up?'

Symptom onset

- Date and time of symptom onset.
- Speed of onset: was it acute or insidious?
- Presence of precipitating and relieving factors such as trauma, other illnesses, medication use, etc.

Pain, swelling and stiffness

It is important to establish the following points:

- Site and radiation.
- Character, e.g., whether it is sharp or dull.
- Periodicity: is it continuous or intermittent?
- Exacerbating and relieving factors.
- Timing: is it worse at any particular time of day?

As a rule, pain and stiffness due to inflammatory conditions such as rheumatoid arthritis are worse first thing in the morning and improve as the day progresses. The duration of early morning stiffness (minutes–to–hours) is a good guide to the severity of the inflammation. By contrast, pain due to mechanical or degenerative problems tends to be worse later in the day, is associated with less severe stiffness and is worse with activity.

Warmth/erythema

Inflamed joints may appear red and feel warm to touch.

Deformity

Some patients consult their doctor because they have developed deformity and are concerned. These often occur in patterns associated with specific conditions. This may or may not be associated with pain.

Weakness

It is important to ascertain whether any weakness is localized or generalized. Localized weakness suggests a focal problem, such as a peripheral nerve lesion, whereas generalized weakness is more likely to have a systemic cause.

Fatigue

Many inflammatory conditions are associated with varying degrees of patient fatigue; this may even be the reason for the patient consulting a doctor in the first place.

Numbness

The distribution of numbness or paraesthesia should be documented, as well as any precipitating factors. For example, if the numbness affects the radial 3.5 fingers and is worse at night, it is probably due to carpal tunnel syndrome. If it affects all the digits, is associated with skin colour changes and is provoked by cold weather, Raynaud phenomenon is more likely.

Functional loss and disability

Loss of function refers to a person's inability to perform an action, such as gripping an object or walking. This is often why a person goes to see their doctor. Disability is a measure of the impact that loss of function has on a patient's ability to lead a full and active life.

HINTS AND TIPS

Always record a patient's functional level in the notes. It is a good marker of progress. Patient assessment questionnaires such as the Health Assessment Questionnaire Disability Index (HAQ-DI) are often used in patients with rheumatoid arthritis.

Any restrictions that a patient's disease has on activities of daily living should be documented.

MEDICAL HISTORY

Ask about all current and past medical and surgical disorders, including musculoskeletal problems. In certain situations it is worth asking about specific illnesses. For example, a patient with carpal tunnel syndrome may have underlying diabetes or hypothyroidism.

DRUG HISTORY

A patient's drug history is always important and sometimes has great relevance to orthopaedic and rheumatological problems. Acute gout can be precipitated by diuretic use and long-term corticosteroids can cause osteoporosis.

SOCIAL HISTORY

Record relevant information about the patient's occupation, their domestic situation, degree of independence, smoking history and alcohol intake. Ask about drugs and sexual history if appropriate. Record the patient's dominant hand.

FAMILY HISTORY

Ask about any family history of musculoskeletal disorders.

SYSTEMIC ENQUIRY

This should be brief but include other symptoms affecting other parts of the body. This is particularly relevant if you think the patient has a connective tissue disease.

● Chapter Summary

- An accurate history is vital to arriving at a correct and sensible differential diagnosis.
- Use open and closed questions to investigate a presenting complaint.
- Remember to ask about pain, swelling and stiffness: these often help to differentiate between mechanical and inflammatory causes.
- Functional questionnaires (such as HAQ-DI) help to quantify the functional impact of a patient's complaint on their activities of daily living.

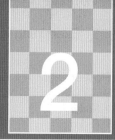
GENERAL PRINCIPLES

It is important to establish a rapport with patients. Dress smartly, be polite and carry identification.

Introduce yourself and start by asking if any areas are painful before you touch the patient. Note any aids such as a wheelchair, Zimmer frame or walking stick.

- Start with adequate exposure of the joint.
- Stand and walk the patient. Watch how they walk. Pathological gait patterns are shown in Table 2.1.
- Position the patient for the joint(s) to be examined. Ensure the patient is comfortable.

Remember that some musculoskeletal conditions are part of multisystem diseases. In the case of polyarthritis and those with inflammatory arthritis, it may be necessary to examine the cardiovascular system, respiratory system and the abdomen. For those with widespread aches and pain, examination of the nervous system may be required.

HINTS AND TIPS

As a general principle, always examine the joints above and below the affected joint.

CLINICAL EXAMINATION

Examination of a patient should be performed systematically and in a structured way. Use the following method:

- Look: check for swelling, muscle wasting, scars, erythema and deformity.
- Feel: palpate the joint, noting any effusions, tenderness and heat. Note any other prominent features.
- Move: demonstrate joint movement actively and passively.
- Examine areas above and below the joints.

Practice this routine on your friends; note how normal joints look, feel and move.

Table 2.1 Pathological patterns of gait

Gait	Features	Cause
Trendelenburg	Waddling gait	Loss of hip abductor function
Antalgic (painful)	The patient tries to offload the painful limb by quickening and shortening the weight-bearing stance phase of the gait cycle	Any painful condition
Short-leg gait	Dipping of shoulder on affected side	Any condition causing significant leg length discrepancy
High stepping	Knee is flexed and foot is lifted high to avoid foot dragging on the floor	Nerve palsy (peroneal or sciatic)
Stiff knee	Knee cleared of floor by swinging out away from the body	Fusion of knee

HINTS AND TIPS

Remember to check active and passive movement. In active movement, the patient moves the joint; in passive movement, the examiner moves the joint.

Peripheral nervous examination

Abnormalities of the structures of the back such as intervertebral disc prolapse can cause abnormalities of the peripheral nerves due to compression of the nerve roots. The most commonly affected are the L5 and S1 nerve roots. In the upper limbs, the most common peripheral neuropathies typically involve compression of the median nerve as it travels through the wrist (carpal tunnel syndrome).

Lower limb

Tone

Lower limb tone is usually normal but is reduced in spinal cord compression (flaccid paralysis).

Power

Power is assessed by Medical Research Council grades:

0: Nothing
1: Flicker
2: Power to move limb with gravity eliminated
3: Power to move limb against gravity
4: Reduced from normal
5: Normal

   Test muscle functions are shown in Table 2.2.

Reflexes

Always compare the reflexes between the two limbs and make sure the patient is relaxed. Reflexes can be present, reduced, brisk or absent.

   Three reflexes are commonly tested:

- Knee L3-L4: flex both knees over the couch or your arm and tap lightly on the patellar tendon.
- Ankle L5-S1: dorsiflex the ankle with the knees flexed and the leg externally rotated. Tap the Achilles tendon.
- Plantar: this is performed by stoking the handle of the tendon hammer up the plantar skin from the heel towards the big toe. If the toe extends, this is abnormal and is 'upgoing', indicating an upper motor neurone lesion.

Sensation

Ask the patient whether the sensation is normal for them and the same as the other side. Dermatomes are shown in Fig. 2.1.

Anal tone and perianal sensation

In cauda equina syndrome, anal tone is lost and perianal sensation reduced; therefore a per rectal examination is an important part of any spinal examination.

Upper limb

Tone

This is usually normal unless there is a lesion in the cervical spine or injury to the brachial plexus.

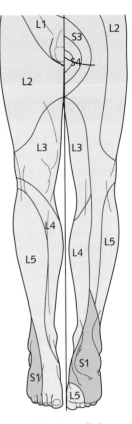

Fig. 2.1 Dermatomes of the lower limb. *L*, Lumbar; *S*, sacral.

Power

Upper limb function can be tested as shown in Table 2.3. The innervation of the upper limb muscles is more complex than in the lower limb.

Reflexes

Three reflexes are commonly tested:

- Biceps C5–C6: place your finger over the biceps brachii tendon as it passes through the cubital fossa at the elbow. Tap your finger with the tendon hammer.

Table 2.2 Testing lower-limb muscle function (myotomes)

Muscle action	Nerve roots tested
Hip flexion (iliopsoas)	L1, L2
Knee flexion (quadriceps)	L3
Ankle dorsiflexion (tibialis anterior)	L4
Great toe extension (extensor hallucis longus)	L5
Ankle plantar flexion (soleus/ gastrocnemius)	S1

Table 2.3 Testing upper-limb function (myotomes)

Muscle action	Nerve root tested
Shoulder Abduction	C5
Shoulder Adduction	C6, C7
Elbow Flexion	C5, C6
Elbow Extension	C7, C8
Wrist Flexion/Extension	C6, C7
Metacarpophalangeal/ interphalangeal flexion/extension	C7, C8
Metacarpophalangeal abduction/ adduction	T1

- Triceps C7: with the elbow at 90 degrees, place your finger over the triceps tendon and tap lightly with the tendon hammer.
- Brachioradialis C6–C7: tap the brachioradialis tendon about 4 inches proximal to the base of the thumb as it inserts into the radial styloid process.

Sensation

Ask the patient if sensation is the same on both sides. Upper limb dermatomes are shown in Fig. 2.2.

EXAMINATION OF THE HIP

Hip disease is common and examination follows the pattern of look, feel, move. True hip pain is often felt in the groin and may radiate to the knee on movement.

The examiner starts by observing the patient walk from the waiting area. A Trendelenburg (waddling) gait is due to failure of the hip abductors to elevate the pelvis on weight bearing, causing a dipping or rolling gate (Fig. 2.3). To compensate for this, the trunk is thrown over the weight-bearing hip, which maintains balance.

Failure of hip abduction can be due to pain or as a complication following surgery.

The patient may also have an antalgic gait (see Table 2.1).

Look

Scars from previous surgery could be present anteriorly, laterally or medially. Look for erythema, obvious deformity and muscle wasting, particularly over the quadriceps

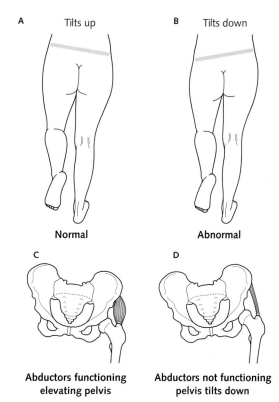

Fig. 2.3 The Trendelenburg test.

muscles. As the hip is a deep joint, swelling can be difficult to see. Look at both sides of the hip by turning the patient to the prone position.

True leg-length discrepancy

Ensure the patient is lying comfortably on the examination couch with both knees straight. Measure both limbs from the anterior superior iliac spine to the medial malleolus and compare the values.

Flexing the hips and knees and placing them together can give an idea of where the discrepancy occurs. Look from side to side to determine the position of knees.

If one knee is higher than the other, this suggests tibial shortening. However, if one knee lies behind the other, it suggests a femoral discrepancy (Fig. 2.4).

Feel

The hip is deeply situated and few features are palpable. The greater trochanter is easily felt laterally, over which bursitis may be present.

Move

Normal movements are shown in Fig. 2.5.

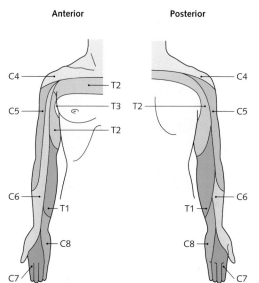
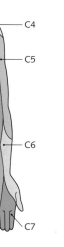

Fig. 2.2 Dermatomes of the upper limb. *C,* Cervical; *T,* thoracic.

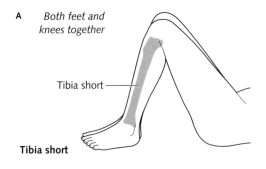

A *Both feet and knees together*

Tibia short

Tibia short

B

Femur short

Femur short

Fig. 2.4 Assessing leg-length discrepancy.

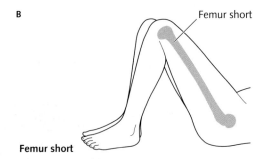

HINTS AND TIPS

When assessing hip movements, remember to stabilize the pelvis with the hand to ensure that pelvic tilting does not occur.

Trendelenburg test

This is used to assess the function of the hip abductors.

Stand face-on to the patient and put your hands on the patient's pelvis, then ask the patient to place their hands on your forearms lightly to steady themselves. Ask the patient to lift each leg in turn and watch for pelvic tilting. Remember that you are testing the standing leg and the patient should lift their other leg up behind them by flexing the knee. Flexing the hip can tilt the pelvis.

If the abductors on the standing leg are not working properly, the pelvis tilts towards the unsupported leg (Figs 2.3B and D).

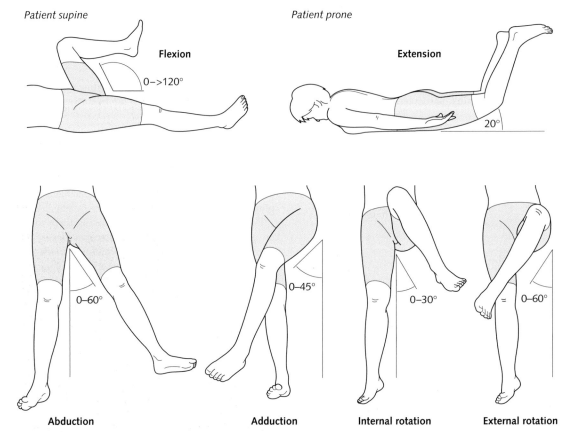

Patient supine

Flexion

$0->120°$

Patient prone

Extension

$20°$

Abduction $0–60°$

Adduction $0–45°$

Internal rotation $0–30°$

External rotation $0–60°$

Fig. 2.5 Movements of the hip (note that all ranges are approximate and vary from patient to patient).

Thomas test

This is a test for fixed flexion of the hip.

The purpose of the test is to abolish the natural lordosis of the lumbar spine and to visualize the true degree of flexion deformity at the hip.

To perform the test, the patient is positioned supine (flat on the back) and the opposite hip is flexed fully. The manoeuvre fully corrects the lordosis that is felt by placing the hand under the spine. Now simply observe any degree of flexion (if any) in the opposite hip (Fig. 2.6).

EXAMINATION OF THE KNEE

The knee lies superficially and many landmarks are easily palpable.

Look

- Look for quadriceps wasting, which can be assessed by measuring the thigh circumference and comparing with the other side.
- Localized swelling anteriorly and posteriorly may be visible.
- Note any effusions (which can be seen by loss of the normal skin dimples at the joint line), scars, erythema or evidence of psoriasis.
- Look for surgical scars.
- Ask the patient to stand and walk; note any gait abnormalities.
- Deformities (varus, valgus and fixed flexion) are more obvious on standing.

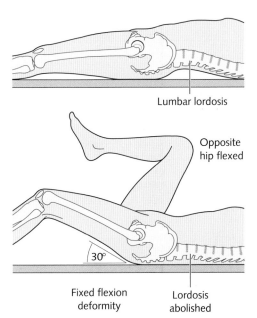

Lumbar lordosis

Opposite hip flexed

30°

Fixed flexion deformity

Lordosis abolished

Fig. 2.6 The Thomas test for fixed flexion of the hip.

COMMON PITFALLS

Posterior swelling of the knee is easily missed. Ask the patient to stand and examine them from behind.

Feel

Flexing the knee to 90 degrees allows structures to be palpated more easily. Feel for warmth in the knees with the back of the hand.

Be methodical, starting distally over the tibial tuberosity and moving proximally, palpating in turn the patellar tendon, proximal tibia, medial and lateral joint lines, femoral condyles, patella and quadriceps tendon (Fig. 2.7). The collateral ligaments are also palpable.

RED FLAG

Remember to palpate the posterior aspect of the knee. A Baker's cyst or bursa may be present!

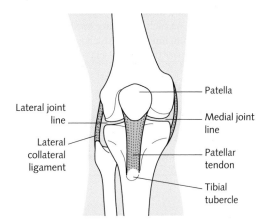

Patella

Lateral joint line

Medial joint line

Lateral collateral ligament

Patellar tendon

Tibial tubercle

Fig. 2.7 Anatomical structures easily palpated around the knee.

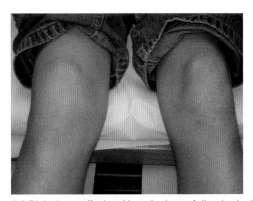

Fig. 2.8 Right knee effusion. Note the loss of dimples in the thigh and under the patella.

It is important to recognize a knee effusion (Fig. 2.8), as it always indicates pathology. There are two tests commonly used to confirm this: the patellar tap and the swipe test.

Patellar tap

Fluid is forced from the suprapatellar pouch, which lifts the patella away from the femur. The patella is then pushed down on the femur, producing a palpable tap (Fig. 2.9).

Swipe test

Fluid is forced out of the medial compartment. The examining hand then sweeps fluid from the lateral side of the knee, refilling the medial compartment with a visible bulge.

Move

Both active and passive movements should be tested. The normal range of movement is 0–150 degrees (Fig. 2.10). Note any fixed flexion or hyperextension of the knee. Feel for patellar crepitus during flexion.

Medial and lateral collateral ligaments

Patients have differing degrees of laxity of the ligaments. It is therefore important to compare your findings with the healthy side. Flex the knee to 15 degrees and alternately stress the joint line on each side. Place one hand on the opposite side of the joint line to that which is being tested and apply force to the lower tibia (Fig. 2.11).

Anterior cruciate ligament

Anterior draw test

This is a test for anterior cruciate ligament (ACL) deficiency but can be misleading because it can also be positive after medial meniscectomy or in posterior cru-

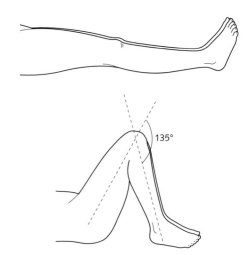

Fig. 2.10 Range of movement of the knee.

ciate ligament (PCL) deficiency. The knee is flexed to 90 degrees and the hamstrings are relaxed. The examiner carefully sits on the patient's foot and both thumbs are placed on the proximal tibia and over both joint lines. The tibia is pulled forward and, if movement is excessive, the test is positive.

COMMUNICATION

Testing the anterior cruciate ligament can be uncomfortable for patients. Remember to explain clearly the test before performing it.

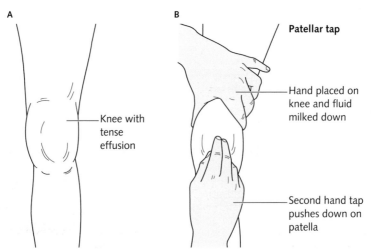

A

Knee with tense effusion

B

Patellar tap

Hand placed on knee and fluid milked down

Second hand tap pushes down on patella

Fig. 2.9 The patellar tap sign.

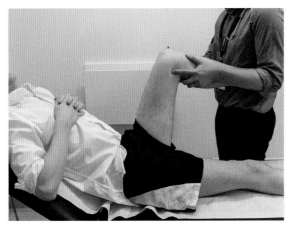

Fig 2.11 Collateral ligament examination.

Posterior cruciate ligament

The posterior drawer test is performed exactly the same way as the anterior drawer test, but the knee is pushed backwards.

The classic sign of PCL rupture is posterior sag. This is demonstrated by flexing both knees to 90 degrees and comparing the knee contour (Fig. 2.12). A sag occurs because the tibia falls posteriorly and the tibial tuberosity becomes less prominent.

EXAMINATION OF THE ANKLE AND FOOT

Look

Inspect the ankle and foot with the patient in both resting and weight-bearing positions. Observe nails and skin for psoriatic changes. Look at the distribution of any swelling. Synovitis of the ankle usually produces diffuse swelling, obscuring the contours of the medial and lateral malleoli. Swelling in the region of the Achilles tendon is more likely to be due to Achilles tendinopathy or tendon rupture.

Disease of the subtalar joint or abnormalities of the longitudinal arch of the foot may disrupt the alignment of the heel and Achilles tendon. This should be vertical and is easily seen when observing from behind a standing patient. Pes planus (flat foot) can cause pronation of the foot and valgus deformity of the heel (Fig. 2.13).

Forefoot issues are common. Hallux valgus is a deformity of the great toe, which becomes abducted at the metatarsophalangeal (MTP) joint. Excessive pressure on the medial side can lead to formation of a bursa, often called a bunion. Look at the patient's footwear for signs of excessive wear. Fig. 2.14 shows other common forefoot deformities.

Feel

Feel for warmth. Palpate the ankle joint, subtalar joint, forefoot and squeeze the MTP joints to elicit any discomfort.

HINTS AND TIPS

Do not forget to feel the Achilles tendon and check its integrity. This can be done by elevating the leg and gently squeezing the calf muscle, observing for plantarflexion of the foot.

Move

Test plantar flexion and dorsiflexion of the ankle with the knee flexed. The subtalar joint allows inversion and eversion of the hindfoot. This is tested by stabilizing the tibia with one hand and turning the calcaneus inward and outward with the other.

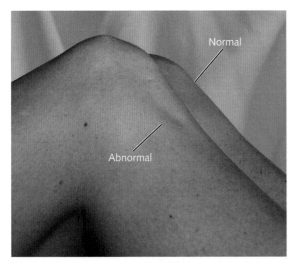

Normal

Abnormal

Fig. 2.12 Posterior sag sign. The right knee shows the positive sign. Note that the tibial tuberosity is more prominent on the left.

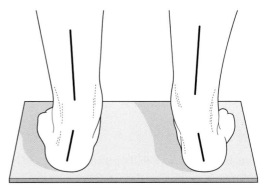

Fig. 2.13 Pes planus with pronation of the feet and hindfoot valgus.

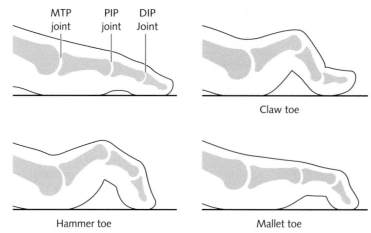

Fig. 2.14 Common deformities of the forefoot.
DIP, Distal interphalangeal; *MTP*, metatarsophalangeal; *PIP*, proximal interphalangeal.

Midtarsal movements contribute to plantar flexion, dorsiflexion, inversion and eversion. These are tested by stabilizing the heel with one hand and moving the foot with the other. Movements of the MTP joints, proximal interphalangeal (PIP) joints and distal interphalangeal (DIP) joints are best examined actively while the patient is lying or sitting.

EXAMINATION OF THE SPINE

When examining the spine, remember to perform a peripheral nervous system examination.

Look

Assess the patient's posture. Check for cervical lordosis, thoracic kyphosis and lumbar lordosis. If the patient has sciatica, the affected leg is often flexed and the posture stooped. Muscle wasting, asymmetry and scoliosis may be present.

HINTS AND TIPS

In scoliosis, the rib hump deformity is more clearly seen when the patient bends forward (see Fig. 9.11).

Feel

Palpation is performed with the patient standing and lying prone.

Feel the spinous processes, the paraspinal muscles and the sacroiliac joints for tenderness.

Move

Cervical spine

Movements of the cervical spine (Fig. 2.15) are usually stated as percentage loss when compared with normal.

Flexion

Ask the patient to bend their head forward to put their chin on their chest.

Extension

Ask the patient to look towards the ceiling.

Lateral flexion

Ask the patient to put their ear down towards their shoulder.

Rotation

Ask the patient to look to either side.

Thoracolumbar spine (Fig. 2.16)

Flexion

Patients are often reluctant to flex the spine if it is acutely tender. Ask the patient to bend over, keeping their knees extended, and reach as far as they can.

Look and feel for movement of the lumbar spine. This can be done by marking two points on the lumbar spine and observing the increase in distance between them on flexion. This is known as the Schrober test (discussed further in Chapter 13).

Extension

Ask the patient to arch their back backwards. In conditions such as spinal stenosis, this can exacerbate pain.

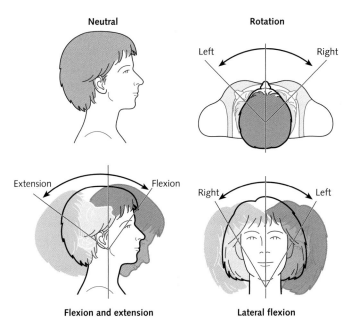

Neutral

Rotation

Left   Right

Extension   Flexion

Right   Left

Flexion and extension

Lateral flexion

Fig. 2.15 Movements of the cervical spine.

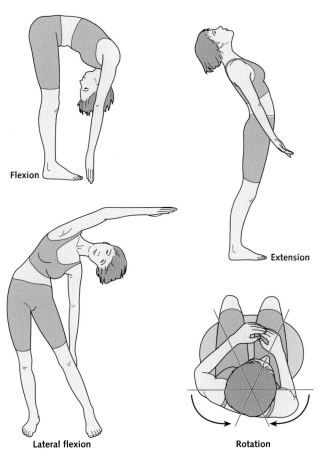

Flexion

Extension

Lateral flexion

Rotation

Fig. 2.16 Thoracolumbar spinal movements.

Rotation

With the patient sitting on a bed to fix the pelvis and with their arms crossed in front, ask the patient to turn from side to side.

Lateral flexion

Ask the patient to slide one hand down the side of their leg and observe.

Special tests

Straight-leg raise

Straight-leg raising is a test for radiculopathy (nerve root irritation).

With the patient supine, elevate the affected leg passively, keeping it straight. If the patient complains of pain down the leg, look at the angle that the leg makes with the couch, e.g., 30 degrees. The next step is to bend the knee, as this will abolish the symptoms by relieving tension on the nerve.

For the test to be positive, the pain must radiate to the foot (often patients will complain of back pain when raising the leg).

EXAMINATION OF THE SHOULDER

Movement of the shoulder is complex and occurs at four joints (Fig. 2.17). The majority of the total range of movement arises from the glenohumeral and scapulothoracic joints.

Look

Look at the position and contours of the shoulder from the front, side and behind and compare with the opposite side.

- Swelling of the shoulder is uncommon but is best seen anteriorly.

- Muscle wasting may occur due to chronic shoulder pathology, such as rotator cuff tendinopathy.
- Scars from shoulder replacement are usually anterior.

Feel

Palpate for tenderness over the acromioclavicular, sterno-clavicular and glenohumeral joints. A gap on palpation of the acromioclavicular joint indicates dislocation. Feel for warmth, comparing both sides. Palpate the surrounding muscles for tenderness.

Move

Examine active and passive movements, looking at the range of abduction, forward flexion, and internal and external rotation.

A quick way to evaluate active shoulder movements is by asking the patient:

- To put their hands behind their head with the elbows back (external rotation/abduction, flexion).
- To reach behind their back, as if to fasten a bra strap (internal rotation, adduction, extension).
- To raise their arms behind them (extension) and to the front (flexion).

A normal range of passive movements means glenohumeral disease is unlikely.

HINTS AND TIPS

Normal passive movement with painful or restricted active shoulder movements suggests a muscle or tendon problem.

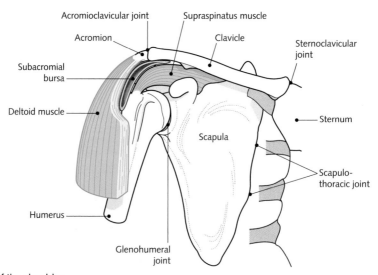

Fig. 2.17 Anatomy of the shoulder.

A hitch-up of the shoulder on active abduction of the arm is a sign of reduced glenohumeral range (Fig. 2.18).

- Loss of passive external rotation and abduction are highly indicative of adhesive capsulitis (frozen shoulder).
- Scapular movements should be assessed from behind during the range of movements. 'Winging' is a common sign of serratus anterior dysfunction, caused by damage to the long thoracic nerve.

The rotator cuff

The supraspinatus, infraspinatus, teres minor and subscapularis muscles make up the rotator cuff. They hold the head of the humerus in the glenoid cavity, maintain stability and initiate shoulder abduction. Rotator cuff inflammation, injury and degeneration are common. Disease of the supraspinatus especially causes pain on abduction when the tendon becomes depressed beneath the acromion. The pain is felt at between 60 and 120 degrees of abduction. This is what is referred to as a 'painful arc' (see Fig. 2.19).

Resisted shoulder movement should be examined. Pain or weakness on resisted movements suggests involvement of the rotator cuff muscles and tendons.

- Supraspinatus is tested with the arm abducted to 30 degrees, flexed to 30 degrees and internally rotated with the thumb pointing down. Abduction is then resisted.
- Subscapularis is tested with resisted internal rotation.
- Infraspinatus and teres minor are tested with resisted external rotation.

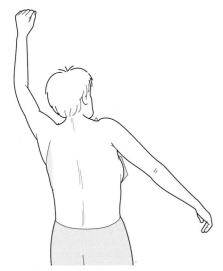

Fig. 2.18 A 'hitched' shoulder. The patient is unable to elevate the arm to the side properly and is 'cheating' by shrugging the right shoulder.

EXAMINATION OF THE ELBOW

The elbow consists of two articulations. The first is between the humerus, radius and ulna, which allows flexion to 150 degrees. The second is the superior radioulnar joint, which allows rotation of the wrist through 180 degrees.

Look

Examine the elbow in flexion and extension looking for scars, muscle wasting, fixed flexion, swelling, erythema, rheumatoid nodules and psoriatic plaques. Olecranon bursitis may be seen as a 'golf-ball' swelling over the elbow.

Feel

Feel for warmth. Palpate the olecranon process and medial and lateral epicondyles. The medial will be tender in golfer's

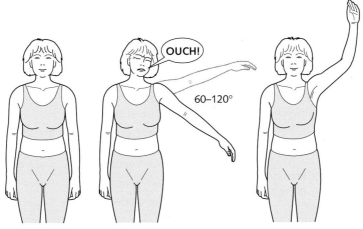

Fig. 2.19 Demonstration of the painful arc.

elbow; the lateral is tender in tennis elbow. The radial head is usually felt easily in the lateral aspect of the joint and its movement can be assessed in pronation and supination.

Move

Test flexion and extension, pronation and supination. Extension of the elbow to 180 degrees and beyond is normal. The inability to straighten the elbow to 180 degrees is therefore considered pathological, even if pain-free. Many people can extend a further 5–10 degrees, therefore true hypermobility is defined as extension beyond 190 degrees.

It is best to assess pronation and supination with the elbow flexed at 90 degrees and held close to the body. If you suspect the patient may have epicondylitis, examine resisted movements of the wrist for pain.

EXAMINATION OF THE WRIST AND HAND

Rest the patient's hands on a pillow for comfort.

Look

Inspection of the hands is an important part of the musculoskeletal examination. Look at the skin, nails, joints and muscles.

Skin
Check for psoriasis, rheumatoid nodules and tightening of the skin (scleroderma) or skin thinning (steroid use). Nail fold infarcts, haemorrhages and digital ulcers can occur as a consequence of vasculitis and systemic sclerosis. Scars from carpal tunnel decompression are seen on the volar aspect of the wrist. Redness, or erythema, is often seen when inflammation is present.

Nails
Look for pitting or onycholysis in psoriasis and splinter haemorrhages in vasculitis.

Joints
Look for deformity, swelling and scars of joint replacement. The pattern of deformity aids in diagnosis:
- Osteoarthritis tends to affect the DIP/PIP joints.
- Rheumatoid arthritis mainly affects the PIP/MCP and wrist joints.

Muscles
Wasting of the thenar and hypothenar eminences suggests median (carpal tunnel) or ulnar nerve pathology respectively, or disuse due to joint disease.

Atrophy of the dorsal interossei occurs in rheumatoid arthritis.

Feel

Palpate each joint systemically for the boggy and spongy feeling of synovitis. Bony overgrowth, such as osteophytosis, will feel hard. A bimanual approach is best with the examiners fingertips placed at either side of the joint, feeling for soft-tissue swelling.

Tenosynovitis of the finger flexors can be associated with tendon nodules, which can be felt moving on finger flexion.

Remember to feel the metacarpophalangeal joints for warmth and to squeeze them to elicit tenderness.

Check sensation in the distribution of the radial, median and ulnar nerves (Chapter 10).

Move

It is important to assess hand function. Active and passive movements of the wrist and digits should be performed and the patient's ability to perform certain tasks should be assessed. The muscles responsible for various movements are shown in Table 2.4.

- The prayer sign is useful when assessing hand and wrist function. Ask the patient to extend both wrists and place the palms together as if praying (see Fig. 2.20). Patients with limited wrist extension, deformities

Table 2.4 Muscles responsible for hand and wrist movements

Movement	Muscle(s) responsible (nerve supply)
Wrist flexion	Flexor carpi radialis (median) Flexor carpi ulnaris (ulnar) Palmaris longus (median)
Wrist extension	Extensor carpi radialis longus and brevis (both radial) Extensor carpi ulnaris (radial)
DIP joint flexion	Flexor digitorum profundus (median and ulnar)
PIP joint flexion	Flexor digitorum superficialis (median)
MCP joint flexion and IP joint extension	Lumbricals (median and ulnar)
Finger abduction	Dorsal interossei (ulnar)
Finger adduction	Palmar interossei (ulnar)
Extension of MCPs, PIPs and DIPs	Extensor digitorum (radial)
Thumb abduction	Abductor pollicis brevis (median)
Thumb adduction	Adductor pollicis (ulnar)
Thumb opposition	Opponens pollicis (median)
Thumb extension	Extensor pollicis longus (radial)

DIP, Distal interphalangeal; IP, interphalangeal; MCP, metacarpophalangeal; PIP, proximal interphalangeal.

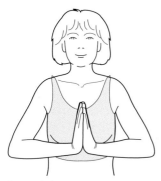

Fig. 2.20 The 'prayer' sign.

and synovitis of the MCP or PIP joints will find this difficult. Next 'reverse' the prayer sign so that the fingers point down towards the floor.

- Ask the patient to make a fist, tucking fingers into the palm.
- Ask the patient to straighten their fingers against resistance.

HINTS AND TIPS

Ask the patient to pick up a penny from the table or fasten a button. This will give you a good idea of the hand function.

- Abduct fingers and check power with the corresponding finger of the examiner's hand pressing against the patient's finger.
- Check interossei by asking the patient to hold a sheet of paper between the fingers.
- Abduction of the thumb against resistance checks median nerve function.

Special tests

Tinel and Phalen tests should be performed in patients who have symptoms suggestive of carpal tunnel syndrome. These are described in Chapter 10.

Chapter Summary

- Joint examination should be undertaken using a look, feel and move approach.
- You should always consider examining the joints above and below the affected joint.
- Gait observation gives vital clues to pathology in the lower limbs.
- When examining the hip, remember to stabilize the pelvis during movement.
- Examination of the knee should always involve testing for an effusion, which can be done using the patellar tap and swipe tests.
- Testing ligament stability using the anterior and posterior draw test can be painful, but it is necessary during knee examination.
- The straight-leg raise test is a quick way to test for nerve root irritation in the lumbrosacral spine.
- A painful shoulder arc is typical of a supraspinatus rotator cuff injury, which is a common cause of shoulder pain.
- The patterns of joint involvement in the small joints of the hands give vital clues to the aetiology: PIP and DIP joint involvement in osteoarthritis, PIP, MCP and wrist joint involvement in rheumatoid arthritis.

FURTHER READING

Douglas, G., Nicol, F., Robertson, C., 2013. Macleod's Clinical Examination, thirteenth edition. Elsevier, Edinburgh.

Regional examination of the Musculoskeletal System (REMS) handbook, Available online at www.arthritisresearchuk.org.

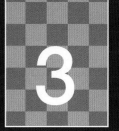
BLOOD TESTS

Many different blood tests are taken when evaluating rheumatic and orthopaedic problems. The following are most useful:

Full blood count

Full blood count (FBC) is a measure of the different constituent cells of the blood sample.

- Anaemia may be found in chronic inflammatory conditions or with blood loss from trauma. A normocytic anaemia usually indicates acute blood loss or chronic inflammation. A microcytic anaemia is found in iron deficient states, such as that caused by non-steroidal anti-inflammatory drug (NSAID) use with chronic gastrointestinal blood loss. Haemolytic anaemia can occur as a result of autoinflammatory disease and is typically macrocytic anaemia.
- A high white cell count may be due to infection, inflammation or due to steroid use.
- A leukopenia can be a feature of systemic lupus erythematosus (SLE), connective tissue disease or from bone-marrow suppression from antirheumatic drugs.
- Thrombocytosis often occurs in active inflammatory disease. In this case, it is referred to as a reactive thrombocytosis. Thrombocytopenia can be seen in SLE and antiphospholipid syndrome.

RED FLAG

A normal or low white cell count does not exclude infection if the clinical situation suggests otherwise. Patients who are immunosuppressed, or who are elderly, often present in this way.

Erythrocyte sedimentation rate

Erythrocyte sedimentation rate (ESR) is the rate at which red blood cells sediment over an hour and is a marker of inflammation.

- The measurement increases with higher levels of plasma proteins such as immunoglobulins and fibrinogen.
- The upper limit of ESR increases with advancing age and in overweight women.

C-Reactive protein

C-Reactive protein (CRP) is an acute phase protein that is manufactured in the liver.

- Its level rises in a nonspecific way as a result of inflammation and infection.
- It typically takes 6–10 hours after an inflammatory event to increase.

HINTS AND TIPS

C-Reactive protein responds more rapidly than erythrocyte sedimentation rate to changes in inflammation.

Urea and electrolytes

Renal impairment may occur in gout or connective tissue disease. NSAIDs can cause interstitial nephritis.

Liver function tests

- Alkaline phosphatase is found in both the liver and bone; some tests can differentiate between the isoenzymes.
- A raised alkaline phosphatase is seen in Paget disease
- Some drugs used for musculoskeletal problems are hepatotoxic, such as methotrexate and sulfasalazine, and require routine monitoring.

Uric acid

Uric acid levels are high in many patients with gout, but they can be normal during an attack of gout.

Calcium

- Hypocalcaemia occurs in osteomalacia and vitamin D deficiency.
- Hypercalcaemia can be a feature of malignancy, sarcoid and excess parathyroid hormone production.

Creatine kinase

Creatine kinase is a muscle enzyme that increases in response to muscle injury (trauma, hypoperfusion or inflammation).

Procalcitonin

Procalcitonin is a relatively new test performed when a patient's joint is hot. It can be useful in combination with ESR, CRP and the FBC to establish whether patients have joint infections or joint inflammation. A high procalcitonin is indicative of bacterial infection and sepsis.

Rheumatoid factor

Rheumatoid factor is an antibody directed against the Fc fragment of human immunoglobulin G (IgG). It may be of any class, but IgM anti-IgG is the most commonly measured. Around 75% of patients with (RA) have a positive rheumatoid factor antibody.

Cyclic citrullinated peptide antibody

Cyclic citrullinated peptide antibody (antiCCP) is an antibody found in patients with RA. It is more specific than rheumatoid factor and when strongly positive, it has a high predictive value in the risk of developing RA. AntiCCP is associated with an increased risk of joint erosions and more aggressive disease.

Antinuclear antibodies

Antinuclear antibodies (ANAs) are antibodies to nuclear antigens. They are detected in blood using labelling methods such as indirect immunofluorescence. A positive ANA means there are antibodies present in the blood that will bond to a sample cell used in the test.

If an ANA test is positive, it is important to examine which nuclear antigens the antibodies bind to. The pattern of immunofluorescence gives a clue, such as speckled, nucleolar or homogenous. The titre of the antibody also offers valuable information; the significance of the positive result is increased if the antibody is detectable after multiple dilutions (e.g., 1/2560 is more significant than 1/40).

Table 3.1 shows the ANAs directed against specific nuclear antigens and the diseases they are associated with. Antibodies to double-stranded DNA are very specific for SLE and are useful measures of disease activity.

Antineutrophil cytoplasmic antibodies

Antineutrophil cytoplasmic antibodies (ANCA) are antibodies directed against enzymes present in neutrophil granules. They are associated with inflammatory and vasculitic conditions. Two main immunofluorescent patterns are seen: cytoplasmic (c-ANCA) and perinuclear (p-ANCA).

c-ANCA and p-ANCA bind to several neutrophil enzymes, the most common being proteinase-3 (PR3) and myeloperoxidase (MPO). Antibodies to PR3 are found in around 80% of patients with granulomatosis with polyangiitis (GPA), formerly known as Wegener's granulomatosis. Those against MPO are found in microscopic polyangiitis and eosinophilic granulomatosis with polyangiitis (EGPA, formerly Churg-Strauss syndrome).

Table 3.1 Antinuclear antibodies against specific nuclear antigens and their associated diseases

Autoantibody	Associated disease
Anti-double stranded DNA (anti-dsDNA)	SLE
Histone	Drug induced lupus
Ro, La	Sjorgen syndrome, SLE
Anticentromere	Limited cutaneous systemic sclerosis
Scl-70 (topoisomerase)	Diffuse systemic sclerosis
RNP	Mixed connective tissue disease
Jo-1	Antisynthetase syndrome (polymyositis & dermatomyositis)

SLE, Systemic lupus erythematosus.

Antiphospholipid antibodies

Lupus anticoagulant and anticardiolipin antibodies are found in antiphospholipid syndrome. There is an association with venous and arterial thrombosis and recurrent miscarriages.

Complement

Complement molecules are small proteins activated in response to injury and inflammation. They bind to vessel walls and tissue when activated. This can lead to low serum levels of C3 and C4, as seen in SLE and some forms of vasculitis.

Urine tests

- A quick urine dip test gives a guide to protein and blood in the urine.
- Microscopic haematuria is often seen in vasculitis affecting the kidneys.
- Proteinuria can suggest glomerulonephritis found in connective tissue disease, vasculitis and amyloidosis.
- Free light chains can be detected in multiple myeloma.
- Antistreptolysin-O (ASO) titre can be a useful way of detecting recent streptococcal infection in cases of reactive arthritis.

SYNOVIAL FLUID ANALYSIS

Synovial fluid analysis is the most useful test for investigating potential cases of septic or crystal arthropathies. Synovial fluid can be aspirated from most peripheral joints and many departments have microscopy facilities for quick analysis.

Macroscopic appearance

Normal fluid is a pale yellow, straw-like colour. Changes in the colour of the fluid can give clues to the underlying pathology (see Table 3.2).

Gram Stain and culture

This should be performed if there is any suspicion of septic arthritis.

> **RED FLAG**
>
> The absence of organisms on microscopy does not exclude infection. It may be more difficult to detect organisms if antibiotics have been given before an aspirate is obtained.

Polarized light microscopy

To assess accurately the presence of crystals in fluid, the sample should be examined under polarized light. Urate crystals are needle-shaped and show strong negative birefringence: this means that crystals parallel to the plane of light appear yellow, while those at right angles appear blue. Calcium pyrophosphate dihydrate crystals are small and rhomboid-shaped and show weak positive birefringence.

Table 3.2 Macroscopic appearance of synovial fluid and associated pathology

Synovial fluid appearance	Pathology
Yellow and clear	Normal
Blood-stained	Haemarthrosis or trauma from aspiration
Cloudy	Increased numbers of white cells from infection or inflammation
Frank pus	Infection or occasionally crystal arthropathy
Chalky	Gout crystals, occasionally cholesterol crystals

NERVE CONDUCTION STUDIES AND ELECTROMYOGRAPHY

Nerve conduction studies (NCS) and electromyography (EMG) are electrophysiological tests used to diagnose and assess neuromuscular problems. They help to differentiate between primary muscle disease and neuropathic disorders, for example, carpal tunnel syndrome, myositis and steroid myopathy. NCS measure the velocity of motor and sensory nerve signals and can localize and assess the severity of peripheral nerve lesions. EMG records the spontaneous and voluntary electrical activity of muscles.

BIOPSY

Biopsies are occasionally performed to help with the investigation of musculoskeletal disorders. They are important in the assessment of bony lesions in suspected cancer. Vasculitis can often be diagnosed based on skin, blood vessel or nerve biopsies. Muscle biopsies are sometimes necessary in cases of suspected myositis. Occasionally, synovial biopsies are undertaken in cases of unexplained monoarthritis.

IMAGING

X-ray examinations

A plain X-ray (radiograph) examination is usually the first line of investigation in most musculoskeletal disorders. X-rays are good at visualizing bone, but not soft tissue. To investigate ligaments and tendons, an ultrasound or MRI is often required.

Using X-rays involves the use of electromagnetic radiation produced by electrons striking a rotating metal target in an X-ray tube. A narrow beam of X-rays is produced, which then passes through the patient, and the image is formed when these rays hit an X-ray sensitive film placed behind the patient (Fig 3.1).

Two views are required to assess for fractures, usually taken at 90 degrees to each other (usually anteroposterior and lateral). Sometimes specific views are required, such as a scaphoid view.

Ultrasound

Ultrasound is widely used and has the advantage of being safe, cheap and portable. It allows a dynamic assessment of joints and surrounding structures.

The image is produced using a transmitter that emits a beam of high-frequency sound (ultrasound) and detects the sound waves reflected from the soft tissues of the patient.

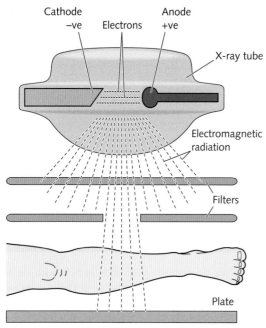

Fig. 3.1 Taking a radiographic image.

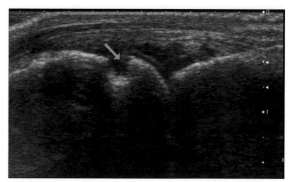

Fig. 3.3 Ultrasound image showing early erosion on the head of the metacarpal bone at the metacarpophalangeal joint in a patient with rheumatoid arthritis. The arrow indicates the 'bitten out' appearance of the erosion. (Provided by Dr Anna Ciechomska, Consultant Rheumatologist, Wishaw General Hospital.)

The different tissues absorb and reflect varying amounts of the beam and the reflections are analysed to produce a greyscale image.

Over recent years, the detection of synovitis and early erosions by ultrasound has helped to tailor therapy in RA (see Figs. 3.2 and 3.3). Other commonly imaged areas include shoulders looking for rotator cuff tears and the hip joint looking for evidence of effusions.

Ultrasound can also be used for guidance in joint injection and aspiration.

Computed tomography

Computed tomography (CT) uses the principles of an X-ray machine but the images are obtained when the X-ray tube is circled around the patient. Instead of an X-ray plate, the CT scanner has detectors within the machine to collect images. A large number of images are required by the computer software to build up the cross-sectional images taken in different planes.

The main role of CT in musculoskeletal disorders is in the study of bones, although contrast studies can be useful in conditions such as vasculitis.

CT scans also allow three dimensional images to be reconstructed, which can be useful in complex fractures.

COMMUNICATION

Remember computed tomographies and X-rays can carry a significant radiation exposure, dependent on the anatomical site to be imaged. Always communicate clearly why an investigation is required and gain consent.

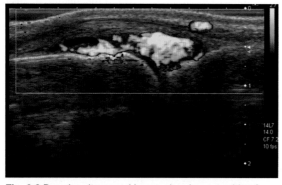

Fig. 3.2 Doppler ultrasound image showing synovitis of a metacarpophalangeal joint in a patient with rheumatoid arthritis. The high orange/yellow signal indicates increased blood flow within the synovium. (Provided by Dr Anna Ciechomska, Consultant Rheumatologist, Wishaw General Hospital.)

Magnetic resonance imaging

Magnetic resonance imaging (MRI) gives excellent imaging of soft tissues and bone marrow.

Images are generated using a powerful magnet and radio waves. The electromagnetic field of the scanner causes the protons in the body to line up with the field. Short bursts of radio waves are then directed at certain parts of the body, causing the protons to be knocked out of alignment. When the radio waves are turned off, the protons realign, sending out radio waves that are picked up by the receiver within the machine. Different tissues protons realign at differing speeds, which allows the computer to generate detailed images.

As the machine uses a large magnet, caution must be taken with metal components. Patients with cardiac pacemakers, intracranial aneurysm clips or with a suspicion of intraocular foreign bodies must not have an MRI examination unless first discussed with a radiologist.

MRI is commonly used to look at the knee (Fig. 3.4), the shoulder and the spine. In rheumatology, it can be used to assess synovitis and erosive damage (see Chapter 12, Fig. 12.11).

Isotope bone scan

An isotope bone scan involves the use of radioactive tracers injected into the body and taken up physiologically by bone. The most commonly used tracer is technetium-99m and its decay is measured using a gamma camera. The procedure is divided into three stages: blood flow (initial), blood pool (30 minutes) and delayed (4 hours).

The images show an outline of the body with areas highlighted where the isotope has accumulated.

Bone scans are a useful tool for identifying the presence of a disease process in bone (sensitive) but not in giving a diagnosis (nonspecific). Increased uptake typically occurs in growth plates, arthritis, fractures, metastases, infection and Paget disease. Fig. 3.5 shows multiple metastatic deposits. Fig. 3.6 shows active lesions in Paget disease.

Decreased uptake occurs in some tumours (haemopoeitic) and also in avascular bone.

Bone mineral density assessment

Bone densitometry (DEXA scanning) uses two X-ray beams to determine the density of bone relative to age- and sex-matched controls and is used in assessing and diagnosing osteoporosis. It is further explained in Chapter 15.

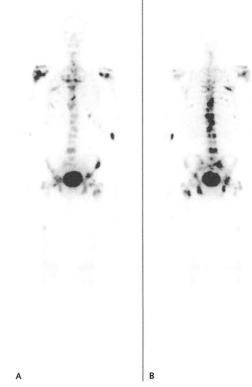

A   B

Fig. 3.5 Bone scan showing metastatic deposits. (A: anterior view; B: posterior view.)

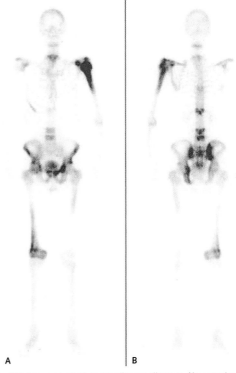

A   B

Fig. 3.6 Bone scan showing Paget disease (A: anterior view; B: posterior view.)

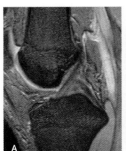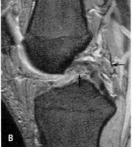

Fig. 3.4 Magnetic resonance imaging scans of the knee. (A) Normal. (B) Rupture of both cruciate ligaments (*arrows*).

Positron emission tomography

Positron emission tomography (PET) is a nuclear medicine scanning technique that can be used to observe metabolic activity within the body. Radiolabelled tracers are injected into patients who are then scanned to observe specific concentrations within the tissues. This can be a very useful imaging modality for identifying active inflammation in specific tissues, such as large vessel vasculitis or for localizing occult infections.

● Chapter Summary

- Various blood tests are used in investigating rheumatological and orthopaedic disorders.
- Many autoantibodies are disease-specific, such as antiCCP antibody for rheumatoid arthritis and anti-double stranded DNA antibody for SLE.
- Joint aspiration with fluid microscopy is the gold-standard test for a hot, swollen joint.
- Plain X-rays are useful for visualizing bone, while MRI and ultrasound are useful for examining soft tissues.
- Ultrasound has an emerging role in the detection of early synovitis and erosions in inflammatory arthropathies.

BACK, HIP AND LEG PAIN

Patients commonly present to general practitioners and accident and emergency with back, hip or leg pain. 80% of people will suffer from back pain in their lifetime and 30%–50% of people will suffer from chronic back pain.

History and examination of patients presenting with pain in this region are very important. Many patients do not appreciate the anatomy of the hip and commonly point to the greater trochanter or iliac crests when describing pain! Because of the complex anatomy of the spinal cord, pain signals can be referred to other regions and a detailed clinical examination is therefore required to evaluate.

Differential diagnosis

- Simple lower back pain (see Chapter 9)
- Osteoarthritis (see Chapter 11)
- Prolapsed intravertebral disc/degenerative disc disease (see Chapter 9)
- Inflammatory spondyloarthropathy (see Chapter 13)
- Vertebral crush fracture (see Chapter 15)
- Spinal stenosis/spondylolisthesis (see Chapter 9)
- Malignancy (see Chapter 21)
- Infective discitis (see Chapter 9)
- Avascular necrosis of the hip
- Trochanteric bursitis
- Paget disease (see Chapter 15)
- Abdominal pathology: referred pain (e.g., pancreatitis, bleeding/dissecting aortic aneurysm).

History focusing on back pain

There are four common patterns to consider:

- Back pain
- Back and leg pain
- Hip pain, with or without leg pain
- Leg pain

Fig. 4.1 shows the different patterns of pain around the back, hip and leg.

Back pain

Mechanical lower back pain

This is the most common cause of acute back pain, usually preceded by a history of lifting or straining the lower back. The pain is band-like, severe and does not usually radiate into the legs.

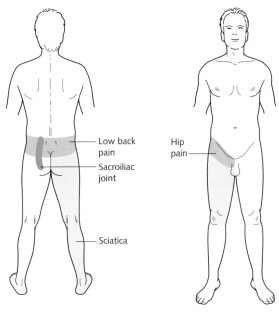

Fig. 4.1 Patterns of pain around the back, leg and hip.

Sinister back pain

Night sweats and weight loss with back pain should trigger concerns over 'sinister causes' of back pain (See Fig. 21.10). Have a low threshold for intensive investigation in patients presenting with these signs. Referred back pain is associated with nonmusculoskeletal diseases such as pancreatic cancer (weight loss, jaundice and back pain).

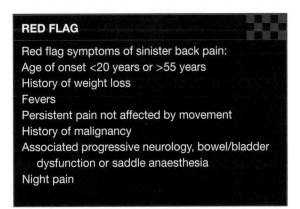

RED FLAG

Red flag symptoms of sinister back pain:
Age of onset <20 years or >55 years
History of weight loss
Fevers
Persistent pain not affected by movement
History of malignancy
Associated progressive neurology, bowel/bladder dysfunction or saddle anaesthesia
Night pain

Back and leg pain

Back pain radiating to the legs suggests nerve root entrapment.

Sciatica

Sciatica originates from the lower back and radiates down the leg, past the knee and into the foot. Weakness or numbness may also occur. It might result from an acute event, such as a disc prolapse onto the nerve root or from chronic degenerative back-disease causing compression at the exiting foramen. The pain is usually severe, sharp or shocking and is constant but with exacerbations. Positions such as standing or coughing can worsen the pain. Over time it usually settles.

Spinal stenosis

Pain from spinal stenosis is made worse by walking and relieved by rest and leaning forward, which opens up the spaces in the back. This is what is referred to as spinal claudication. Patients often adopt a stooped gait.

Facet joint osteoarthritis

Osteoarthritis can result in breakdown of the cartilage between the facet joints in the back and when the joints move the lack of cartilage causes pain and stiffness with loss of motion. The pain occurs in the back and may radiate to the top of the leg but does not extend below the knee.

Hip pain, with or without leg pain

True hip pain is felt in the groin and may radiate down to the knee.

Hip osteoarthritis

The onset of pain is insidious with restricted movement. It feels deep and gnawing.

Hip fracture

This is a common complication of falls in the frail and elderly. The leg appears shortened and internally rotated. Pain is severe and sharp and the patient cannot bear weight on that leg.

Leg pain

Occasionally sciatica presents with leg pain only, without the lower back discomfort.

Muscular conditions such as myositis or muscular dystrophy can present with muscle pain, weakness and gradual loss of function.

Peripheral vascular disease causes cramping leg pain on walking (claudication), which is relieved with rest. Skin changes and ulceration may be present.

Loss of function and disability

It is important to explore how pain impacts patients' functional abilities and whether there are limitations on certain activities. Patients may need ergonomic adjustments within the workplace.

Associated symptoms

It is essential to perform a neurological examination of the back and legs and to ask about associated symptoms such as bowel and bladder disturbance. Incontinence suggests a cauda equina syndrome requiring urgent magnetic resonance imaging (MRI) and decompression.

Weight loss, night sweats and a previous history of cancer suggest a tumour.

Investigations

A full set of blood tests including bone profile (calcium, phosphate and albumin) is important. Certain tests, such as a myeloma screen, are important in those over 55 years of age with sinister features.

X-ray examination of the back, when suspecting mechanical back pain, is not useful. It exposes the patient to a significant amount of radiation and has a low diagnostic yield. When sacroiliac joint disease or inflammatory spondyloarthropathy are suspected, MRI is the investigation of choice.

Where red flags are found, the following findings are significant and warrant further investigation:

- Osteoarthritis changes in the hip and spine.
- 'Squaring' of the vertebral bodies and bridging syndesmophytes in ankylosing spondylitis (see Chapter 13).
- Spondylolisthesis
- Lytic lesions of the vertebral body, classically the pedicle (winking owl sign; see Fig 4.2), indicating malignancy.
- Fracture
- Erosion of the vertebral body around the disc due to infection.

Computed tomography (CT), isotope bone scanning and MRI remain available for situations where doubt remains, especially for infection, malignancy and cord compression.

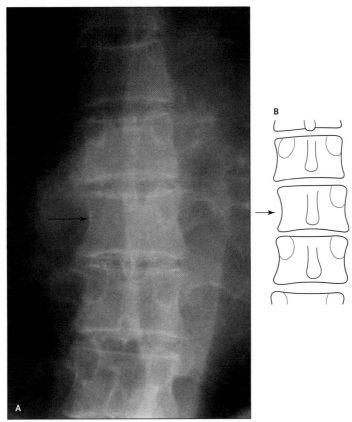

Fig. 4.2 Malignancy of the spine. (A) The 'winking-owl sign' *(black arrow)* occurs when the pedicle is destroyed due to metastasis. (B) The missing 'eye' *(black arrow)* represents bony destruction of the pedicle by tumour, so always look closely at the pedicles.

KNEE PAIN

Knee pain accounts for over a third of all referrals to orthopaedic surgeons.

Differential diagnosis

- Osteoarthritis
- Meniscal injuries
- Ligament injuries
- Bursitis
- Osteochondrosis
- Rheumatoid arthritis or other inflammatory arthritis
- Septic arthritis
- Patellofemoral disorders
- Referred pain from the hip/spine

History focusing on knee pain

Consider the patient's age, occupation and activity levels. A young athletic patient with a recent injury is unlikely to have rheumatoid arthritis (consider meniscal or ligament injury). An elderly patient with gradually worsening pain will most likely have osteoarthritis.

Character of the pain

In osteoarthritis, the onset of pain is gradual over months or years. Sudden onset pain is usually due to ligament or meniscal injury or a fracture if there is trauma. Spontaneous severe pain is most likely due to septic arthritis or a crystal arthropathy.

Pain and stiffness in the morning that gets better as the day goes on suggests inflammatory arthritis.

Pain originating from the knee rarely radiates, but children commonly experience pain referred from the hip as knee pain.

Nature of the pain

- Meniscal tear and soft tissue injuries produce sharp, stabbing pains.
- Osteoarthritis causes a deep gnawing pain.
- Constant pain that is not affected by movement is often a feature of anterior knee pain.

Aggravating/relieving factors

Osteoarthritis pain is often worse on movement and relived by rest; inflammatory pain gets better with use of the joint.

Pain from meniscal injury is worse on full flexion or on twisting.

Patellofemoral pain is worse when walking up or down stairs.

In acute crystal arthropathy or septic arthritis, any movement of the joint produces severe pain.

Pain from prepatellar bursitis is worse on kneeling.

Site of pain

Pain can be generalized or localized. Generalized pain suggests an arthritis process affecting the whole joint. Large, tense effusions, such as after an injury or septic arthritis, also produce pain all over the joint.

Localized pain causes depend on the site of pain. Common painful areas are shown, with anatomy of the knee joint, in Fig. 4.3.

- Anterior: patellofemoral pain is felt here. Pain above or below the knee cap may be due to prepatellar or infrapatellar bursitis respectively.
- Medial or lateral: localized pain to either side of the joint may be due to osteoarthritis (particularly so in the medial joint line), collateral ligament injury or from meniscal tears.
- Posterior: pain here is less common, but typically caused by Baker cyst or bursitis.
- Pain down the front of the thigh and into the knee is typical of referred hip pain.

Loss of function

Patients may have significant disabling symptoms from knee pain. Injuries that affect the ligaments often lead the patient to tell you they 'don't trust the knee': a hallmark of joint instability.

Associated symptoms

Ask about general symptoms of health, such as fever, lethargy and malaise.

Any history of injury is important, therefore ask some closed questions:

- Ask if the patient heard a snap.
- How long did any swelling take to appear?
- Is there a history of locking? (This might suggest meniscal injury.)

HINTS AND TIPS

Remember the mnemonic **SOCRATES** when describing pain:

- **s**ite
- **o**nset
- **c**haracter
- **r**adiation
- **a**ssociations
- **t**iming
- **e**xacerbating/relieving factors
- **s**everity

Investigations

Fig. 4.4 provides an algorithm for investigating knee pain.

Further imaging

This is only warranted in certain conditions:

- MRI: useful for ligament or meniscal pathology.
- CT: gives detailed imaging of bony structures.
- Isotope bone scan: useful in showing 'hot spots' of increased bone metabolic activity, but does not

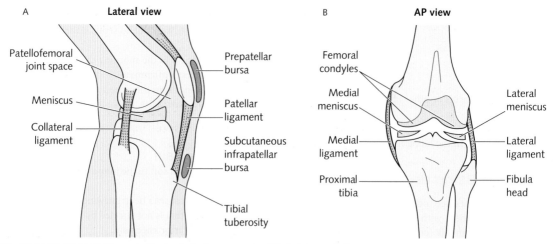

Fig. 4.3 Anatomical structures in the knee that cause pain. *AP*, Anteroposterior.

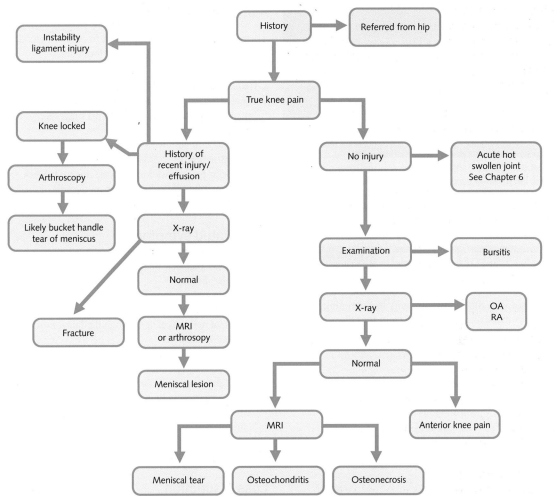

Fig. 4.4 Algorithm for the investigation of knee pain. *MRI*, Magnetic resonance imaging; *OA*, osteoarthritis; *RA*, rheumatoid arthritis.

given an exact diagnosis (nonspecific). It can be useful for rarer conditions such as bone tumours and osteomyelitis.

- Ultrasound: useful for examining for synovitis, effusions and for guided injections.

- Blood-stained fluid is usually from haemarthrosis after injury or occasionally spontaneously (e.g., patients on warfarin). Blood and fat globules (lipohaemarthrosis; Fig. 4.5) indicate a fracture or anterior cruciate ligament rupture.

Aspiration

Aspirating a joint is a simple way of getting some specific clues about diagnosis.

Using aseptic technique, feel the upper and lower border of the patella. From the midpoint, feel laterally until you can identify the patellofemoral joint space. This is the easiest landmark to use and the needle should be inserted at 90 degrees to the lateral aspect of the knee, angled slightly proximally. Inject local anaesthetic and aspirate fluid.

Examine the fluid obtained:

- Normal fluid is yellowish/straw coloured.
- Slightly clouded yellow fluid indicates inflammation.
- Greenish or pus-like fluid indicates infection.

HINTS AND TIPS

Always send fluid for microscopy, culture and sensitivity testing and ask the laboratory to examine for crystals.

Arthroscopy

This involves keyhole surgery into the joint. This is discussed further in Chapter 24.

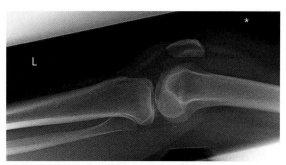

Fig. 4.5 A lipohaemarthrosis in the suprapatellar pouch of the left (L) knee secondary to a subtle tibial plateau fracture. A fluid level is seen as the fat 'floats' on the blood *(white arrow)*. (Courtesy of Dr Aziz Marzoug, Radiology Specialist Trainee, Aberdeen Royal Infirmary.)

ANKLE AND FOOT PAIN

The unique complexity of the structure of the foot and ankle combined with the relative difficulty in examining individual joints make diagnosis of ankle and foot disorders more challenging. Biochemical factors play a particularly important role in ankle and foot problems.

Differential diagnosis

The differential diagnosis of pain in the ankle and/or foot is shown in Fig. 4.6.

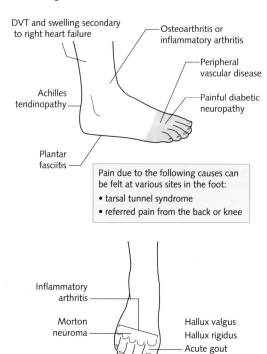

Fig. 4.6 Differential diagnosis of ankle and/or foot pain. *DVT,* Deep vein thrombosis.

History focusing on the ankle

The following points are important to cover when taking a history from patients with ankle or foot pain.

Character of the pain
• Severe, recurrent self-limiting pain (especially of the first metatarsophalangeal joint) suggests crystal arthropathy.
• Chronic dull pain with soft tissue swelling suggests inflammation.
• Posterior pain on walking may be due to Achilles tendinopathy, while discomfort on the sole of the foot suggests plantar fasciitis.

Associated symptoms
• Back or knee pain may suggest referred pain.
• Coldness, pallor or ulcers may be due to peripheral vascular disease.
• Burning and numbness can occur with Morton neuroma, tarsal tunnel syndrome (compression of the tibial nerve passing through the tarsal tunnel) or diabetic neuropathy.
• Plantar fasciitis is associated with spondyloarthropathies so ask about back pain, psoriasis and inflammatory bowel disease.
• Repetitive trauma such as running, jumping or other athletic injuries can result in Achilles tendinopathy. Quinolones, such as ciprofloxacin, can cause spontaneous Achilles tendon rupture.
• A recent illness or starting diuretic therapy can trigger gout.

Loss of function
It is important to enquire about the impact of pain in the foot and ankle on a patient's function and lifestyle. Achilles tendinopathy can ruin the career of an athlete, but a sedentary older patient may not feel significantly impacted by this.

Examination

Examination of the foot and ankle joint is described in Chapter 2.

Investigations

Standard blood tests are a useful screening tool in all patients.

Radiological investigations
• Plain X-ray images may show inflammatory erosions or degenerative changes.
• Ultrasound images can identify synovitis, effusions, osteoarthritis, tendinopathy and ligament damage and Morton neuromas.
• MRI can also be used to assess the above and is less user-dependent but more expensive.

Synovial fluid analysis

See the earlier section on knee pain.

Nerve conduction studies

These are useful for confirming tarsal tunnel syndrome or peripheral neuropathy.

NECK AND/OR UPPER ARM PAIN

A detailed history of the problem is required due to the wide differential of causes, which include cardiac and neurological issues.

Differential Diagnosis

The following boxes give the differential diagnoses that should be considered when patients present with neck, shoulder, elbow or wrist and hand pain.

DIFFERENTIAL DIAGNOSIS OF NECK PAIN

Mechanical neck pain

Cervical spondylosis

Ankylosing spondylitis

Cervical disc prolapse

Metastatic vertebral deposits

Referred pain from

    Local structures (e.g., carotid dissection, lymphadenopathy, thyroiditis)

    Distant structures (e.g., ischaemic heart disease, subphrenic abscess)

DIFFERENTIAL DIAGNOSIS OF SHOULDER PAIN

Rotator cuff pathology (impingement, tear or tendinopathy)

Capsulitis

Arthritis of the acromioclavicular joint

Arthritis of the glenohumeral joint

Bicipital tendinopathy

Polymyalgia rheumatica

Referred pain from

    Neck pathology

    Cardiac ischaemia

    Pancoast tumour

    Intraabdominal pathology, Kehr sign (e.g., subphrenic abscess, splenic rupture)

DIFFERENTIAL DIAGNOSIS IN ELBOW PAIN

Lateral epicondylitis (tennis elbow)

Olecranon bursitis

Crystal arthropathy

Osteoarthritis

Inflammatory arthritis

Medial epicondylitis (golfer's elbow)

Referred pain from the neck or shoulder

DIFFERENTIAL DIAGNOSIS IN WRIST AND HAND PAIN

Osteoarthritis

Inflammatory arthritis

Carpal tunnel syndrome

De Quervain tenosynovitis

Crystal arthropathy

Ulnar nerve entrapment

Raynaud phenomenon

Complex regional pain syndrome

Referred pain from the cervical spine, shoulder or elbow

Neck pain

History

Trauma or high impact injuries to the neck require careful assessment to exclude neurological damage or fracture. Carotid artery dissection produces a severe, anterior sharp/tearing pain secondary to trauma. Chronic stiffness may suggest inflammation. Shooting pain radiating down the arms suggests nerve entrapment. Weakness or clumsiness in the legs and bladder or bowel disturbance suggests cord compression.

Dizziness may occur in severe degenerative disease due to vertebral artery compression. Fever, weight loss and general malaise raise the prospect of malignancy, infection or sepsis. A chronic bilaterally ache in the neck and shoulder with high erythrocyte sedimentation rate (ESR) suggests polymyalgia rheumatica.

Examination

Examination of the neck is described in Chapter 2. Any patient with neck pain should have a full neurological examination of the cranial nerves and all limbs.

Shoulder pain

History

Shoulder pain is a common complaint, but referred pain is common at the shoulder. Reduction in movement and functional ability with pain may occur in frozen shoulder and painful arc syndrome, the latter being worse on abduction. The site of pain may give a clue to the origin of the pain. Fig. 4.7 shows how the site of shoulder pain varies depending on the cause.

Examination

Shoulder examination is described in Chapter 2. Anterior dislocation produces an obvious bulge to the front, while frozen shoulder gives a globally restricted joint. Wasting of the shoulder muscles can occur in chronic rotator cuff injuries.

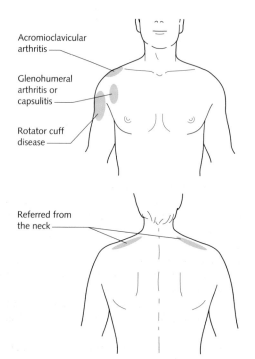

Fig. 4.7 Many structures can give rise to shoulder pain. These diagrams show how the site of pain varies with the origin.

A reduction in passive movement and active movement suggests osteoarthritis or capsulitis of the joint. A reduction in active movement with normal passive movement suggests a rotator cuff problem.

Elbow

History

Repetitive movements can trigger lateral epicondylitis (tennis elbow). Acute, egg-like swelling suggests olecranon bursitis. Inflammatory arthritis produces pain that is worse on waking and eases on movement/use of the joint.

Examination

Elbow examination is also described in Chapter 2. Resisted dorsiflexion commonly exacerbates the pain of tennis elbow.

Wrist and hand

History

Triggers for symptoms may be important:

- Cold weather triggers Raynaud phenomenon
- Changes in medication may trigger gout
- Repetitive use (e.g., using a keyboard) may exacerbate osteoarthritis

Examination

Look for:

- Heberden or Bouchard nodes, seen in osteoarthritis
- Synovial swelling of the small joints of the hand or tendon sheaths, seen in rheumatoid arthritis
- Rheumatoid nodules
- Psoriatic plaques
- Gouty tophi
- Changes to the nails
- Colour changes to the digits or ulceration as seen in Raynaud phenomenon
- Changes in skin colour with atrophy and reduced hair growth as features of complex regional pain syndrome
- Wasting of the thenar and hypothenar muscles resulting from median and ulnar nerve compression respectively

As well as helping to identify tendon structure, palpation helps in assessing causes of swelling. Osteoarthritis causes hard bony swelling and is easily distinguishable from the soft, boggy synovial swelling of inflammatory arthritis. The presence of heat and erythema is also important. Inflamed tendon sheaths feel thickened and irregular and may produce crepitus. Fig. 4.8 shows a suggested algorithm for examining the wrist and hands.

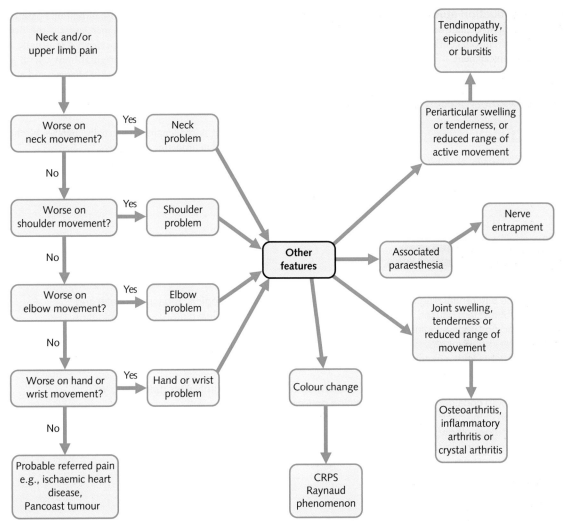

Fig. 4.8 Algorithm for the diagnosis of neck and/or upper-limb pain. *CRPS*, Complex regional pain syndrome.

Investigations

The choice of investigations depends on the clinical history and examination findings. Many diagnoses can be reached without further investigation, such as dull aching hands in a 75-year-old man with Heberden nodes and carpometacarpal (CMC) joint pain, indicating osteoarthritis. Plain X-ray images will confirm the diagnosis but will not alter the management.

Blood tests
- ESR and C-reactive protein may be elevated in inflammation, infection or malignancy.
- A positive rheumatoid factor and CCP-antibody in a patient with synovitis is highly suggestive of rheumatoid arthritis.

Radiological investigations
- Plain X-ray images may show signs of osteoarthritis or rheumatoid arthritis, calcification due to tendinopathy, periosteal reactions due to enthesitis or bony metastasis.
- Ultrasound images can demonstrate thickening and oedema of the tendon sheaths in tendinopathy and can identify synovitis, effusions and early erosions.
- MRI is useful in examination of the cervical cord and nerve root and in detecting rotator cuff inflammation and degeneration.
- Isotope bone scans can help to identify hot spots due to metastasis, infection, inflammation or fracture. These should then be followed up with CT or MRI examinations.

Nerve conduction studies

These can help to exclude cervical radiculopathy in patients with neck pain or can confirm the presence of median and ulnar nerve entrapment.

COMPLEX REGIONAL PAIN SYNDROME

This is also known as reflex sympathetic dystrophy and is a long-term complex pain syndrome that worsens over time. It is an uncommon cause of regional pain that typically affects the upper limb, particularly the distal forearm and hand. The pain experienced is usually severe and out-of-context of the original injury, with key features of pain, hypersensitivity, skin changes and autonomic disturbance. Allodynia is often present (pain from a stimulus that would not normally produce pain, e.g., light touch).

Treatment is challenging but usually involves bisphosphonates and neuropathic pain killers.

● Chapter Summary

- Back pain is a common complaint with many varied causes.
- The differential diagnoses from regional pain include neurological, musculoskeletal and multisystem causes. Thought must be given to both the clinical history and examination findings in developing a sensible differential diagnosis.
- The important red-flag features of neck and back pain must be considered, particularly in patients with a history of trauma or those whose histories suggest malignancy, cord compression or infection.
- Knee and ankle pain can often be referred from distant proximal sites (back/hip). You should consider this when examining patients.
- Pain in the neck, arms and hands typically follows patterns of involvement (neck, shoulder, elbow, and wrist and hand).
- Complex regional pain syndrome is an uncommon but debilitating cause of nonspecific regional pain.

FURTHER READING

NICE Guideline (NG59), 2016. Low back pain and sciatica in over 16s: assessment and management. Available at https://www.nice.org.uk/guidance/ng59.

Goebel, A., Barker, C.H., Turner-Stokes, L., et al., 2012. Complex regional pain syndrome in adults: UK guidelines for diagnosis, referral and management in primary and secondary care. RCP, London.

Widespread musculoskeletal pain

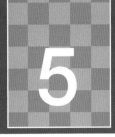

Widespread musculoskeletal pain can be distressing for patients. The differential diagnosis is varied and requires careful examination and investigation to separate causes (see below):

THE DIFFERENTIAL DIAGNOSIS OF WIDESPREAD MUSCULOSKELETAL PAIN

Inflammatory arthritis
Fibromyalgia
Systemic lupus erythematosus
Myositis
Polymyalgia rheumatica
Metabolic bone disease (osteomalacia, Paget disease)
Paraneoplastic rheumatic syndrome
Widespread skeletal metastases
Vitamin deficiency: B12/folate
Hypothyroidism

The patient's age, gender and race might give important clues about the diagnosis. For example, polymyalgia rheumatica (PMR) rarely affects people under the age of 60 years, fibromyalgia and systemic lupus erythematosus (SLE) are more common in women than men and osteomalacia is more prevalent in the Asian than the Caucasian population.

INVESTIGATING WIDESPREAD PAIN

History

A history should be taken covering the following points:

Onset of pain
Widespread pain is usually insidious and progressive, but in rare cases SLE and PMR can produce pain that develops over a few days.

Timing of pain
Generally, pain that is worse in the morning and eases as the day progresses is typical of inflammation.

Site
Patients may struggle to localize pain. Pay close attention to whether pain is felt in the muscles, joints or whether it follows nerve tracts.

Stiffness
Stiffness that is worse in the morning and lasts more than 30 minutes is suggestive of SLE or PMR.

Associated symptoms
- Temporal headaches, jaw claudication and blurred vision suggest giant cell arteritis in association with PMR.
- Rashes, mouth ulcers and Raynaud phenomenon raise the possibility of SLE.
- Psychiatric problems, anxiety and depression can be features of fibromyalgia.
- Abdominal pain and confusion can be present in hypercalcaemia.

Examination and investigation

Fig. 5.1 gives a suggested algorithm for the examination and investigation of patients with widespread musculoskeletal pain.

Examination
Examination is useful in determining whether pain is coming from the bones and joints or from muscles and soft tissues. Carefully examine the joints for signs of inflammation and palpate the muscles and soft tissues for tenderness. Examination of other systems may be required if the history is suggestive of more atypical causes.

Investigations
These are guided by examination findings. It is important to note that many tests can be normal in the early stages of a disease.

Blood tests
- Erythrocyte sedimentation rate (ESR) and C-reactive protein (CRP) may be elevated in PMR, SLE or inflammatory arthritis
- Calcium levels may be high if there are bony metastases or low in cases of osteomalacia.
- Parathyroid hormone (PTH) levels should be checked in hypercalcaemia to exclude hyperparathyroidism.
- Low vitamin D levels are found in osteomalacia.
- Serum alkaline phosphatase may be elevated in Paget disease.
- An immune screen including antinuclear antibody (ANA), anti-dsDNA antibodies and complement, may be abnormal in SLE.

Fig. 5.1 Algorithm for investigation of widespread musculoskeletal pain. *ANA,* Antinuclear antibody; *CRP,* C-reactive protein; *ESR,* erythrocyte sedimentation rate; *SLE,* systemic lupus erythematosus.

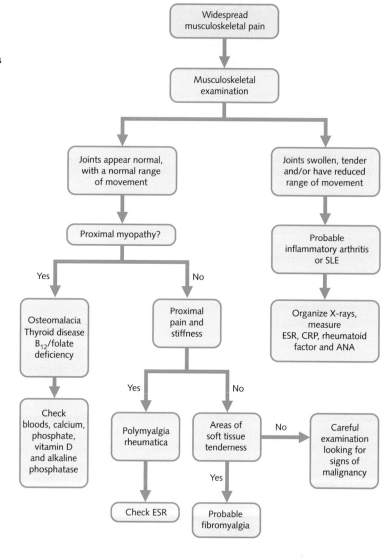

Radiology

Small joint X-ray images may show erosive changes. X-ray examination of the long bones can be useful in osteomalacia, where Looser zones may be seen.

Other radiological tests (chest X-ray examination, bone scans, computed tomography scans) may be required if there is a strong suspicion of malignancy.

FIBROMYALGIA

Definition

Many patients who present to the Rheumatology Department with chronic widespread pain cannot be readily diagnosed. The spectrum of symptoms associated with fibromyalgia are often nonspecific and many patients suffer for a long time between onset of symptoms and establishing a diagnosis. Associated symptoms of fatigue, depression, insomnia, altered bowel habits and poor concentration are accompanied by a widespread soft tissue tenderness localized over a number of trigger points. However, the existence of fibromyalgia as an organic disease remains controversial. Many clinicians recognize the above symptoms and clinical features but feel that labelling patients may reinforce their illness. However, there is evidence that referral rates and investigations lessen once patients have been diagnosed.

Prevalence

Fibromyalgia is common: the prevalence is estimated at between 2% and 5%.

Aetiology

The aetiology of fibromyalgia is poorly understood. Several theories exist, including a postviral trigger and up-regulation of pain receptor sensitivity. Elements recognized to be indicative of being at risk include:

- Women
- Middle age
- Stressful life events

There is considerable overlap between fibromyalgia and several other conditions that have a functional component (Fig. 5.2).

Pathogenesis

The roles of various neurotransmitters, pain receptor pathways, hormones and peptides have been examined in fibromyalgia. Unfortunately, in spite of much research, the pathogenesis remains poorly understood.

Clinical features

Fibromyalgia predominantly affects women between the ages of 30 and 60 years. Patients complain of a long history of severe widespread pain that is exacerbated by minimal exertion and responds poorly to analgesia. Other common symptoms are shown in the box below.

COMMON SYMPTOMS IN FIBROMYALGIA

- Fatigue
- Sleep disturbance
- Poor concentration, sometimes referred to as 'fibro fog'
- Headache
- Paraesthesia
- Anxiety/depression
- Altered bowel habit
- Widespread pain

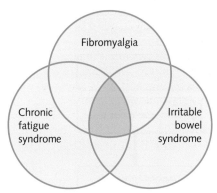

Fig. 5.2 Overlap between fibromyalgia and other syndromes.

The only significant finding on examination is the presence of soft-tissue tenderness, usually in multiple sites. Common sites of tenderness are shown in Fig. 5.3.

Investigations

Fibromyalgia is a clinical diagnosis based on recognition of symptoms and tender points. The only role of investigations is in the exclusion of other conditions.

Management

There is no specific treatment, but some general approaches are advised (Fig. 5.4). Poor quality of life and significant socio-economic impact remain an issue. Addressing social stressors and depression is essential if better outcomes are to be achieved. The following treatment strategies may help:

COMMUNICATION

It is important to explain a diagnosis of fibromyalgia carefully to patients. Explain that the pain is real and not simply 'in their heads'. Although activity can be painful, reassure them that exercise will not damage their joints.

Education

- Inform patients about their condition.
- Reassure them they do not have a destructive arthritis.
- Explain why further investigations might not be useful.
- Emphasize that exercise will not cause harm to their joints.

Physiotherapy/exercise

A graded exercise programme can improve fitness and reduce pain and fatigue.

Cognitive behavioural therapy

This encourages patients to develop coping mechanisms to deal with their symptoms.

Drug therapy

Many types of drugs have been trialled with varying success. Tricyclic antidepressants such as amitriptyline, dual reuptake inhibitors (duloextine), anticonvulsants (pregabalin, gabapentin) and analgesics such as tramadol are all used with varying success. There is no role for antiinflammatory drugs.

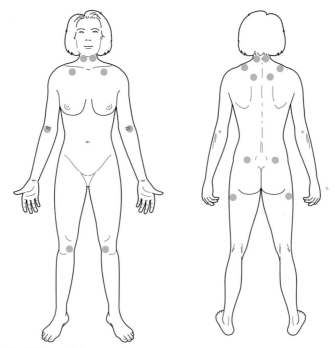

Fig 5.3 The tender points of fibromyalgia.

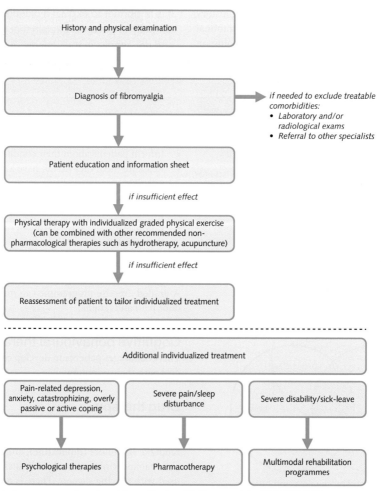

Fig. 5.4 Recommended management protocol for patients with fibromyalgia; EULAR 2016.

PARANEOPLASTIC RHEUMATIC SYNDROME

This is a rare but serious cause of widespread musculoskeletal pain. Patients with lymphoma, leukaemia or other malignancies might present with rheumatic symptoms. These can mimic inflammatory arthritis or PMR. Patients who fail to respond to typical treatment or who have other red flag features should be investigated to rule out an occult malignancy.

Equally, widespread bony metastases can present with widespread, or whole body, pain. Primary tumours that frequently metastasize to bone include breast, lung, kidney, thyroid and prostate cancers.

FURTHER READING

Macfarlane GJ, Kronisch C, Dean LE, et al. EULAR revised recommendations for the management of fibromyalgia. *Annals of the Rheumatic Diseases.* Published online: 04 July 2016. doi: 10.1136/annrheumdis-2016-209724
Fibromyalgia Action UK, www.fmauk.org.
The Pain Society Britain, www.britishpainsociety.org.

● Chapter Summary

- Widespread musculoskeletal pain is a common reason for referral to a rheumatologist.
- Causes are varied, but fibromyalgia is common, particularly amongst middle-aged women.
- Symptoms that are difficult to investigate are often found in conjunction with fibromyalgia, including chronic headache, fatigue, low mood and irritable bowel syndrome.
- Education, reassurance and graded exposure to exercise are key in helping to rehabilitate patients.
- Paraneoplastic rheumatic syndromes are rare, but it is important to consider in patients presenting with apparent inflammatory arthritis that fails to respond to typical therapies.

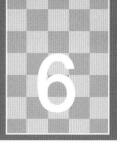
DIFFERENTIAL DIAGNOSIS

The phrase 'acute hot swollen joint' implies that the patient has presented as an emergency with an acute onset of symptoms and with a large effusion. Differentials include:

- septic arthritis
- crystal arthropathy
  - gout
  - pseudo-gout
- inflammatory arthritis
- haemarthrosis
- transient synovitis

> **RED FLAG**
>
> Whilst there are many causes of a swollen and hot joint, the most important to exclude in an acute setting is septic arthritis. This can cause life-threatening sepsis.

HISTORY FOCUSING ON THE ACUTE HOT SWOLLEN JOINT

Pain

Patients with septic arthritis or acute gout classically present with severe pain. However, it is difficult to differentiate between these conditions because the majority of patients will present with severe pain that is worse on movement.

Patient's age and sex

All the above conditions can present in adults, whereas only septic arthritis, reactive arthritis and inflammatory arthritis are likely causes in children.

Gout is more common in men and rheumatoid arthritis is more common in women.

Site

Certain joints are more commonly affected by specific disorders (Fig 6.1):

- Gout most commonly affects the first metatarsophalangeal joint of the foot.

- Pseudo gout is common in the wrist and knee.
- If multiple joints are affected, an inflammatory disorder such as rheumatoid arthritis or juvenile idiopathic arthritis is possible.

Is the patient unwell?

Fever, night sweats, rigors and general flu-like symptoms suggest an infection. A severe flare-up of inflammatory arthritis may cause severe fatigue and patients sometimes feel 'flu-like', but fevers and rigors are unlikely.

History

Patients with a history of gout are likely to have recurrent episodes (up to 90%), as are those with inflammatory arthritis. Conditions such as septic arthritis are usually solitary episodes, unless the patient has a predisposing risk factor such as immunosuppression, diabetes mellitus or sickle cell disease.

> **HINTS AND TIPS**
>
> Be careful! Patients with known inflammatory or crystal arthritis can present with joint infections. Patients on immunosuppressants may not present the usual inflammatory responses and the joint or the patient's blood tests may not have features typically associated with infection.

Associated symptoms

Patients with an inflammatory disorder may have other systemic features of their disease process, such as sacroiliitis in ankylosing spondylitis or painful metacarpophalangeal joints in rheumatoid arthritis.

Symptoms affecting the eyes can occur in:

- Reiter syndrome (conjunctivitis)
- Rheumatoid arthritis (keratoconjunctivitis, episcleritis, scleritis)
- Juvenile idiopathic arthritis (uveitis)

Patients with a history of recent sexually transmitted infection or diarrhoea may have Reiter syndrome. Always consider gonococcal arthritis in patients with a history of sexually transmitted disease or a recent change in sexual partner.

A recent viral illness can also cause a reactive arthritis.

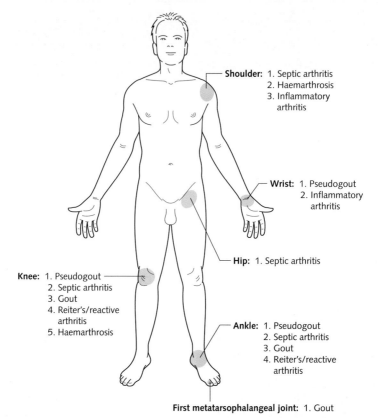

Shoulder: 1. Septic arthritis
2. Haemarthrosis
3. Inflammatory arthritis

Wrist: 1. Pseudogout
2. Inflammatory arthritis

Hip: 1. Septic arthritis

Knee: 1. Pseudogout
2. Septic arthritis
3. Gout
4. Reiter's/reactive arthritis
5. Haemarthrosis

Ankle: 1. Pseudogout
2. Septic arthritis
3. Gout
4. Reiter's/reactive arthritis

First metatarsophalangeal joint: 1. Gout

Fig. 6.1 Likely diagnosis for each joint in a patient presenting with an acute hot swollen joint.

Medical history

Patients with diabetes mellitus are at risk of septic arthritis, as any other infection.

Gout is linked with increased cell turnover and therefore any catabolic illness can predispose to a flare. Haematological diseases are particularly likely to cause gout, as are cancers where the patient is given chemotherapy, killing vast numbers of cells.

Patients with bleeding disorders (such as haemophilia) or those taking anticoagulants such as warfarin or DOACs are at risk of developing acute haemarthrosis (acute bleeding into the joint). These patients can present with large tense effusions from a seemingly trivial injury.

Drug history

Diuretics, particularly thiazides, and low-dose aspirin can increase uric acid levels, predisposing to gout.

Patients on steroids or other immunosuppressants are at increased risk of infection.

Social history

Alcohol excess and a high-purine diet predispose to gout.

EXAMINATION OF AN ACUTE HOT SWOLLEN JOINT

General

- Most patients presenting will be in pain, look uncomfortable and may be agitated.
- Pyrexia suggests infection, although a mildly elevated temperature can be seen in both gout and inflammatory arthritis.
- In severe cases of sepsis, the patient may show signs of cardiovascular instability such as tachycardia and hypotension (septic shock).
- The patient should be examined for signs of inflammatory arthritis.
- Patients with gout may have tophi. Look at the extensor surfaces of the elbow and fingers.

The joint

- The knee is the most common joint affected.
- Any affected joint will have a tense effusion and be tender to palpation and active and passive movement. Typically, a septic joint will be extremely tender and the patient will avoid movement. Other causes of arthropathy, whilst tender, tend not to be as severe.

- A full examination of the joint is often not possible on account of pain.
- A thorough examination of other joints should be performed to make sure the patient only has monoarthritis.

INVESTIGATION OF AN ACUTE HOT SWOLLEN JOINT

An algorithm for investigating a patient with an acute hot swollen joint is shown in Fig. 6.2.

Blood tests

The aim of initial investigations is to confirm or to exclude septic arthritis. Do not rely on blood tests alone because they can be normal:

- A raised white cell count (WCC) suggests infection but can be due to inflammatory causes. WCCs tend not to be elevated, or only very slightly elevated, in cases of crystal arthropathies.
- Inflammatory markers, erythrocyte sedimentation rate (ESR) and C-reactive protein (CRP), can be elevated in all conditions due to inflammation or infection.
- In cases of immunosuppression, the usual increases in WCC and inflammatory markers may not be seen. Interpret these results with caution.
- Serum urate may be elevated or normal in patients with acute gout.

- Serum calcium should be checked if pseudogout is suspected, especially if hyperparathyroidism is present.
- If haemarthrosis is suspected, a clotting screen should be checked and patients on warfarin should have their international normalized ratio (INR) checked.
- A procalcitonin test is useful to determine between infective and inflammatory causes of a hot swollen joint. Procalcitonin levels are high in the presence of a bacterial infection.

X-ray examinations

X-ray images may show:

- Normal appearance
- Chondrocalcinosis (found in pseudogout)
- Bony erosions due to gout or inflammatory arthritis
- Periosteal reaction

Aspiration/synovial fluid analysis

- A superficial joint such as the knee is simple to aspirate, particularly if a tense effusion is present.
- Deeply situated joints such as the hip must be aspirated using ultrasound or X-ray guidance.
- Aspiration should ideally be performed before antibiotics are given to increase the diagnostic yield of the test. Always ask for an urgent Gram stain of the fluid and request culture, sensitivity and microscopy to establish the presence of crystals.
- The general appearance of synovial fluid should be described (see Chapter 3).

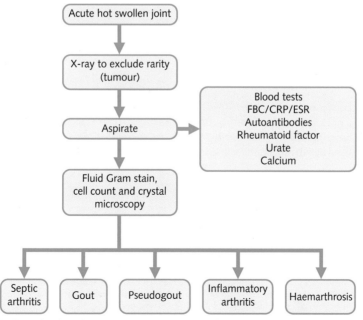

Fig. 6.2 Algorithm for the investigation of an acute hot swollen joint. *CRP*, C-reactive protein; *ESR*, erythrocyte sedimentation rate; *FBC*, full blood count.

Of all the investigations, joint aspiration is the most important for reaching a diagnosis.

Ultrasound

This can be useful in showing an effusion, particularly in the hip.

Chapter Summary

- There are many possible causes for an acute hot swollen joint: the most important cause to exclude is septic arthritis.
- Patient history, clinical examination and various investigations are useful in assessing an acute hot swollen joint.
- The suggested investigation algorithm should be followed when investigating a hot swollen joint.
- Joint aspiration with urgent Gram-staining and crystal microscopy is the gold-standard diagnostic test for an acute hot swollen joint.
- Procalcitonin is a relatively new test, which is useful for differentiating infective and inflammatory causes of acute hot swollen joints.

A child with a limp

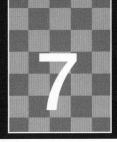

A child can limp for many reasons, but the most important condition to identify is septic arthritis, which can cause major morbidity or even result in death if missed.

DIFFERENTIAL DIAGNOSIS

- Septic arthritis
- Irritable hip
- Slipped upper femoral epiphysis (SUFE)
- Developmental dysplasia of the hip (DDH)
- Perthes disease
- Osteomyelitis
- Occult trauma
- Neuromuscular causes
- Juvenile idiopathic arthritis (JIA; see Chapter 17)
- Malignancy (very rare)

Table. 7.1 Diagnosis by age in a child with a limp

All ages	Infection Juvenile idiopathic arthritis Nonaccidental injury
Infant (1–3 years)	Late-presenting DDH Irritable hip Neuromuscular Occult trauma (including nonaccidental injury)
Childhood (3–11 years)	Perthes disease (3–7 years old) Irritable hip Neuromuscular SUFE Nonaccidental injury
Adolescence (12–16 years)	SUFE Infection

DDH, Developmental dysplasia of the hip; SUFE: slipped upper femoral epiphysis.

FOCUSED HISTORY

There is a big difference between an infant aged 15 months and an adolescent aged 15 years. Infants will not give an accurate history and if very unwell, they may be distressed and uncooperative. The majority of children do, however, give a good history.

Age

The most important factor in assessing a child with a limp is their age. Table 7.1 shows the likely differential diagnosis depending on the age of the child.

Gender

The gender of the child can also give clues to the diagnosis; for example, Perthes disease is much more common in boys than in girls.

Is the child ill?

To answer this question, the general state of the child must be noted. Systemically unwell children will show little interest in play or food and simply will not be themselves. Fever, rigors and night sweats should be noted as well as duration of symptoms. An unwell child suggests infection or JIA (see Chapter 17).

Pain

Most children limp because of a history of pain:

- Trauma or infection: rapid onset of pain is more likely.
- Perthes disease: often a vague gradual onset of pain and limp.
- SUFE: often a background of hip or knee pain for weeks followed by sudden increase in pain.
- Transient synovitis of the hip: pain in the groin and mimics septic arthritis.
- Any child complaining of knee pain must be suspected of having hip pathology.
- Malignancy: to be considered in cases of pain at night or gradually increasing pain not relieved by analgesia (see Chapter 21).

Painless limp

- Late-presenting DDH: limp and leg length discrepancy.
- Neuromuscular disorders: poor gait due to muscle imbalance rather than pain. Cerebral palsy can present as developmental delay but milder forms can present later in childhood as the weakness becomes more apparent. Muscular dystrophy can also present with gradual onset of weakness and limp.

Associated symptoms

History of injury may be elicited in trauma but in non-accidental injury this may not be forthcoming. Systemic features of ill health such as pyrexia, drowsiness and irritability should be noted and will point towards infection as the cause. Multiple joint problems may be obvious initially, suggesting JIA. Neuromuscular disorders may be obvious or detected on neurological examination.

RED FLAG

NONACCIDENTAL INJURY

Carefully consider nonaccidental injury in any child where history is incongruous. Signs may include:

- Multiple/delayed presentations
- Fractures not in keeping with normal childhood patterns
- Inconsistent or changing history
- Any concerns should be acted on immediately
- See Chapter 17, Paediatric joint disease

A recent history of upper respiratory tract infection, otitis media or any system infection is often found in patients with transient synovitis.

Multiple joint aches and pains suggest juvenile arthritis. In JIA, the child's eyes can be involved as part of the systemic effects of the disease. If left untreated, blindness can result (see Chapter 17).

Medical history

Any history of Perthes disease or SUFE is very important as these patients are at increased risk of developing disease in the opposite hip.

Family history

A family history of Perthes disease, DDH and SUFE also leads to an increased risk.

See 'Clinical notes' for summary of features of a limp requiring urgent assessment in the emergency department.

CLINICAL NOTES

Reasons to refer urgently to emergency department if seen in community

- Age <3 years
- Unable to bear own weight
- Fever/systemic symptoms

- Severe pain
- Maltreatment
- >9 years old with painful hip movements (Internal rotation), SUFE

FOCUSED EXAMINATION OF A CHILD WITH A LIMP

Inspection

Gait

- An antalgic gait is present in painful conditions.
- A Trendelenburg gait (see Chapter 2) is present in a toddler with late DDH or some neuromuscular conditions.
- Neuromuscular disorders give a variety of patterns of gait abnormality.
- A worrying sign is if a child is too ill or in too much pain to bear their own weight.

Standing

- An abnormal single large posterior skin crease is present in DDH.
- In SUFE or infection, the hip is often held in an abnormal position of external rotation and flexion (Fig. 7.1).

Further inspection could reveal scars, swelling or erythema.

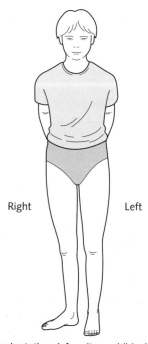

Right   Left

Fig. 7.1 External rotation deformity: a child with externally rotated right leg in slipped upper femoral epiphysis.

Fixed flexion

If the Thomas test is positive (a fixed flexion deformity), a significant problem should be considered, such as advanced Perthes disease, DDH or SUFE.

Limb length discrepancy

- A short leg is typical of DDH.
- Apparent shortening will be present if there is any fixed flexion deformity.

Palpation

Palpate any tender areas for effusion, warmth and localized pain.

The hip joint cannot be palpated directly because it is a deep joint; it is important to palpate the groin and greater trochanter for tenderness.

Palpation around the knee will reveal joint line tenderness in conditions such as osteochondritis or, in older children, meniscal tears.

Tenderness over the tibial tubercle is likely to be due to Osgood-Schlatter disease.

Movement

- Loss of hip movements indicates pathology.
- DDH results in loss of abduction compared with the other side.
- Perthes disease results in loss of abduction and flexion. Complete loss of abduction is a worrying sign in Perthes as this may indicate subluxation of the joint.
- In septic arthritis, any movement causes extreme pain. A child will hold a joint rigid to avoid pain.

COMMUNICATION

Listening to the child's parents and observing the child at play or rest is a key part of deciding whether a child is unwell. Play may be the only way to examine their painful limb.

INVESTIGATING A CHILD WITH A LIMP

Blood tests

Markedly elevated white cell count (WCC), erythrocyte sedimentation rate (ESR) and C-reactive protein can indicate the presence of infection, but these inflammatory markers can also be mildly increased in transient synovitis or JIA.

Very rare causes of abnormal blood tests include leukaemia. Creatinine kinase is elevated in muscular dystrophy.

X-ray examinations

A plain X-ray image is often unremarkable in the younger child, particularly in cases of transient synovitis.

A hip radiograph may show:

- Subluxation in the case of DDH
- Perthes disease
- SUFE
- Evidence of infection (remember, X-ray images are initially normal)
- A fracture

HINTS AND TIPS

If hip pathology is suspected, request anteroposterior pelvis and frog leg lateral view. If knee pathology is expected, anteroposterior and lateral images should be taken.

Knee radiographs may show:

- Osgood-Schlatter disease
- Osteochondritis dissecans
- A fracture

Ultrasound examination

Ultrasound examination is very useful for suspected joint problems, particularly of the hip, which is deeply situated, and is also helpful in aspiration.

The scan will show an effusion in:

- Septic arthritis
- Transient synovitis
- Perthes disease (early)

Magnetic resonance imaging

Magnetic resonance imaging (MRI) is not a first-line investigation in children. It is difficult for a young child to stay still for the scan. However, if necessary, an anaesthetic can be given to facilitate scanning. MRI is useful in:

- Diagnosis of knee disorders (see Chapter 17)
- Bone and soft-tissue tumours
- Osteomyelitis

Kocher criteria can be extremely useful clinically for diagnosing septic arthritis.

HINTS AND TIPS

Kocher criteria can be used as a tool to help differentiate transient synovitis from septic arthritis in children with hip pain. Four criteria are assessed and a score out of four is then calculated, giving a prediction regarding the likelihood of septic arthritis:

- White cell count >12,000 cells/mm^3
- Inability to bear weight
- Fever >38.5°C
- Erythrocyte sedimentation rate >40 mm/h

Predictive value of Kocher criteria (Kocher et al., 1999).

Score	Chance of septic arthritis as cause for hip pain (%)
1	3
2	40
3	93
4	99

Chapter Summary

- Examine the child thoroughly and assess their gait, carefully assessing whether it is painful or painless.
- Elicit whether the pain is coming from the hip, knee or ankle before investigating further.
- Be sure to rule out any malignant or infective cause and decide whether the child is unwell before considering the more common diagnoses.
- Carefully sort the common diagnoses according to age as shown in Table 7.1. Suspect Perthes disease in those aged 3-7 years, but think more of SUFE in older children.
- An irritable hip is a common problem but should be a diagnosis of exclusion, not your first thought.
- Carry out relevant investigations: blood tests, X-ray examinations and further imaging to rule out serious conditions, particularly septic arthritis.
- Ultrasound scan can be useful in these cases, but magnetic resonance imaging is rarely performed and difficult to achieve in young children.
- Seek expert help if uncertain with these diagnoses as they can be challenging even for experienced staff.

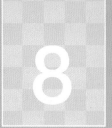

A discrete swelling on a limb may be a sign of underlying disease. Whilst a lesion may have an obvious and simple pathology (e.g., lipoma), all swellings should be considered thoroughly and investigated appropriately.

DIFFERENTIAL DIAGNOSIS

It is helpful to consider differential diagnoses in relation to the anatomical location:

Skin or subcutaneous:

- Cyst
- Lipoma
- Rheumatoid nodule
- Bursitis
- Neurofibroma
- Ganglion
- Neuroma

Joint:

- Joint effusion
- Ganglion
- Baker cyst

Bone:

- Osteophytes
- Bone tumour

Muscle/deep soft tissues:

- Sarcoma
- Lipoma

Patients commonly present with lumps, bumps and swellings. The majority of these are benign; when diagnosing these, the main consideration is to rule out malignant causes.

HISTORY FOCUSING ON A SWELLING

Duration

How long has the patient had the lump or swelling and when did the patient first notice the lump?

Increase in size

Has it grown rapidly or recently increased in size? Malignant tumours may present in this way.

Solitary or multiple

Does the patient have more than one lump or swelling and if so, where? Neurofibromata or rheumatoid nodules are often multiple. Multiple lipomas may represent a hereditary lipomatosis.

Variability

Does the swelling come and go and, if so, over what period? Classically, a ganglion will disappear and then recur. A joint effusion will be larger during an exacerbation of the underlying joint disease.

Is it painful?

The majority of lesions away from weight-bearing areas are not painful. A tense effusion will be painful, as may bursitis. Deep pain related to a bony or soft-tissue mass may be sinister. Constant deep bony pain and pain worse at night are symptoms suspicious of malignancy.

Loss of function

Does the swelling or lump inhibit the patient in any way? Swellings around the hand can be a nuisance to patients and those on the foot can rub when shoes are worn.

Associated symptoms

Usually there will be no associated symptoms.

The general health of the patient should be ascertained and red flags for malignancy should be explored if the rest of the history indicates.

RED FLAG

Assessment of a lump yielding any suspicious features should be asked red flag questions for malignancy:

- Weight loss
- Fatigue
- Night sweats
- Loss of appetite

Large swellings or masses can very occasionally compress vessels or nerves, e.g., in the case of malignant lesions, and can be a cause of whole limb swelling.

Patients presenting with joint swelling may have other symptoms related to the underlying disease process, such as pain in the joint if arthritic.

A patient may have painless joint swelling as a presenting feature of a more generalized inflammatory condition. It is important therefore to ask about other joints such as those in the hand.

A patient with a Baker cyst may have pain in the knee.

Occupational history

Patients who kneel frequently, such as carpet fitters, are very prone to developing prepatellar bursitis.

COMMUNICATION

Patients are often aware of the potential for lumps to be malignant and will often be looking for reassurance rather than removal. Many people do not mind living with their lump as long as they can be reassured that it is benign: let them know as soon as you are sure.

EXAMINATION FOCUSING ON A SWELLING

The affected area or joint and the local lymph nodes should be examined.

The following points relate to a swelling or mass rather than a joint effusion, which should be examined as part of full knee examination.

When examining a lump or swelling, the following points should be elicited.

Site

Which limb is affected and where is the lesion?

Size

Sinister pathology should be suspected in any lump larger than 5 cm.

Depth of lesion

- Is the lesion within the skin, in the subcutaneous tissue, tethered or deep to the fascia? Painful deep lesions are suspicious and need investigation.
- Is the skin inflamed or abnormal over the lesion?

Consistency

Is the lesion soft, firm or hard? A lipoma is often described as firm.

Diffuse or discrete

Some swellings are large without clear margins and appear to merge with the surrounding structures, whereas others are more easily palpable.

Surface

Is the surface of the lesion smooth or irregular?

Mobile or fixed

A discrete mass may be fixed to the underlying structures, e.g., a ganglion, or more mobile, e.g., a lipoma.

Fluctuance

Fluctuant lesions contain fluid, such as a Baker cyst.

Pulsatile

Pulsatile and expansile lesions are vascular aneurysms.

Transillumination

Fluid-filled lesions (e.g., ganglion) will transilluminate when tested with a pen torch if the fluid is clear.

The patient presenting with joint swelling only

Occasionally a patient will present with swelling of a single large joint and this can be the onset of a generalized condition such as rheumatoid arthritis.

Therefore it is important to examine other joints, such as the hand (if rheumatoid arthritis is suspected) or the spine (if ankylosing spondylitis is suspected).

INVESTIGATION OF A PATIENT WITH A SWELLING

We will consider joint swelling as a separate condition from a discrete swelling or mass.

Joint swelling (effusion)

Exclude infection (see Chapter 20).

Blood tests should be carried out to include inflammatory markers, urate, rheumatoid factors and autoantibodies to look for inflammatory arthritis.

X-rays may show osteoarthritis or rheumatoid arthritis or be normal.

Fluid aspiration and synovial fluid microscopy is performed looking for crystals indicating gout and pseudogout.

A limb swelling or lump

Further investigation may be unnecessary. For example, a patient has a cystic lesion on the volar aspect of the wrist, which comes and goes and is fixed to deep structures. The lesion is firm and smooth and transilluminates. This patient probably has a ganglion, which can be confirmed by aspirating jelly-like fluid or proceeding directly to surgical excision.

Further investigation is necessary if there is doubt about a diagnosis:

- If bony pathology is suspected, an X-ray examination of the affected limb should be performed. A benign or malignant bony lesion may be found.

- A deeply situated soft-tissue lesion may be a sarcoma and if so, needs urgent further investigation.
- An initial ultrasound scan may be useful to confirm the presence of a mass and whether it is fluid-filled or solid.
- However, a magnetic resonance imaging scan with contrast gives detail regarding the exact nature of the lesion.
- If doubt still exists, the patient should be referred to a specialist musculoskeletal oncology service and the next step would be a biopsy.
- An algorithm for the investigation of a limb swelling is given in Fig. 8.1.

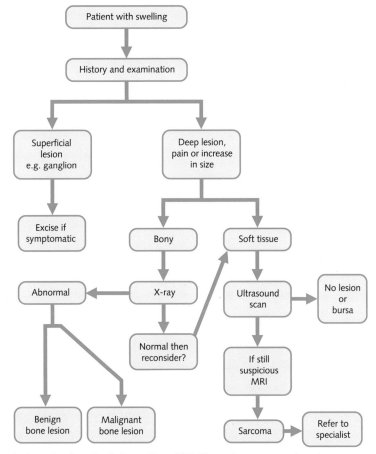

Fig. 8.1 Algorithm for the investigation of a limb swelling. *MRI*, Magnetic resonance imaging.

Chapter summary

- Important features in the history are rapidity of onset, size, presence of night pain and associated red flag symptoms.
- Lumps that are a cause for concern come on rapidly, grow in size and have associated symptoms of night pain and systemic upset.
- Examining the lump should focus on whether it is a deep or superficial mass and its relation to any joints.
- Pulsatile masses should be investigated urgently as should those with any suspicious features
- The aim when investigating a lump is always to rule out malignancy or infection before considering common benign causes.
- If in doubt, further imaging is always indicated in the form of ultrasound scan or magnetic resonance imaging.

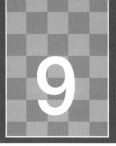
Back pain, or leg pain secondary to pathology in the spine, is extremely common. In fact, as many as 80% of the population will have an episode of back pain in their life. The patient may present with back pain, leg pain or both, and it is important to take a detailed history and perform a detailed examination to try to elicit the cause of the patient's symptoms. There are many pitfalls when assessing a patient with back pain; however, the most important thing is to distinguish the common musculoskeletal pains from the less frequent but more sinister and urgent pathologies. Any history must aim at distinguishing whether problems are truly arising from the spine or from the hip, abdomen or other causes.

DIFFERENTIAL DIAGNOSIS

Mechanical low back pain:

- Osteoarthritis of the spine
- Prolapsed intervertebral disc
- Vertebral crush fracture
- Spinal stenosis/spondylolisthesis
- Malignancy

Infection:

- Discitis
- Vertebral osteomyelitis
- Vascular insufficiency

Hip causes:

- Osteoarthritis
- Avascular necrosis

Abdominal causes

- Pancreatitis
- Dissecting aortic aneurysm
- Renal disease

HISTORY FOCUSING ON BACK AND LEG PAIN

- Age: older patients are less likely to have disc disease and malignancy is more common
- Elicit the timescale of symptoms: traumatic event?
- Leg pain: bilateral or unilateral?
- Numbness and distribution if present
- Weakness
- Change in bowel/bladder habits

- Weight loss or systemic upset: for red flags alerting to serious spinal pathology see Chapter 4
- Previous surgical intervention/injection

A focused history for back pain should clearly define the timespan of the symptoms and initially aims to rule out spinal pathology requiring urgent intervention. A clearer history of mechanical back pain may be useful once this is done.

EXAMINATION FOCUSING ON BACK AND LEG PAIN

General examination

Look at the patient: weight loss, anaemia and general ill health may suggest malignancy. Look at the patient's posture and gait:

- A stooped posture with flexion of the knee can suggest sciatica.
- A frail elderly woman with a stooped posture may have osteoporotic fractures.
- A very stiff spine may be ankylosing spondylitis or simple low back pain requiring analgesia to relieve spasm.
- Fixed flexion of the hip with an antalgic or Trendelenburg gait is likely to be hip pathology. There may be a limb-length discrepancy.
- Look for deformity of the spine, previous scars, wasting and any lower-limb deformity.

If hip pathology is suspected, a full hip examination and Trendelenburg and Thomas tests should be performed as described in Chapter 2.

Palpation

- With the patient standing, palpate the spine centrally and surrounding muscles for tenderness. In simple low back pain, the area around the posterior superior iliac spine and sacroiliac joint is often tender.

Movement

- Assess movements of the spine. Diminished movement is likely if pathology is present. It may be impossible for the patient to comply because of pain.

Special tests

If the nerve root is irritated by a prolapsed disc or spinal stenosis, a positive sciatic stretch test (Lasègue test) will show that straight-leg raising is diminished.

A peripheral nervous system examination may show weakness and sensory loss in a single nerve root pattern.

A digital rectal examination is mandatory in all patients with suspected cauda equina syndrome. This should assess for tone and the ability to distinguish sharp and dull touch.

INVESTIGATION OF A PATIENT WITH BACK PAIN

Blood tests

Blood tests are not always necessary but should be performed to exclude sinister causes in patients over 55 years of age or as guided by clinical suspicion. Full blood count and biochemistry may reveal:

- Elevated white cell count if infection is present, such as in discitis.
- Anaemia or high calcium levels in malignancy.
- Erythrocyte sedimentation rate (ESR) and C-reactive protein (CRP) are elevated in infection and malignancy. Immunoglobulin and urinary Bence Jones protein should be checked to exclude myeloma.
- Patients presenting with metastatic disease and an unknown primary need thorough investigation. Biopsy specimens taken at surgery may identify the primary cause.

Plain X-ray

Plain X-ray images of the spine should only be taken routinely after trauma.

Normal appearances are seen in simple low back pain, prolapsed disc and even in malignancy or infection if early in the disease process (it is therefore not a useful test).

However, they can be helpful in identifying:

- Osteoarthritic changes in the spine.
- A spondylolisthesis.
- Destruction of the vertebral body, classically the pedicle (winking-owl sign; see Chapter 4, Fig. 4.2), indicating malignancy.
- Fracture.
- Erosion of vertebral body around the disc due to infection.

Further special tests are often needed if there is doubt about the diagnosis or to plan surgery:

- Magnetic resonance imaging (MRI): this is the most common imaging for soft-tissue structures, including identification of disc prolapse and nerve root prior to surgery and early detection of malignancy and infection.
- Computed tomography (CT) scanning: Useful for looking at bony structures in detail, e.g., spondylolisthesis or fracture in trauma setting.
- Isotope bone scanning: hot spot in infection and malignancy.

An algorithm for the investigation of sinister back pain is provided in Fig. 9.1.

MECHANICAL LOW BACK PAIN

Back pain is extremely common and causes a significant burden on the resources of westernized societies in terms of lost working days.

Definition

Musculoskeletal back pain is not a single specific disease entity but rather a collection of ill-defined conditions presenting with low back pain. This diagnosis should only be made after other pathological conditions have been excluded.

Incidence

Of the population, 80% will have back pain at some stage in their lives.

Aetiology and pathology

As back pain is so common, it is difficult to define clear aetiological factors for its occurrence.

A lot of the pathological changes seen on imaging will also be present in the healthy, normal population with no symptoms.

- Facet joint arthritis shows the typical features of osteoarthritis with joint space destruction and osteophyte formation.
- Degenerative disc disease occurs with ageing and is related to decreased water content in the nucleus pulposus. The disc space narrows and the segment is said to become more mobile. This abnormal movement, together with an inability to distribute load, causes pain.

Patients rarely present with mechanical back pain after 60 years of age and as they enter old age the symptoms usually subside. This is said to be due to stiffening of a mobile spine.

Clinical features

There are two typical clinical scenarios: acute back pain over days or weeks and chronic unrelenting back pain for many years.

Acute back pain over days or weeks

Pain is usually solely located in the back, possibly following a precipitating incident. Pain is severe and the patient may have difficulty getting into a comfortable position. Sometimes the patient has pain referred down the back of the leg but this differs from true radicular pain in that back pain is still the predominant feature and the pain does not typically radiate beyond the knee. The pain is mechanical (i.e., worse on movement).

Clinical examination will show muscle spasm with loss of lumbar lordosis. The patient may find it difficult to walk and spinal movements will be minimal.

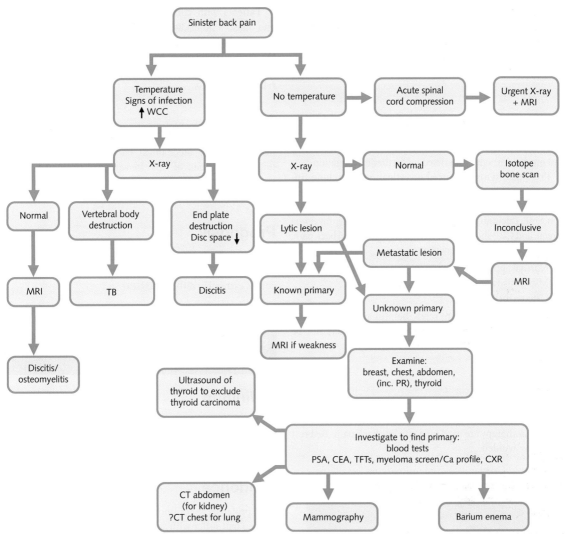

Fig. 9.1 Algorithm for the investigation of sinister back pain.
Ca, Calcium; *CEA*, carcinoembryonic antigen; *CT*, computed tomography; *CXR*, chest X-ray; *MRI*, magnetic resonance imaging; *PR*, per rectum; *PSA*, prostate-specific antigen; *TB*, tuberculosis; *TFTs*, thyroid function tests; *WCC*, white cell count.

Sciatic stretch testing and peripheral nerve examination will be negative.

Chronic unrelenting back pain for many years

The patient will be unable to work and often has seen numerous doctors, physiotherapists and other allied health workers, including alternative medical practitioners.

The back pain is usually unrelenting and does not have any relieving factors. Leg pain may or may not be present.

Clinical examination rarely shows any significant features other than reduced movements. Inappropriate signs (Waddell signs) may be present (see Clinical notes box describing these signs).

CLINICAL NOTES

WADDELL SIGNS FOR NONORGANIC COMPONENT TO LOW BACK PAIN

- Superficial tenderness and tenderness not in keeping with the anatomy in question.
- Regional pain not conforming to known neuroanatomy.
- Pain on movements not affecting the lower back, e.g., axial loading and simulated rotation.
- Lack of pain after distraction, e.g., patients being unable to lift a leg straight but able to sit

on the examination couch with legs straight and hips flexed to 90 degrees.
- Overreaction to pain. This is very subjective and should be used with caution.

Diagnosis and investigation

The majority of patients with a short history (less than 6 weeks) and mechanical symptoms need no further investigation.

Prolonged symptoms need investigation to exclude sinister causes of back pain.

Blood tests including full blood count, ESR, liver function tests, calcium/phosphate/alkaline phosphatase, myeloma screen, and CRP should all be normal in mechanical back pain.

X-ray examination may show:

- Normal appearances
- Minor disc narrowing
- Osteoarthritis (Fig. 9.2)

MRI and CT scanning are rarely helpful and may be misleading if they highlight an abnormality that may not be significant.

Treatment

Conservative

Analgesia, nonsteroidal antiinflammatory drugs (NSAIDs) and physiotherapy are used for acute low back pain. Bed rest should be avoided.

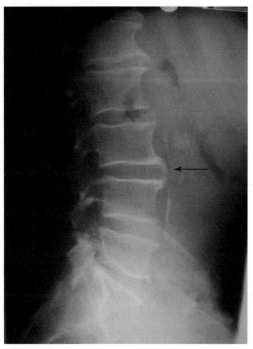

Fig. 9.2 Osteoarthritis of the spine (*black arrow*).

Patients with chronic pain are very difficult to treat and need a multidisciplinary approach to try to break the pain cycle. Psychological input may be required and the pain management team might have to be consulted. Occasionally, facet joint injections for localized disease can relieve symptoms.

Surgical

In the vast majority of patients, surgery has no role in the management of mechanical back pain and the patient must be informed of this. In very few selected patients, some surgeons will advocate surgery in degenerative disc disease.

Prognosis

Most acute back pain episodes settle spontaneously and the patient returns to normal. Once chronic, the condition becomes extremely difficult to treat.

PROLAPSED INTERVERTEBRAL DISC

Definition

A disc prolapse occurs when part of the nucleus pulposus herniates through the annulus fibrosus and presses on a spinal nerve root.

Incidence

Disc prolapse is common: up to 3% of men and 1% of women will suffer with sciatica related to a prolapsed intervertebral disc. Usual presentation is between the ages of 30 and 50 years.

Aetiology and pathology

There is good evidence that manual workers involved in heavy lifting have increased incidence of disc prolapse. Regular automobile use is also said to be a risk factor.

The herniation of disc material tends to occur posterolaterally where the annulus is thinner. Central disc prolapse can occur and press on the combined nerve roots, including those supplying the bladder and bowel (cauda equina syndrome). Prolapse can occur without spinal root involvement, in which case the patient will have symptoms of back pain but not true sciatica.

Disc prolapse most commonly occurs at L4–L5 or L5–S1 level but can occur at any level (including cervical and rarely thoracic). The nerve root crosses its space before exiting the spine beneath the pedicle: L4–L5 disc presses on L5 nerve root (Fig. 9.3).

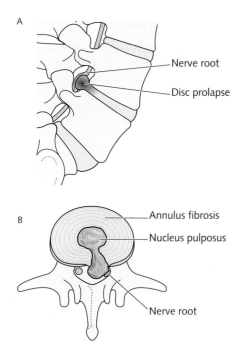

Fig. 9.3 (A and B) Prolapsed intervertebral disc.

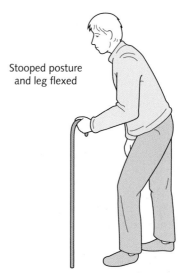

Fig. 9.4 Posture in prolapsed intervertebral disc.

Clinical features

Sciatica is a symptom of lower lumbar or sacral nerve root irritation. The patient complains of severe pain radiating down the leg as far as the toes. There may be numbness and tingling or weakness of the foot. Patients find it very uncomfortable to sit, and either stand or lie down.

CLINICAL NOTES

SYMPTOMS OF CAUDA EQUINA SYNDROME SUGGEST IMMEDIATE MRI

- Altered bladder/anal function: urinary retention or incontinence
- Perineal paraesthesia: due to compression of the nerves within the cauda equine, which supply motor function to the bowel and bladder sphincters, and sensation to the perineum.
- Bilateral leg pain
- Bilateral paraesthesia
- Bilateral motor deficit
- Perineal pain

Clinically, a patient will have an abnormal posture, stooping to the affected side and standing with the knee flexed to relieve pressure on the dura (Fig. 9.4).

Nerve root tension signs such as straight-leg raising will be positive.

The crossover sign may be positive (elevation of the opposite or normal leg gives pain shooting down the affected leg).

Numbness in a dermatomal distribution and weakness with loss of reflexes may be present.

Check for any sinister features (see Fig. 4.2).

Diagnosis and investigation

In older patients, blood tests, described above, should be performed to exclude any sinister causes.

X-ray images are usually normal and are performed to exclude bony pathology such as spondylolisthesis.

MRI scanning is now the investigation of choice in patients with persistent symptoms (Fig. 9.5).

Treatment

Conservative

A short period of bed rest followed by gentle physiotherapy with adequate analgesia (including NSAIDs) is the initial treatment for most discs.

Surgical

Lumbar nerve root injection can provide diagnosis and treatment for nerve root compression.

The only indications for urgent surgical discectomy are cauda equina syndrome and progressively worsening neurological deficit.

If patients have prolonged intractable back pain (>3 months), surgery is considered. However, patients are informed that back pain is rarely improved and only leg symptoms can be reliably treated.

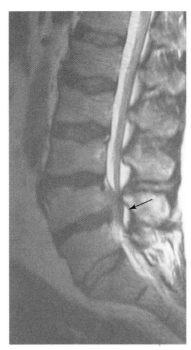

Fig. 9.5 Magnetic resonance imaging scan of prolapsed intervertebral disc at L4–L5 level (*black arrow*).

Prognosis

Ninety-seventy per cent of acute disc prolapses settle spontaneously with conservative treatment. It is important to let your patient know acute disc prolapses are usually a self-limiting condition.

SPONDYLOLISTHESIS

Definition

This means one vertebral body slipping on another.

> **COMMUNICATION**
>
> It is easy to confuse the terminology. A *spondylolysis* is a defect in the pars interarticularis that may allow the vertebra to slip forward, causing a *spondylolisthesis* (forward slippage of one vertebra on another).

Incidence

The condition is common (approximately 5% of the population) but most are asymptomatic. It is more common in Caucasian males.

Aetiology and pathology

Certain sports predispose to spondylolysis (gymnasts and fast bowlers in cricket). Spondylolisthesis can be caused by spondylolysis and numerous other pathologies.

The slip usually occurs at the L5–S1 level. The degree of slip is normally assessed as a percentage (0%–25%, 25%–50%, 50%–75% or >75%) and graded 1–4. There can be an associated kyphosis or scoliosis.

Clinical features

Spondylolisthesis is the most common cause of persistent back pain in children.

Initially, back pain is the sole presentation but if the slip becomes severe, nerve root irritation will occur, causing sciatica. Radicular symptoms are more common in adults.

There may be central spinal tenderness. Movement is usually preserved, but classically hyperextension is painful.

Diagnosis and investigation

Oblique X-rays may show the classic 'collar on Scottie dog' appearance of spondylolysis (Fig. 9.6) and the lateral X-ray image will show the degree and angle of slippage (Fig. 9.7).

CT scans clearly demonstrate the lesion.

MRI should be performed if nerve root irritation is suspected.

Treatment

Conservative

Initial rest and restriction of activities may allow a spondylolysis to heal before a slip occurs.

In adult patients, a trial of conservative treatment is advised with physiotherapy, analgesia and activity modification.

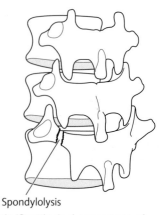

Spondylolysis

Fig. 9.6 Classic 'Scottie dog' appearance of spondylolisthesis.

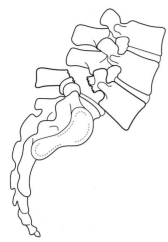

Fig. 9.7 An L5–S1 spondylolisthesis with a pars defect.

Surgical

Persistent pain, radiculopathy and significant deformity are indications for surgery.

Fusion with or without metalwork and bone graft is commonly performed.

Prognosis

The outcome is variable, depending on the type and degree of slip.

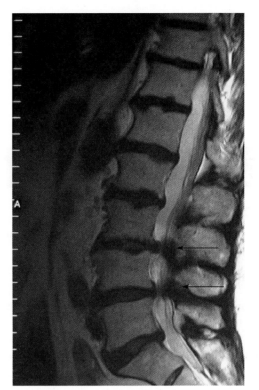

Fig. 9.8 Magnetic resonance imaging scan of spinal stenosis (*arrows*).

SPINAL STENOSIS

Definition

Spinal stenosis is caused by degenerative changes narrowing the spinal canal and causing compression of the nerve roots.

Incidence

This is a common disorder, mainly affecting men over 50 years of age.

Aetiology and pathology

Spinal stenosis is more common in heavy manual labourers.

It is usually secondary to degenerative changes. Thickening of ligaments, osteophytes and posterior disc bulge encroach into the spinal canal (Fig. 9.8).

It is thought that ischaemia of the spinal nerves during exercise produces the classic symptoms.

Clinical features

Typically, patients present with discomfort when walking, with pain referred to the buttock, calves and feet. The pain can be claudicant in nature and relieved by rest; it must be distinguished carefully from vascular claudication. The 'shopping cart sign' may highlight spinal stenosis, whereby patients who normally suffer severe pain are able to walk greater distances when they have a flexed spine whilst leaning on their shopping trolley. Flexion is thought to open up the spinal canal a little, relieving some of the stenosis. Back pain is usually present. Pain is worse on extension and relieved by rest and flexion of the spine.

Examination will reveal stiffening of the spine but sciatic stretch testing may be normal.

It is important to examine the peripheral vascular system to confirm whether the cause is spinal or vascular in origin.

Diagnosis and investigation

X-ray examination will usually reveal degenerative changes.

MRI shows the degree of stenosis and nerve root involvement. If suspected, exclude peripheral vascular insufficiency with Doppler scans.

Treatment

Conservative

Weight loss, physiotherapy, activity modification and NSAIDs may relieve symptoms sufficiently to avoid surgery.

Surgical

Severe symptoms not responding to conservative measures require surgical decompression.

Prognosis

The condition tends to be progressive.

DISCITIS/VERTEBRAL OSTEOMYELITIS

Definition

Discitis is infection of the disc space and vertebral osteomyelitis is infection of a vertebral body.

Incidence

The incidence is approximately 1/100,000, but the condition is more common in less developed countries.

Aetiology and pathology

Conditions associated with other bone and joint infection (see Chapter 20), particularly intravenous drug use, immunocompromised patients and those with diabetes are predisposed to spinal infection. Patients with recent sepsis from pneumonia or urinary tract infection can subsequently develop discitis by seeding of infection. It can occur following surgery to the disc.

Common infecting organisms are staphylococci and streptococci in adults and staphylococci and *Haemophilus* in children. Tuberculosis should also be considered (Pott disease).

Clinical features

Patients are unwell with pyrexia and complain of severe, unrelenting back pain.

Clinical examination may reveal swelling and, in severe cases, an angular scoliosis or kyphosis (gibbus). There is pain on palpation, reduced movement and possible abnormal neurology.

Discitis commonly presents late: patients often have 6–12 weeks of symptoms before the correct diagnosis is made.

Diagnosis and investigation

The white cell count, ESR and CRP are elevated.

X-ray examination reveals narrowed disc space (discitis) and bony destruction (osteomyelitis) (Fig. 9.9).

An isotope bone scan will show that the affected area is hot.

MRI scanning should be performed to detect any epidural abscess: 50% of patients with neurological symptoms will have this.

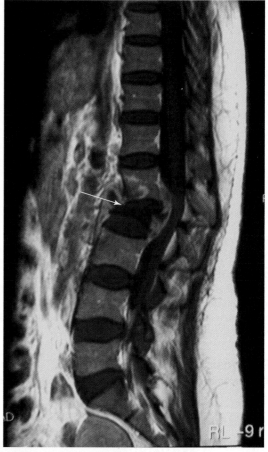

Fig. 9.9 Magnetic resonance imaging showing tuberculosis of the spine. There is complete collapse of the vertebra (*white arrow*) with resultant kyphosis.

CT-guided biopsy should be obtained for culture and sensitivity tests.

Treatment

Conservative

Intravenous antibiotics are given for 6 weeks, with a prolonged course of oral/ IV antibiotics if required. Follow-up MRI scanning at 6 weeks is usually indicated.

Surgical

Any abscess should be drained and an unstable spine with significant deformity needs stabilization.

Prognosis

Prognosis is variable: childhood cases respond well and should return to normality; severe adult infections can be life-threatening and surgery carries significant risk.

SCOLIOSIS

Definition

This is a lateral deviation and rotational abnormality of the spine.

Incidence

Up to 2.5% of the population are affected by idiopathic scoliosis.

Aetiology and pathology

Causes of scoliosis are listed in Table 9.1. Curves are thoracolumbar (Fig. 9.10).

Table 9.1 Causes of scoliosis

Type	Pathology	Example
Congenital	Abnormal development of spine	Hemivertebra
Idiopathic	Unknown	Adolescent idiopathic scoliosis
Neuromuscular	Abnormal muscle forces acting on the spine	Cerebral palsy
Secondary	Curve develops secondary to another process	Leg-length discrepancy

Clinical features

Pain is not usually a feature; rather the patient or relatives complain of deformity, in the form of an asymmetrical rib hump, spinal curve and limb length inequality. For clinical examination, the rib hump is more prominent on forward flexion (Fig. 9.11).

Very severe deformity reduces chest expansion, which can be life-threatening.

Diagnosis and investigation

Standing X-ray images show the curve and serial films are important to monitor the progress of the curve.

A significant increase in the severity of the curve is often an indication for surgical stabilization.

MRI scans are performed to exclude any associated spinal cord abnormality.

Treatment

Conservative

The treatment depends on the angle of the curve measured on the X-rays. In idiopathic scoliosis, the initial treatment is bracing for mild to moderate curves.

Surgical

All congenital, most neuromuscular and severe or progressive idiopathic curves will require surgical stabilization, fusion and correction.

Thoracic spine

Lumbar spine

Pelvis

Fig. 9.10 Thoracolumbar curve in scoliosis.

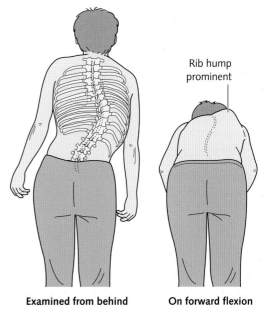

Rib hump prominent

Examined from behind   **On forward flexion**

Fig. 9.11 Examination of a patient with scoliosis.

Prognosis

The majority of curves are minor and require little treatment.

Very severe neuromuscular curves can lead to death due to cardiorespiratory compromise.

CLINICAL NOTES

Metastatic cord compression should be considered in patients with known metastatic disease and back pain. If imaging confirms this, urgent treatment is usually with radiotherapy under the oncology team.

● Chapter Summary

Back pain should be investigated carefully, ruling out any pathological causes before thinking that it is simple back pain, despite this being the most common cause.

- Chronic back pain has an unpredictable course but comes and goes in the majority of cases.
- Differentials that are cause for concern are tumours, metastases, cauda equina and infection.
- It is essential to ask about red flags.
- The difference between spinal and vascular claudication can be elicited with a good history, with spinal claudication more likely positional.
- Spondylolysis is pain coming from the discs, whereas spondylolisthesis is one vertebra slipping on another.
- Discitis and vertebral osteomyelitis should be treated with aggressive antibiotic treatment and require further imaging to diagnose.

The most likely malignant cause for back pain is metastatic spread from a distant primary.

- If in doubt, further imaging of back pain is always indicated in the form of CT or MRI, with MRI being better for analysing discs or nerve roots and CT for bony pathology.

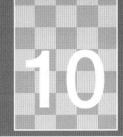
Neurological symptoms occur when there is irritation to a nerve. This may be due to chronic compression or an acute injury. Patients may complain of numbness, pins and needles, electric shock-type pain, burning, hypersensitivity, dysaesthesia and weakness. The pattern of these symptoms will help diagnose which nerve is causing the problem.

DIFFERENTIAL DIAGNOSIS

Peripheral nerve lesions:

- Carpal tunnel syndrome (CTS)
- Ulnar nerve entrapment
- Tarsal tunnel syndrome

Spinal pathology:

- Disc prolapse
- Spinal stenosis
- Osteoarthritis
- Cervical rib
- Malignancy
- Morton neuroma
- Nerve tumours, e.g., neurofibroma, schwannoma
- Medical causes, e.g., multiple sclerosis or stroke
- Postsurgery, e.g., superficial radial nerve neuroma
- Peripheral neuropathy, e.g., alcoholism, diabetes mellitus, drugs, vitamin B_{12} deficiency
- Complex regional pain syndrome (see Chapter 4).
- Vibration white finger

HISTORY

The following points should be covered.

Site

The site of the neurological problem is very important in determining which nerve is affected (Fig. 10.1) or whether it is a global change.

Onset of symptoms

- Acute onset usually occurs with disc prolapse, where pain may be the main feature.
- There is a gradual onset in nerve compression, e.g., spinal stenosis, CTS.

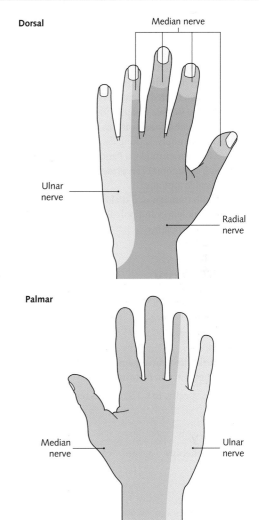

Fig. 10.1 Median, ulnar and radial nerve innervation of the hand.

- Onset of symptoms may occur after trauma, e.g., CTS after distal radius fracture.
- Accidental laceration to a nerve during surgery can result in paraesthesia in the distribution of the affected nerve or a painful neuroma.

Nature of symptoms

Exacerbating features

Sneezing and coughing often exacerbate symptoms of leg pain with disc prolapse.

Relieving features

- Patients with CTS often get night pain, which is relieved by hanging their hand down off the bed.
- Patients with lumbar spinal stenosis suffer pain and numbness in their legs after walking short distances (spinal claudication), which is relieved by bending forward.

Associated features

- Loss of bowel or bladder function in patients with back pain should be treated as cauda equina syndrome until proven otherwise (see Chapter 9).
- Check for constitutional features such as weight loss, malaise or haemoptysis (lung cancer) if malignancy is suspected. For example, a Pancoast tumour (an apical lung carcinoma) can present with upper-limb neurological symptoms.
- Patients with undiagnosed diabetes mellitus may have weight loss, polyuria and polydipsia associated with peripheral neuropathy.

Medical history

The following can predispose to nerve lesions:

- Malignancy
- Previous surgery
- Trauma
- Osteoarthritis and rheumatoid arthritis
- Systemic lupus erythematosus

A list of causes specific to CTS can be seen later.

Drug history

Some chemotherapy agents can cause peripheral neuropathy.

Social history

Manual jobs may trigger ulnar or carpal tunnel symptoms. A history of alcohol use may be relevant.

Family history

For example, a family history of neurofibromatosis (von Recklinghausen disease) or diabetes.

Examination

Knowledge of myotomes and dermatomes will help determine the level of a spinal cord lesion. For peripheral nerve lesions, establish the sensory distribution and motor function. Some special tests may reproduce nerve symptoms such as tapping a nerve (Tinel test). Café-au-lait spots are characteristic of neurofibromatosis.

COMMUNICATION

Sleep is affected in severe carpal tunnel syndrome. Patients look tired, unhappy and even depressed. When using their hands, they may be struggling to complete complex tasks and be dropping things. Pain might be more severe when using the phone or typing. Simple splints may allow them a good night's sleep and to function at work.

Investigation

Plain radiographs of the spine may show osteophytes causing nerve root compression, the presence of a cervical rib or osteoarthritis (OA) in the wrist. Magnetic resonance imaging (MRI) provides very detailed soft-tissue images and is commonly used to investigate spinal pathology such as a disc prolapse. Ultrasound scans or MRI can diagnose a Morton neuroma. Nerve conduction studies are used routinely to confirm CTS and can be used to diagnose other peripheral nerve lesions. Blood tests may demonstrate the cause of a peripheral neuropathy, e.g., fasting glucose, thyroid function tests, haematinics.

CARPAL TUNNEL SYNDROME

Definition

CTS results from compression of the median nerve as it passes through the carpal tunnel at the wrist. The carpal tunnel is formed by the space between the transverse carpal ligament and the carpal bones.

Incidence

CTS is very common, especially in middle-aged and elderly women.

Aetiology

CTS is usually idiopathic but can be associated with several underlying conditions (see Clinical Notes).

CLINICAL NOTES

CONDITIONS PREDISPOSING TO CARPAL TUNNEL SYNDROME

- Diabetes mellitus
- Hypothyroidism
- Rheumatoid arthritis
- Pregnancy
- Acromegaly
- Trauma, e.g., wrist fractures

Clinical features

CTS presents with pain and/or paraesthesia in the median nerve distribution (Fig. 10.1). These symptoms can radiate distally to the fingers or proximally towards the elbow. They are often worse at night, waking the patient. It is important to try to distinguish this from other peripheral neuropathy causes such as alcoholic or diabetic neuropathy. The presence of bilateral fingertip numbness in all digits should raise doubt about CTS being the cause.

Examination may reveal sensory loss in the median nerve distribution but can be unremarkable. The strength of the thenar muscles should be tested; they may be weak and wasted in advanced disease. Carpal tunnel compression testing with Phalen and Tinel tests may reproduce the symptoms (Fig. 10.2).

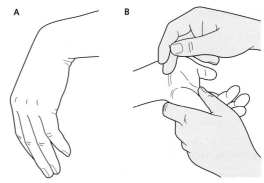

Fig. 10.2 Provocation tests for carpal tunnel syndrome may reproduce the patient's symptoms. (A) Phalen test: the wrist is held in maximal palmar flexion. (B) Tinel test: tap over the median nerve proximal to the transverse carpal ligament in the wrist.

 CLINICAL NOTES

MEDIAN NERVE MUSCLE SUPPLY IN HAND (MNEMONIC: LOAF)

Lateral (1st and 2nd) lumbricals
Opponens pollicis. Ask patient to touch the thumb to the little finger and resist attempts to separate the two.
Abductor pollicis brevis. With dorsum of hand flat on table ask patient to abduct thumb and then resist adduction force.
Flexor pollicis brevis. Flexes thumb at MCP joint.

 COMMUNICATION

Patients with carpal tunnel syndrome do not always complain of pain radiating from the wrist to their thumb, index and middle fingers. They often find it difficult to localize their symptoms and they may complain that their whole forearm and hand feel painful and/or numb.

Investigations

Nerve conduction studies show reduced nerve conduction velocities across the wrist. This will be very helpful in distinguishing entrapment from cervical disc pathology where the distal nerve conduction will be intact or uniformly reduced. Investigations such as serum glucose and thyroid function tests should be performed to exclude underlying medical conditions.

Management

The most successful treatment is surgical decompression of the carpal tunnel by division of the transverse carpal ligament. This is a very effective procedure and can be performed under local anaesthetic. In less severe cases, wrist splints may help nocturnal symptoms and corticosteroid injection of the carpal tunnel may bring some relief. In cases associated with pregnancy, the patient should be assessed postdelivery as symptoms may disappear.

 CLINICAL NOTES

VIBRATION WHITE FINGER

Also known as hand arm vibration syndrome **(HAVS)**

- A secondary form of Raynaud syndrome believed to be caused by continual industrial exposure to vibration.
- Leads to tingling or numbness in digit tips, excessive whiteness in cold and re-perfusion pain, possible reduced dexterity.
- Frequency reduced by industrial safety procedures.

ULNAR NERVE ENTRAPMENT

Definition

The ulnar nerve can become compressed as it passes behind the medial epicondyle or through Guyon canal in the wrist.

Incidence

Ulnar nerve damage at the elbow is fairly common due to its superficial position.

Aetiology

Ulnar nerve entrapment may be idiopathic or due to a precipitating cause.

CLINICAL NOTES

PRECIPITATING FACTORS FOR ULNAR NERVE ENTRAPMENT

- Local trauma, e.g., fractures of the elbow
- Prolonged leaning on the elbow
- Elbow synovitis

Clinical features

Patients develop pain and/or paraesthesia in the medial side of the elbow, which radiates to the medial forearm and the ulnar nerve distribution in the hand (see Fig. 10.1). The pain is often exacerbated by elbow flexion.

Examination usually reveals reduced sensation in the ulnar nerve distribution. Palpation of the nerve behind the medial epicondyle may provoke the symptoms. Motor dysfunction may result in atrophy of the hypothenar eminence and intrinsic muscles, the majority of which are supplied by the ulnar nerve. Due to intrinsic weakness, abduction and adduction of the fingers may be weak and in severe cases there may be clawing of the hand (Fig. 10.3).

Investigations

Nerve conduction studies confirm the diagnosis and establish the site of compression.

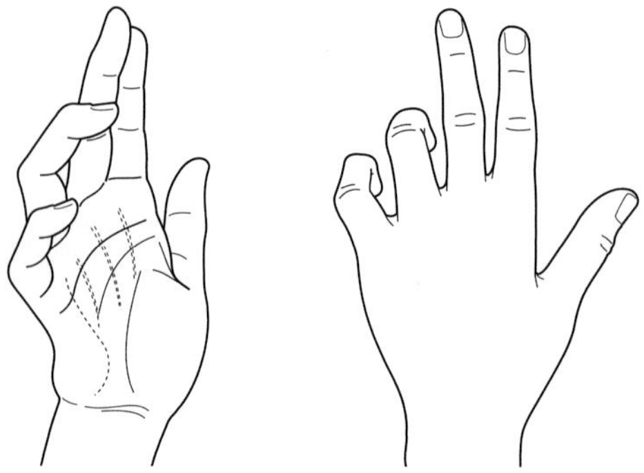

Management

Ulnar nerve compression due to elbow synovitis may respond to corticosteroid injection of the elbow. Surgical decompression should be performed if sensory symptoms cannot be tolerated or if there is muscle weakness or wasting.

RADIAL NERVE INJURIES

Aetiology

Radial nerve compression at the axilla is typically seen in an inebriated person who falls asleep with an arm hanging over the back of a chair ('Saturday night palsy'). The radial nerve may also be injured by fractures of the humeral shaft.

Clinical features

The wrist extensors are paralysed, resulting in wrist drop. Grip strength is dramatically reduced because the finger flexors do not function well with the wrist in a flexed position. Nerve injury in the axilla will also lead to paralysis of the triceps. Due to nerve overlap, sensory loss is best detected in the small area of skin on the dorsum of the hand between the first and second metacarpals.

Management

The wrist should be splinted immediately and the cause of the radial nerve palsy should be assessed. Fracture or dislocation reduction can help with nerve entrapment relief and may sometimes need to be performed surgically. If there is no resolution, tendon transfer or nerve grafting may be indicated.

COMMON PERONEAL NERVE INJURIES

Aetiology

The common peroneal nerve winds around the neck of the fibula and is in a vulnerable position. It may be damaged by fractures of the neck of the fibula or pressure from a tight bandage, plaster cast or intraoperative pressure points.

Clinical features

Common peroneal nerve injury results in paralysis of the ankle and foot extensors. Unopposed action of the foot

Fig. 10.3 Clawing of the hand due to ulnar nerve palsy.

flexors and inverters cause the foot to be plantar flexed and inverted. This is referred to as 'foot drop'. Patients develop a high-stepping gait, flicking the foot forwards to avoid tripping over it. There is also loss of sensibility over the anterior and lateral sides of the leg and the dorsum of the foot and toes.

Management

Pressure on the nerve should be relieved and a splint should be applied. If the foot drop does not resolve, an ankle–foot orthosis can be used to maintain some degree of dorsiflexion. Nerve conduction studies are done to assess nerve status.

● Chapter Summary

- Entrapments can be differentiated from other patterns of neurological deficit through medical history and examination.
- For neurological symptoms affecting the upper and lower limbs, we should first think of central conditions such as stroke and brain conditions and then gradually move distally to find the diagnosis.
- Common causes distally are spinal nerve entrapments and peripheral nerve entrapments such as carpal or ulnar nerve entrapment.
- Common investigations used to investigate neurological conditions will include MRI for the spine and nerve conduction studies.
- Pregnancy, diabetes and rheumatoid arthritis are common factors in carpal tunnel syndrome.
- It is not uncommon to release the carpal tunnel at the time of distal radius fracture surgery if acute nerve symptoms are present.

Release of distal nerve entrapments such as carpal tunnel is commonly performed under local anaesthetic.

FURTHER READING

Nashel, D.J., 2003. In: Hochberg, M.C. (Ed.), Entrapment neuropathies and compartment syndromes.

Silman, A.J., Smolen, J.S., et al. (eds.), Rheumatology, third ed. Mosby, London, pp. 713–724.

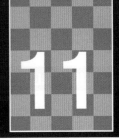
DEFINITION

Osteoarthritis (OA) is a disorder of synovial joints characterized by articular surface damage, formation of new bone and secondary inflammation. It is sometimes known as degenerative joint disease. It causes joint pain, stiffness, swelling and deformity.

INCIDENCE

OA is the most common chronic joint disease, with incidence and prevalence increasing with age. At some point, up to 80% of the population will be affected by OA. However, it is often asymptomatic and the prevalence of true symptoms in the Western world is somewhere around 20%.

PATHOLOGY AND AETIOLOGY

Histologically, repeated microtrauma or abnormal biomechanical forces cause damage to the weight-bearing cartilage surface, which eventually wears away completely exposing the subchondral bone (Fig. 11.1). Chondrocytes attempt repair by releasing degradative enzymes. Cysts occur and new bone is laid down (sclerosis) as a result of microfracturing of the articular surface. Disorganized new bone formation occurs at the joint margins (osteophytes) and the synovial lining becomes thickened and inflamed, producing excess synovial fluid (effusions).

HINTS AND TIPS

These changes explain the four cardinal features found on X-ray examination of osteoarthritis joints:

- Joint space narrowing
- Sclerosis
- Cyst formation
- Osteophytes

OA is described as primary when no single underlying cause is identified. Risk factors can be found in the previous box. Secondary OA occurs when a clear cause is identified; it can include trauma, congenital/developmental issues and metabolic diseases.

Early changes

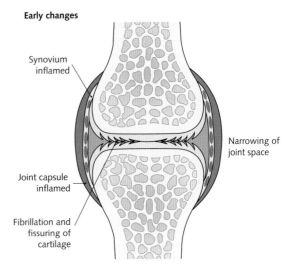

Changes secondary to loss of cartilage

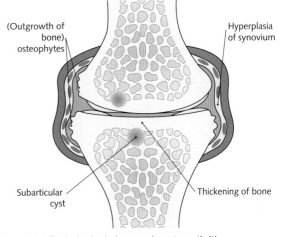

Fig. 11.1 Pathological changes in osteoarthritis.

RISK FACTORS FOR OSTEOARTHRITIS

- Increasing age
- Female gender
- Occupation
- Muscle weakness
- Obesity
- Inflammatory joint disease
- Lack of osteoporosis

CLINICAL FEATURES

Pain is the predominant symptom of OA. It is usually described as an aching or burning pain within the affected joint but may be referred distally. The onset is gradual and worse on or after activity. As the disease progresses and the joints develop secondary inflammation, night pain can become a feature. Stiffness is often reported.

Joints are usually affected in an asymmetrical pattern with single or multiple joints involved.

Occasionally a rapid, destructive pattern of OA can occur that may mimic inflammatory or septic arthritis.

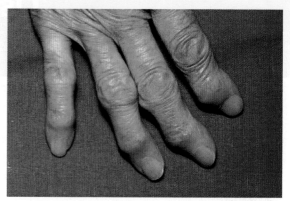

Fig. 11.3 Osteoarthritis of the hand, showing Heberden nodes at the distal interphalangeal joints and Bouchard nodes at the proximal interphalangeal joints. (Reproduced with permission from Ralston, S.H., McInnes, I.B. (eds) Davidson's Principles and Practice of Medicine, 22nd ed. Edinburgh: Churchill Livingstone, 2014.)

HINTS AND TIPS

Remember that pain from the hip can be referred to the knee.

Other symptoms can include swelling, deformity and weakness (usually secondary to muscle wasting). Certain activity can become increasingly difficult; for example, a patient with OA in the hip might not be able to put on their own socks.

Almost any synovial joint can become affected by OA, most commonly the knees, hips and hands. Within the hands, the first carpometacarpal joint, distal interphalangeal (DIP) joints and proximal interphalangeal (PIP) joints are usually affected. The wrists, shoulder and elbows are also susceptible (Figs. 11.2 and 11.3).

EXAMINATION

Examination should start in the joint where the patient complains of symptoms. Here are some useful general tips:

- Watch as the patient gets out of a chair and comes into the examination room. Do they limp or use a stick? Is their gait antalgic?
- Do they struggle to use their hands to get undressed?
- Deformity may be obvious but also note previous scars, redness, swelling and wasting of muscles during inspection.
- Palpate effusions and the joint lines for tenderness.
- There may be fixed flexion deformities and movements may be diminished.
- Remember to examine above and below the affected joints.
- Diagnosis and investigation

HINTS AND TIPS

Classical features of osteoarthritis in the hands include Heberden nodes of the distal interphalangeal joints and Bouchard nodes of the proximal interphalangeal joints (Fig. 11.3).

In most cases, the diagnosis is clear from the history and clinical examination and, apart from a plain X-ray examination, further investigations may be unnecessary.

Blood tests and joint aspiration may be undertaken to exclude septic or inflammatory arthritis in uncertain cases.

X-rays will show narrowing of the joint space, sclerosis, osteophyte formation and subchondral cysts (Fig. 11.4).

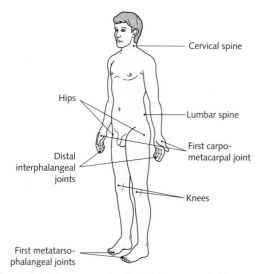

Cervical spine

Hips

Lumbar spine

First carpo-metacarpal joint

Distal interphalangeal joints

Knees

First metatarso-phalangeal joints

Fig. 11.2 Joints commonly affected by osteoarthritis.

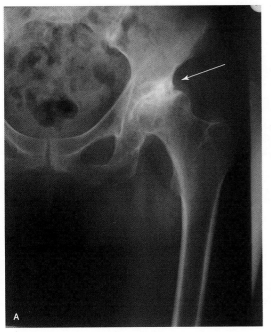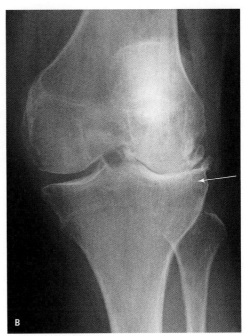

Fig. 11.4 Features of osteoarthritis on X-ray images. (A) Hip joint showing sclerosis, joint space narrowing, cysts and osteophytes. (B) Knee showing OA within the lateral compartment of the femorotibial joint.

MANAGEMENT

There is no cure for OA and treatment is aimed at relieving pain and maintaining function. Treatment options are medical or surgical.

Medical

- Initial lifestyle advice should be given, including with regard to weight loss, regular exercise and avoidance of impact-loading activities. Topical or oral nonsteroidal antiinflammatory drugs such as naproxen are good in the early stages, provided the patient does not have a history of gastrointestinal ulceration. Other regular analgesia such as paracetamol and codeine should be prescribed as required.
- Physiotherapy improves gait and function of an affected limb. Simple measures such as use of a walking stick may improve pain when walking. Orthotic insoles can help with biomechanical off-loading.
- Injections of corticosteroids provide temporary relief from pain and improvement in function. Hyaluronic acid derivative injections may offer relief for those unfit for surgery, but the evidence for this is poor.
- Glucosamine is often tried, but lack of clinical trial data of its benefit means it is not routinely recommended.

The National Institute for Health and Clinical Excellence (NICE) has published guidelines on the care and management of OA in adults (Fig. 11.5).

Surgical

Surgical treatment for OA depends on age, the joint affected, the level of pain and disability experienced. This is dealt with in greater detail in Chapter 24.

There are generally four things a surgeon can do to a joint:

1. Arthroplasty (joint replacement). This is most commonly undertaken for the knee or hip joint. It gives excellent pain relief in 90% of patients for at least 10 years.
2. Arthrodesis (joint fusion). The two sides of the joint are removed and fused together. This is most commonly undertaken in the foot and ankle. When successful, there is good pain relief but movement is lost.
3. Osteotomy (joint realignment). Increased load through a joint because of a deformity often leads to OA. A surgeon can realign the limb by cutting the bone above or below the joint, removing a wedge of bone and correcting the deformity. The most common site for this is at the knee and is often used to correct a varus deformity (bow legs). The tibia is realigned to redistribute the load more evenly, slowing the progression of OA (Fig. 11.6).
4. Joint excision. This involves removal of the failing joint and is less commonly used. It is still undertaken occasionally when other methods have failed.

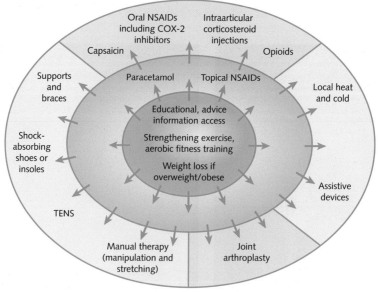

Fig. 11.5 Treatment of osteoarthritis.
COX-2, Cyclooxygenase-2; *NSAIDs,* nonsteroidal antiinflammatory drugs; *TENS,* transcutaneous electrical nerve stimulation. Reproduced from National Collaborating Centre for Chronic Conditions (2008) Osteoarthritis: National Clinical Guideline for Care and Management in Adults (full NICE guidelines). Clinical guideline 59. National Institute for Health and Care Excellence.

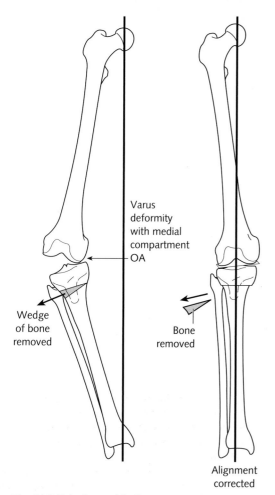

Fig. 11.6 Osteotomy of the knee.
OA, Osteoarthritis.

COMMUNICATION

It is important to explain carefully to patients that joint surgery is not risk-free and, although pain should improve, a replaced joint will never fully function like a healthy native joint. Surgery can also have serious complications for a small number of patients, including joint infection and thromboembolism. This must be explained during the consent process.

Chapter Summary

- Osteoarthritis (OA) is the most common arthritis, with up to 80% of the population affected at some point in their lives.
- It can be primary or secondary, with many alterable lifestyle risk factors.
- The classic X-ray findings of OA are loss of joint space, sclerosis, cyst formation and osteophytes.
- Pain is usually a burning or aching sensation with an asymmetric distribution of joints affected.
- There is no cure for OA and treatment focuses on relieving pain and preserving function either medically or surgically.

FURTHER READING

NICE, 2014. Osteoarthritis: care and management (CG 177). Available online at: www.nice.org.uk/guidance/cg177.

Solomon, L., Warwick, D., Nayagan, D., 2014. Apley and Solomon's Concise Systems of Orthopaedics and Trauma, Fourth edition. CRC Press.

Arthritis Research UK, available online at: www. arthritisresearchuk.org

DEFINITION

Rheumatoid arthritis (RA) is a common autoimmune, inflammatory condition characterized by symmetrical swelling in multiple joints. It typically affects the hands and follows a chronic course that results in disability if left untreated. RA is a multisystems disease, the complications of which can cause reduction in life expectancy.

INCIDENCE AND PREVALENCE

RA affects females more commonly than males, with a female-to-male excess of between two-to-four times. The annual incidence in the UK is 0.1–0.2/1000 for men and 0.2–0.4/1000 for women. RA prevalence in North American and European populations is approximately 1%.

AETIOLOGY

The aetiology of RA remains unclear, but it appears that both genetic and environmental factors have an important influence.

Genetic factors

The most significant genetic predisposing risk factor for RA is in variations of the human leucocyte antigen (HLA) genes. The most significant appears to be the HLA-DRB1 gene.

Environmental factors

Environmental influences on the development of RA are not well understood. The effects of various infections, occupations and lifestyle factors have been examined but no causal links have been found. However, there is an increased risk of the disease in smokers and the disease tends to be more aggressive in these patients.

COMMUNICATION

Remember to ask about smoking history and give advice about smoking cessation.

IMMUNOLOGICAL ABNORMALITIES

In RA, the normal immunological mechanisms that help fight infections and destroy malignant cells target normal tissue, resulting in joint damage. T-lymphocytes play a key role in initiating inflammation in RA (Fig. 12.1) with B-cells and activated macrophages also playing important roles.

The activated cells produce cytokines (intracellular messenger molecules), e.g., tumour necrosis factor-α (TNFα) and interleukin 1 (IL-1). These cytokines have many actions, including those listed in the box 'Actions of cytokines'. Many of these are treated with biologic drugs, which are discussed later.

ACTIONS OF CYTOKINES

- Stimulation of inflammation
- Attraction of other immune cells (chemotaxis)
- Excess synovial fluid production
- Cartilage destruction
- Bone resorption
- Stimulation of B-lymphocyte differentiation and maturation
- Increased antibody production, including production of rheumatoid factor

Rheumatoid factor and anticitrullinated protein antibodies are produced by activated B-cells in the synovium. They are found in approximately 80% of patients with RA. High levels of antibodies are associated with more aggressive disease and the presence of extraarticular features.

PATHOLOGY

The main pathological abnormality in RA is synovitis. As inflammatory cells infiltrate the synovium, it proliferates. Macrophages and osteoclasts create a layer of chronically inflamed tissue, pannus, which extends from the joint margins and erodes the articular cartilage (Fig. 12.2). Extensive erosions of cartilage and bone lead to joint deformity. Ligament insertions (entheses) are a common site of inflammation and the thickened joint capsule distends due to effusion.

A

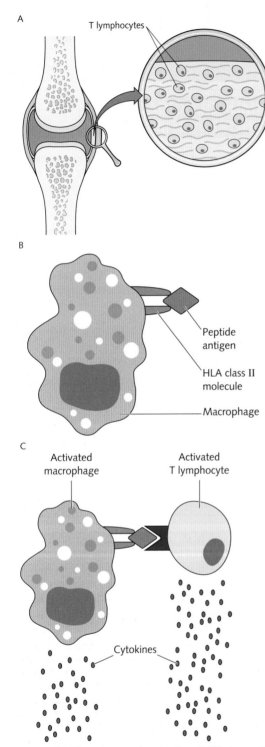

B

C

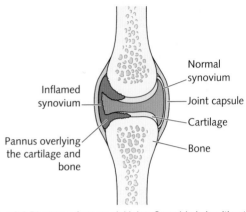

Fig. 12.2 Diagram of a synovial joint. One side is healthy; the other shows the pathological changes of rheumatoid arthritis.

CLINICAL FEATURES

RA can develop at any time of life, but the peak incidence occurs between the ages of 30 and 50 years. Symptoms begin insidiously, developing over weeks and months. Some people may experience a very acute onset. Others can develop monoarthritis or palindromic RA where symptoms are severe but fleeting and affect different joints.

The features of RA can be broadly divided into:

- Articular features
- Extraarticular features

Articular features

Joint pain, stiffness and swelling are the cardinal articular features of RA. Stiffness is typically worse on waking and tends to ease on movement. The duration of this stiffness is a useful guide to disease activity. RA affects mainly small- and medium-sized joints in a symmetrical fashion (Fig. 12.3).

Pain and stiffness lead to varying degrees of functional loss. Even in early disease, the impact on patients' activities of daily living can be profound. By the late stages of the illness, established bony erosions and joint damage further limit a patient's physical abilities.

COMMUNICATION

Patients can feel extremely frustrated and helpless if they suffer loss of function. It is important to listen sympathetically to their concerns, ideas and expectations. Help patients to find a solution. For example, the secretary who struggles to type because of her wrist pain may benefit from occupational therapy input, corticosteroid injections and wrist splints.

Fig. 12.1 (A) T-lymphocytes (predominantly T-helper cells) accumulate in the synovium. (B) Synovial macrophages (antigen-presenting cells) express peptide antigens on their cell surfaces in association with HLA class II molecules. (C) T-lymphocytes with appropriate receptors interact with the macrophages and both cell types become activated. *HLA*, Human leucocyte antigen.

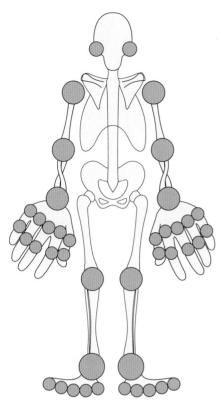

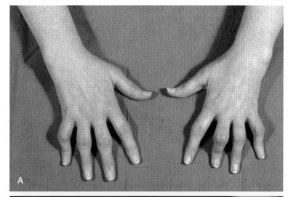

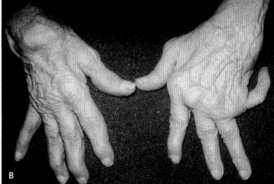

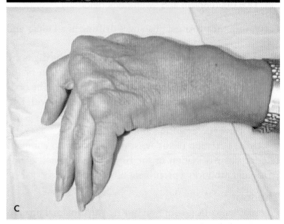

Fig. 12.3 The joints most commonly affected by rheumatoid arthritis.

Synovitis causes 'boggy' joint swelling. The skin overlying an affected joint is usually warm and red due to increased local blood flow. On palpation, the swelling is tender and has a similar consistency to that of a grape.

The effects of RA on specific joint regions

Many of the classical deformities of RA are becoming less common in clinical practice due to more effective therapies being used earlier. Many patients still have long-standing classic joint deformities that need recognition.

> **RED FLAG**
>
> Urgent recognition and treatment is the key to preventing joint damage. Patients with suspected RA should be referred for specialist assessment and treatment within 6 weeks of symptom onset.

The rheumatoid hand and wrist

The hands and wrists are almost always involved in RA (Fig. 12.4). Synovitis typically occurs in the wrists, the metacarpophalangeal (MCP) and proximal interphalangeal (PIP) joints, sparing the distal interphalangeal (DIP) joints.

Fig. 12.4 The hands of a patients with rheumatoid arthritis. (A) Polyarticular swelling of the proximal interphalangeal joints along with wrist deformity. (B) Complete subluxation with ulnar deviation at the metacarpophalangeal joints in a patient with advanced disease. (C) 'Zig-zag' deformity of the hand with radial deviation at the wrist and ulnar deviation at the metacarpophalangeal joints. (With permission from Erickson, A.R., Cannella, A.C., Mikuls, T.R., Clinical Features of Rheumatoid Arthritis, Kelley and Firestein's Textbook of Rheumatology, 10th ed, 2017 Elsevier. (A and B, Courtesy Dr. Iain McInnes; C, Courtesy Dr. Gerald Moore.)

The inflammation can weaken and damage the tendons and ligaments, producing well-recognized deformities.

Ulnar deviation of the fingers results from MCP joint inflammation (Fig. 12.5). Subluxation of the MCP joints can

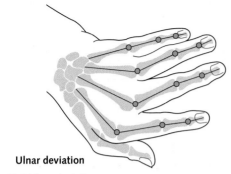

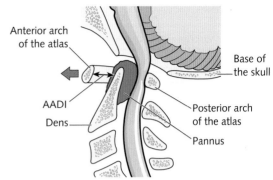

Fig. 12.5 Ulnar deviation.

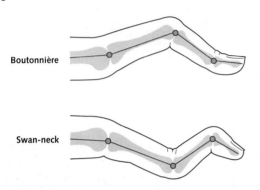

Fig. 12.6 Boutonnière and swan-neck deformity.

Fig. 12.7 In healthy adults, the distance between the anterior arch of the atlas and the dens should not exceed 3 mm. The diagram shows forward subluxation of the atlas on the axis. The spinal cord is compressed between the pannus around the dens and the posterior arch of the atlas. *AADI*, Anterior atlantodental interspace.

This produces neck pain, which radiates to the occiput. Upper motor neurone damage resulting in a spastic quadriparesis is a rare complication. Damage to the articulation between the occiput and the atlas may allow the odontoid peg to move upwards through the foramen magnum. This can threaten the cord and brainstem, sometimes resulting in sudden death after relatively minor jolts to the head and neck. Subaxial subluxation can also occur (below the first cervical vertebra).

HINTS AND TIPS

It is important to take lateral flexion X-ray images or magnetic resonance imaging of the cervical spine in rheumatoid arthritis patients requiring a general anaesthetic. The anaesthetist must be aware of any neck instability so that precautions can be taken during intubation.

---

occur, with the proximal phalanges drifting in an ulnar and solar (palmer) direction.

Boutonnière and swan-neck deformities of the digits are due to PIP synovitis and laxity and/or contraction of the extensor and flexor tendon apparatus (Fig. 12.6). The boutonnière deformity is characterized by PIP flexion with DIP hyperextension. With swan-neck deformity, there is MCP flexion, PIP hyperextension and DIP flexion.

Radial deviation of the wrist occurs partly to compensate for ulnar deviation of the fingers. Subluxation of the wrist joint produces a prominent ulnar styloid.

The foot

Forefoot synovitis is common in RA. The proximal phalanges may sublux dorsally and the metatarsal heads become eroded and displaced towards the floor. They can be easily palpated through the sole of the foot, as the protective fat pad is lost, and can be painful to walk on. Patients often feel as though they are 'walking on marbles'.

Hindfoot involvement can also cause issues with subtalar arthritis. Valgus deformity may develop in patients with longstanding disease. All these deformities are the result of poorly controlled synovitis. The aim of the rheumatologist is to suppress synovitis, limiting bony destruction and reducing disability.

The cervical spine

Inflammation and erosive disease, affecting the first cervical vertebra and stabilizing ligaments of the first two cervical vertebra, can result in atlantoaxial subluxation. The atlas slips forward on the axis, reducing the space around the spinal cord (Fig. 12.7).

Extraarticular features of RA

Rheumatoid nodules

Rheumatoid nodules are firm subcutaneous nodules found in around 20% of rheumatoid patients. They develop in areas affected by pressure or friction, such as the fingers, elbows and Achilles tendon. They are seen in patients who have positive rheumatoid factor antibodies and are more common in smokers. They tend to accompany more severe disease. Unfortunately, methotrexate, often used to treat RA, has the disadvantage of making nodules worse. The cause is unclear, but it is possibly due to a small vessel vasculitis. Histology reveals a shell of fibrous tissue surrounding a centre of fibrinoid necrosis.

Tenosynovitis and bursitis

Tendon sheaths and bursa are lined with synovium, which can also become inflamed in RA. The flexor tendons of the fingers are commonly affected by tenosynovitis, which can result in tendon rupture. The olecranon and subacromial bursae are common sites of bursitis.

Carpal tunnel syndrome

Synovitis can cause entrapment of peripheral nerves. Medial nerve compression resulting in carpal tunnel syndrome is common (see Chapter 10).

Systemic Features of rheumatoid arthritis

As well as causing joint pain and swelling, active RA makes people feel generally unwell. The inflammation can result in systemic symptoms such as low-grade fever, weight loss and lethargy. These symptoms can be prominent, particularly in patients with acute onset RA.

COMMUNICATION

When patients with rheumatoid arthritis first present, they may have felt tired and listless for months. It is reassuring for them to hear that systemic symptoms are common and may improve when the inflammation is treated.

The effects of rheumatoid arthritis on distant organs

RA can affect many different body systems (Fig. 12.8). Extraarticular manifestations can be severe and are associated with an increase in mortality. Some of the more common are explored below.

Anaemia

Anaemia in RA can be due to:

- Anaemia of chronic disease (normocytic)
- Autoimmune haemolysis
- Felty syndrome
- Nonsteroidal antiinflammatory drugs (NSAIDs) can cause iron deficiency anaemia through gastrointestinal inflammation and blood loss.
- Disease-modifying antirheumatic drugs (DMARDs) sometimes potentiate anaemia through bone marrow suppression.

Felty syndrome

Felty syndrome is the associate of RA with splenomegaly and leukopenia. It usually occurs in patients who are rheumatoid-factor positive. The leukopenia leads to bacterial infections. Lymphadenopathy, anaemia and thrombocytopenia can also occur.

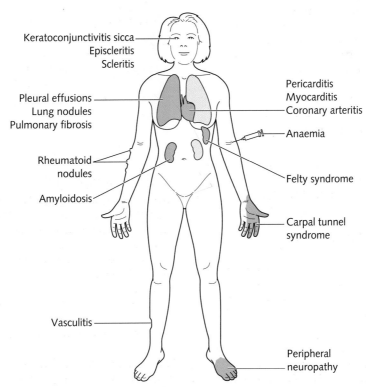

Fig. 12.8 Extraarticular manifestations of rheumatoid arthritis.

Rheumatoid lung disease

Although pulmonary disease is common in RA, it does not always produce symptoms. Men are more commonly affected than women.

Pneumonitis can cause fibrosis and scarring of the lungs leading to pulmonary fibrosis. It may also occur as a reaction to DMARDS and is most commonly associated with methotrexate.

Pleural effusions in RA have become less common with more aggressive early disease management. They occasionally precede arthritis and rheumatoid factors can be detected in the fluid, which is a transudate.

Pulmonary nodules can occur in seropositive patients with subcutaneous nodules. They rarely cause symptoms but may produce a chronic dry cough.

Investigations

Blood tests

Full blood count may show anaemia of chronic disease, thrombocytosis due to chronic inflammation or leukopenia due to Felty syndrome.

Erythrocyte sedimentation rate (ESR) and C-reactive protein (CRP) are usually raised in the presence of synovitis and are useful markers of response to treatment.

Rheumatoid factor is found in the serum of 70%–90% of patients with RA. Patients who lack antibodies are sometimes described as having seronegative rheumatoid arthritis. It is important to remember that rheumatoid factor is found in 5%–10% of healthy individuals, particularly in the elderly. Patients who are rheumatoid-factor positive have a higher rate of systemic disease and a poorer prognosis than those who are not.

Another serological test is available to help in the diagnosis of RA. Anticyclic citrullinated peptide antibodies can be present in patients who are rheumatoid-factor negative and indicate a worse prognosis. They are not associated with systemic features but have a higher specificity for RA.

HINTS AND TIPS

Rheumatoid factor can be present in healthy people. The diagnosis of rheumatoid arthritis can be made on clinical grounds following history, examination and the application of diagnostic criteria.

Radiological investigations

Plain X-ray images should be obtained to look for radiological evidence of RA (Fig. 12.9), which tends to be seen first in the small joints of the hands and feet (Fig. 12.10).

X-ray changes are often not present at diagnosis. It may be many months or even years before changes in the

| Soft-tissue swelling |
| Periarticular osteoporosis |
| Juxta-articular erosions |
| Narrowing of joint space |

Fig. 12.9 The four main radiological signs of rheumatoid arthritis.

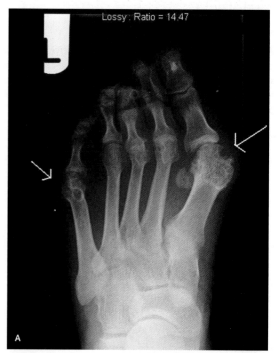

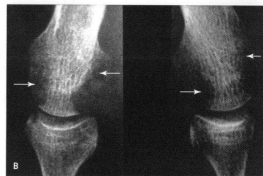

Fig. 12.10 (A) Periarticular osteopenia and erosions of the metatarsophalangeal joints. (B) Large erosions of the two metacarpophalangeal joints.

joint caused by persistent inflammation can be seen on radiological examination, although there is a growing role for the use of ultrasound in detecting synovitis in early arthritis. Magnetic resonance imaging (MRI) can also help in the detection of synovitis and early erosions although this technique is expensive and time-consuming (Fig. 12.11).

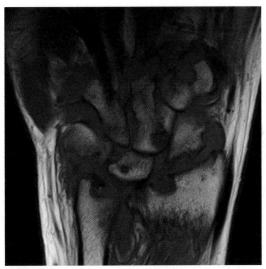

Fig. 12.11 Magnetic resonance imaging of erosions in rheumatoid arthritis.

Management

Patients with RA should be cared for by a multidisciplinary team. Fig. 12.12 lists the professionals involved in the care of RA patients and explains the roles they play.

Drug treatment

There are two main aims of drug treatment in RA:

- Reduction in symptoms.
- Prevention of damage by control of disease.

Nonsteroidal antiinflammatory drugs

NSAIDS can improve joint pain and stiffness but have no effect on disease activity or progression. If a patient does not respond to one NSAID, it is worth trying another.

Disease-modifying antirheumatic drugs

DMARDS suppress inflammation and slow progression of erosive joint disease. They are the mainstay of RA therapy and should be commenced by 6 weeks of disease onset. Some DMARDs suppress the immune system, others inhibit cell replication. However, for many drugs the mechanism of action is not completely understood.

DMARDs are act slowly and take several weeks to produce a clinical effect. If a patient does not respond adequately to one DMARD, a second one can be added or substituted. In patients with poor prognostic markers, several DMARDs may be commenced at diagnosis.

Like many drugs, DMARDs can cause minor side-effects such as nausea, headaches and rashes (Fig. 12.13). More

DMARD	Possible side-effects
Methotrexate	Gastrointestinal upset Oral ulcers Raised liver enzymes Pneumonitis Bone marrow suppression
Sulfasalazine	Gastrointestinal upset Raised liver enzymes Bone marrow suppression
Hydroxychloroquine	Retinal damage
Leflunomide	Hypertension Gastrointestinal upset Bone marrow suppression
Gold	Rash Proteinuria Bone marrow suppression

DMARD, disease-modifying antirheumatic drug.

Fig. 12.13 Some disease-modifying drugs and their side effects.

Professional	Role
Rheumatologist	Monitoring of disease activity. Prescription and monitoring of drug therapy. Identification and management of complications. Referral to other specialists when necessary. Coordination of team. Diagnosis.
Specialist nurse	Patient education. DMARD monitoring. Biologic administration and advice. Joint injections
Orthopaedic surgeon	Replacement of damaged joints. Surgical synovectomy. Tendon repairs
Physiotherapist	Use of physical therapies to combat inflammation. Prescription of exercises to maintain and improve muscular strength and range of joint movement
Occupational therapist	Splinting of acutely inflamed joints Advice on how to function whilst putting as little stress as possible on the joints (joint protection) Provision of aids and appliances to assist with activities of daily living
Podiatrist	Assessment of footwear and advice on choosing suitable shoes Provision of insoles to improve the mechanics of deformed feet Prevention and treatment of skin lesions, such as calluses and ulcers

DMARD, disease-modifying antirheumatic drug.

Fig. 12.12 Professionals involved in the care of rheumatoid arthritis patients and the roles they play.

serious complications, such as bone marrow suppression, abnormal liver function tests and renal impairment are rarer, but well recognized. It is therefore important to monitor closely patients on DMARD therapy. Severity scoring systems, such as the Disease Activity Score-28 (DAS-28), give a guide to response to treatment and may trigger a step-up in therapy.

ETHICS

Serious side-effects to disease-modifying antirheumatic drugs are rare but can cause considerable harm to patients. Ensure patients are given written information of possible side-effects and reactions so that they can make informed decisions on their treatment.

Corticosteroids

Corticosteroids can swiftly improve pain and swelling in RA. Low doses of prednisolone can be used to control the symptoms early in the disease in conjunction with a DMARD, whilst DMARDs take time to exhibit their anti-inflammatory effects. Corticosteroids can be given intraarticularly to treat local synovitis and are sometimes given via the intramuscular route for a generalized flare of RA.

Biological therapies

Biological therapies that target inflammatory mediators to treat RA are now widely used. There are many target molecules in the inflammatory cascade that can be the target site of biologics (Fig. 12.14). The most commonly used are those that target TNF-α, such as entanercept, infliximab and adalimumab. These drugs produce excellent clinical effects but are expensive and carry an increased risk of infection.

Fig. 12.14 Target sites of biological therapies in rheumatoid arthritis. *JAK*, Janus kinase; *STAT*, signal transducers and activators of transcription.

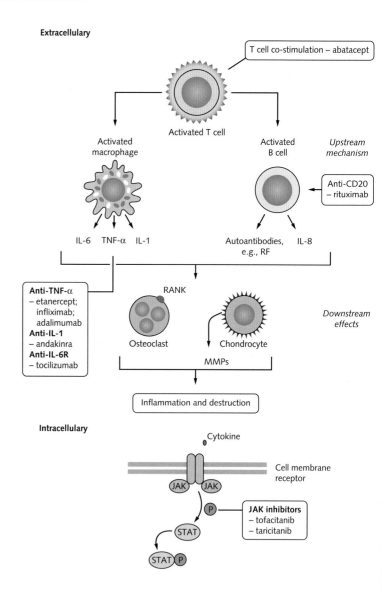

The National Institute for Health and Clinical Excellence (NICE) has issued guidance for their use in the UK. Disease activity scoring systems are employed to select patients for treatment. The development of cheaper generic or biosimilar forms of these drugs will hopefully allow broader access to them.

Other therapies licensed for use include rituximab, a monoclonal antibody against B-cells used in the treatment of RA when one anti-TNF therapy has failed. Abatacept is a T-cell costimulation modulator and Tociluzimab blocks IL-6 to suppress the acute-phase response of inflammation. Recently, janus kinase (JAK) inhibitors such as tofacitinib and baricitinib have been approved by NICE for use in RA: they inhibit the JAK family of enzymes responsible for phosphorylating cytokine receptors. These activated receptors in turn recruit STAT transcription factors, which modulate gene transcription. Blocking this phosphorylation pathway inhibits the actions of various interleukins.

Societal impact

A person's engagement with wider society is affected by the diagnosis of RA. Within 3 years of diagnosis, 25% of patients are no longer working. Personal loss of income, government loss of taxation, drug costs and the impact of disability with associated social care costs all contribute to the financial impact of the disease.

● Chapter Summary

- Rheumatoid arthritis is a multisystems disease characterized by symmetrical polyarticular arthritis, usually involving the hands.
- The typical pattern of involvement includes inflammation of the PIP, MCP and wrist joints, although any synovial joint can be affected.
- Classical deformities include boutonnière and swan-neck deformities.
- Extraarticular features include anaemia, respiratory conditions (pleural effusions, lung nodules and pulmonary fibrosis), pericarditis/myocarditis and inflammation of the eyes.
- The classic radiological features of RA are soft-tissue swelling, periarticular osteoporosis, juxta-articular erosions and narrowing of the joint space.
- Methotrexate, sulfasalazine, lefluonomide and hydroxychloroquine are the most commonly used synthetic DMARDs.
- Biological DMARDs are extremely effective in reducing inflammation and limiting disease activity; they include anti-TNF-α, anti-T cell co-stimulators, anti-IL1, anti-IL-6R, anti-CD20 and JAK-inhibitors.

FURTHER READING

McInnes, I.B., Schett, G., 2011. The pathogenesis of rheumatoid arthritis. N. Engl. J. Med. 365, 2205–2219.

Smolen, J.S., Landewé, R., Bijlsma, J., et al. EULAR recommendations for the management of rheumatoid arthritis with synthetic and biological disease-modifying antirheumatic drugs: 2016 update *Annals of the Rheumatic Diseases*. First published online: 6 March 2017. doi: https://doi.org/10.1136/annrheumdis-2016-210715

SIGN, 2012. Management of early rheumatoid arthritis. Available online at http://www.sign.ac.uk/assets/sign123.pdf.

National Rheumatoid Arthritis Society, www.nras.org.uk.

Spondyloarthropathies | 13

DEFINITION

The term spondyloarthropathy (SPA) describes a group of related and often overlapping inflammatory joint disorders of the spine or vertebral column (see list in box). Spondyloarthropathy with inflammation is commonly referred to as axial spondyloarthritis. It is characterized by enthesitis (inflammation of the insertions of tendons, ligaments and capsules into bone), as well as synovitis, and occurs in patients who are seronegative for rheumatoid factor. For this reason, these disorders are sometimes referred to as seronegative spondyloarthropathies.

THE SPONDYLOARTHROPATHIES	
Ankylosing spondylitis	92%
Psoriatic arthropathy	60%
Reactive arthritis	60%–80%
Enteropathic arthritis	60%
Undifferentiated spondyloarthropathy	25%

AETIOLOGY

All types of SPA are genetically associated with the human leukocyte antigen (HLA) B27, a major histocompatibility complex class I antigen. HLA B27 is more closely linked with some forms of SPA than others. Around 10% of the world's Caucasian population is positive for HLA B27.

The true aetiology of SPAs is unknown. Infection is thought to be important; bacterial infections may trigger an immune reaction in genetically susceptible people. This is particularly true for reactive arthritis. In other forms of SPA, a combination of genetic and environmental factors might trigger inflammation.

PATHOLOGY

The entheses are the key sites of inflammation in SPA. Initial inflammation and erosions are followed by fibrosis and ossification (bone formation), which can result in ankylosis of the joints. In ankylosing spondylitis (AS), the outer fibres of the vertebral discs become inflamed where they attach to the corners of the vertebral bodies. The characteristic squaring of the anterior contour of the vertebra results from destructive osteitis and repair. Ossification leads to formation of syndesmophytes (bony bridges). The sacroiliac joints are commonly affected and become fused. Synovitis is another feature of SPA. Peripheral joints tend to be more commonly affected in psoriatic arthritis and reactive arthritis than in enteropathic arthritis and AS.

Pathological changes are not always confined to the musculoskeletal system (discussed in more detail later).

ANKYLOSING SPONDYLITIS

Clinical features

The prevalence of AS amongst the Caucasian population is 0.5%–1%. It is three times more common in men than women and tends to be more severe in men. It usually develops in the teenage years and early adulthood, with a peak age of onset in the mid-20s. Presentations over the age of 45 years are rare.

Clinical features fall into two groups:

- Musculoskeletal
- Extraskeletal

Musculoskeletal features

Most symptoms in AS are due to spinal and sacroiliac disease. The typical patient presents with gradual onset of lower back or gluteal region pain and stiffness. As symptoms progress, there is loss of anterior flexion, lateral flexion and extension of the spine. The time of onset to diagnosis remains unacceptably high, with many patients having had symptoms for a number of years before referral. Early identification allows for prompt treatment to preserve spinal mobility, limit functional loss and reduce pain and stiffness. Symptoms are worse in the morning and generally improve with exercise. Involvement of the thoracic spine and enthesitis of the costovertebral joints can cause chest pains, reduced chest expansion and breathlessness. Features of inflammatory back pain are showing in the box.

In the early stages of disease, patients may have few clinical signs. In addition to Regional Examination of the

MODIFIED CRITERIA OF INFLAMMATORY BACK PAIN

Chronic back pain (>3 months) with onset of first symptoms before 45 years of age:

- Morning stiffness for at least 30 minutes
- Improves with exercise, but not with rest
- Back pain awakens the patient during the second half of the night
- Alternating buttock pain

Inflammatory back pain is present if two of the above four items are fulfilled.

(Rudwaleit, M., van der Heijde, D., Landewé, R. et al. (2006) Inflammatory back pain in ankylosing spondylitis: a reassessment of the clinical history for application as classification and diagnostic criteria. Arthritis and Rheumatism 54: 569–578.)

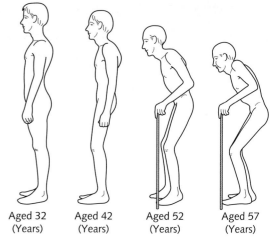

Aged 32 (Years) Aged 42 (Years) Aged 52 (Years) Aged 57 (Years)

Fig. 13.2 Deterioration in posture in ankylosing spondylitis patients over time.

COMMUNICATION

Lower back pain is common and usually due to mechanical or degenerative issues. When assessing a younger person with back pain, always ask about morning stiffness.

Musculoskeletal System (REMS), the following examinations may be useful:

- The sacroiliac joints are often tender and pain can be reproduced by applying pressure to the joints. The sacroiliac squeeze test is achieved by applying pressure on the anterior iliac spines whilst the patient is supine.
- Mobility of the lumbar spine is reduced. The Schober test is used to assess anterior flexion of the lumbar spine (Fig 13.1). With a pen, a mark is made on the skin at the lumbosacral joint, level with the dimples of Venus. A second mark is made 10 cm above. The patient bends forward with the legs straight and attempts to touch the floor. The distance between the marks should increase by at least 5 cm.

Fig. 13.1 The Schober test.

- Lateral flexion of the spine (see Chapter 2) is even more sensitive at identifying AS.

Later in the disease process and in those with severe disease, the spine becomes progressively stiff and immobile and posture deteriorates (Fig 13.2). The normal lumbar lordosis is lost and the thoracic and cervical spines become increasingly kyphotic. The resulting stooped posture restricts chest expansion and causes the abdomen to protrude. It is sometimes referred to as the question mark posture. Measurement of tragus-to-wall distance and chest expansion are helpful indicators of disease progression. The Bath AS Functional Index (BASFI) and Bath AS Disease Activity Index (BASDAI) are two scoring systems commonly used to objectify functional capacity and disease activity.

RED FLAG

Spinal disease can be complicated by atlantoaxial subluxation and fractures. Be sure to perform a full neurological examination in ankylosing spondylitis patients presenting with acute pain.

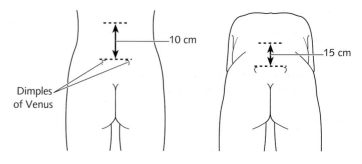

Dimples of Venus   10 cm   15 cm

The peripheral joints are less commonly involved than the axial skeleton in AS. Inflammation tends to target the medium and large joints such as the shoulders, knees and hips. Pain and tenderness due to enthesitis may occur in multiple sites. Achilles tendonitis and plantar fasciitis are common examples of this.

Extraskeletal features

Extraskeletal features are commonly referred to as the four-As:

- *Acute anterior uveitis:* also called iritis, this occurs in approximately one-third of AS patients. The eye becomes red and painful and vision is blurred. It requires urgent assessment by an ophthalmologist as blindness may occur if left untreated. Steroid eye drops are the usual treatment.
- *Aortic incompetence/ascending aortitis*
- *Apical lung fibrosis*
- *Amyloidosis*

In addition, constitutional features such as anorexia, fever, weight loss and fatigue may occur.

> **COMMUNICATION**
>
> Patients suffering from any spondyloarthropathy should be warned of uveitis causing blindness and be advised to seek urgent medical help if they develop a painful red eye or have visual disturbance.

Investigations

Blood tests

- A full blood count may show anaemia of chronic disease.
- Erythrocyte sedimentation rate (ESR) and C-reactive protein (CRP) are often elevated during the active phases of the disease.
- Serological tests for rheumatoid factor are negative.
- Genotyping for HLA B27 is not required for diagnosis but may be useful where doubt exists.

Radiological investigation

The investigation of choice is magnetic resonance imaging (MRI). This technique is able to detect inflammatory back disease in cases where X-ray images may be normal in appearance. MRI also prevents X-ray exposure in the pelvis, which is particularly important in young patients. Sacroiliitis (Figs. 13.3 and 13.4) and bone oedema highlight ongoing inflammation, amenable to therapy. X-ray images have a role in assessing established damage where substantial mechanical change has occurred. Views of the lumbar

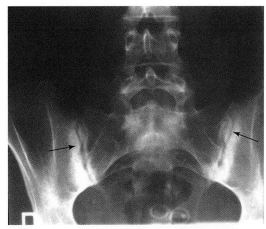

Fig. 13.3 Radiograph showing bilateral sacroiliitis (*arrows*).

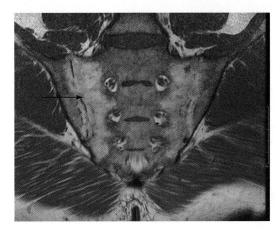

Fig. 13.4 Magnetic resonance image showing sacroiliitis (*arrow*).

spine may show squaring of the vertebrae and formation of syndesmophytes (Fig. 13.5). These are due to ossification of the longitudinal ligaments and produce a bamboo appearance. Radiographs taken at other sites of enthesitis may show erosions, for example at the insertion of the plantar fascia of Achilles tendon.

Management

Patients with AS require a multidisciplinary approach to care (Fig. 12.8).

Physiotherapy

This is an important element in the management of AS. Each patient should follow a long-term exercise programme with the aim of maintaining normal posture and exercise activity. Hydrotherapy is also beneficial.

Drug treatment

Nonsteroidal antiinflammatory drugs (NSAIDs) are the mainstay of initial treatment and provide benefit in the

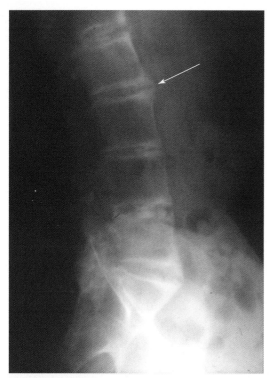

Fig. 13.5 Lateral radiograph showing syndesmophyte formation (*arrow*) in the lumbar spine of a patient with advanced ankylosing spondylitis.

majority of patients. Continuous therapy should occur in patients with ongoing evidence of inflammation. Both NSAID types, cyclooxygenase-1 (COX-1) and COX-2 inhibitors, have shown benefit to patients and may even suppress radiological progression.

Immunosuppressive drugs, such as methotrexate and sulfasalazine, are of less benefit in AS, except where a concomitant peripheral arthritis occurs.

The tumour necrosis factor (TNF) inhibitors, however, have excellent efficacy in treating active axial disease and preventing AS progression. Patients who respond well include those who are young, those who have elevated inflammatory markers and those with a shorter disease progression. Fig. 13.6 shows the general pathophysiology of inflammation in spondyloarthropathies with biological targets of treatment. In AS, anti-IL17 biologics such as secukinumab are licensed for use along with anti-TNFs.

PSORIATIC ARTHRITIS

Clinical features

Psoriatic arthropathy is an inflammatory arthritis associated with psoriasis. Psoriasis occurs in 1%–3% of the population and approximately 10% of those are affected by psoriatic arthritis. It is particularly common in patients with psoriatic nail involvement (Fig. 13.7) and affects men and women with a similar frequency.

Psoriatic arthritis may precede the diagnosis of psoriatic skin disease and does not correlate with the severity of the skin involvement. Differing patterns of joint involvement are listed in the box.

PATTERNS OF JOINT DISEASE IN PSORIATIC ARTHRITIS

- Distal arthritis involving the distal interphalangeal joints
- Asymmetrical oligoarthritis
- Symmetrical polyarthritis indistinguishable from rheumatoid arthritis
- Spondylitis
- Arthritis mutilans

Examination for synovitis is important because patients present with joint pain, stiffness and sometimes swelling. Dactylitis and enthesitis are common features. Involvement of the distal interphalangeal (DIP) joints may be associated with pitting or onycholysis of the nail. Arthritis mutilans is an extremely destructive pattern of joint destruction mainly seen in the hands and feet. Thankfully, it is rare.

Resorption of bone at the metacarpals and phalanges causes telescoping of the digits. They appear shortened but can be passively extended to their original lengths. Psoriatic spondylitis tends to cause milder symptoms than classic AS and sacroiliitis is often asymmetrical and asymptomatic.

The diagnosis is clinical but can be facilitated by using the CASPAR criteria.

THE CLASSIFICATION CRITERIA FOR PSORIATIC ARTHRITIS (CASPAR)

Inflammatory articular disease (joint, spine or entheseal) with ≥3 points from the following:

Evidence of current psoriasis, a personal history of psoriasis or a family history of psoriasis	2 points
Typical psoriatic nail dystrophy, including onycholysis, pitting and hyperkeratosis observed on current physical examination	1 point
A negative test result for the presence of rheumatoid factor by any method except latex	1 point

---

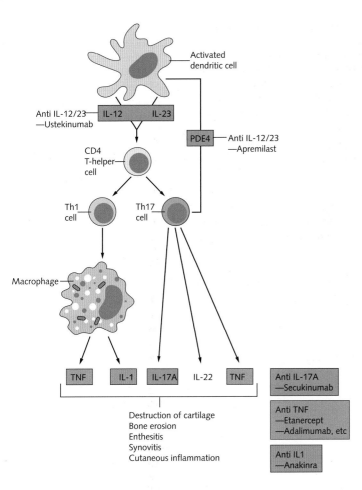

Fig. 13.6 Target sites of biological therapies in spondyloarthritis. *IL,* Interleukin; *Th*, T helper; *TNF*, tumour necrosis factor.

Either current dactylitis, defined as swelling of an entire digit, or a history of dactylitis recorded by a rheumatologist	1 point		

Either current dactylitis, defined as swelling of an entire digit, or a history of dactylitis recorded by a rheumatologist   1 point

Radiographic evidence of juxta-articular new bone formation appearing as ill-defined ossification near joint margins (but excluding osteophyte formation) on plain radiographs of the hand or foot   1 point

Definitions: Current psoriasis is skin or scalp disease present today as judged by a rheumatologist or dermatologist. A personal history of psoriasis is a history of psoriasis that may be obtained from a patient, family physician, dermatologist, rheumatologist or other qualified healthcare provider. A family history of psoriasis is a history of psoriasis in a first- or second-degree relative according to patient report.

(Adapted from Taylor, W., Gladman, D., Helliwell, P. et al. 2006 Classification criteria for psoriatic arthritis: development of new criteria from a large international study. Arthritis and Rheumatism 54: 2665–2673.)

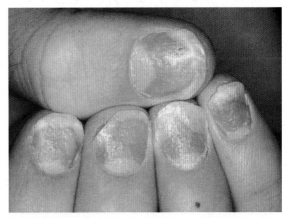

Fig. 13.7 Psoriatic nails with hyperkeratosis. (With permission from Bender AM, Disorders of the Hair and Nails, in: Cohen BA, (ed.) Pediatric Dermatology, 4th ed., 2013, Elsevier.)

Investigations

Blood tests

Full blood count, ESR and CRP show a similar picture to that of AS. Rheumatoid factor is usually absent.

Radiological investigations

The radiological changes of psoriatic arthritis are asymmetrical and target the small joints of the hands and feet, particularly the DIP joints (Fig. 13.8). Changes that can be seen on X-ray images include:

- Erosions with proliferation of the adjacent bone
- Resorption of the terminal phalanges
- Pencil-in-cup deformities
- Periostitis
- Ankylosis
- New bone formation at entheses
- Sacroiliitis is found in up to 30% of cases and is usually asymmetrical (Fig. 13.4).

Management

Treatment depends on the pattern of joint disease:

- Peripheral joint disease is treated with NSAIDS, methotrexate, leflunomide and sulfasalazine. Anti-TNF therapies work well in selected patients where conventional synthetic disease-modifying antirheumatic drugs (DMARDs) have failed.
- Axial disease is treated in a similar way to AS with physiotherapy, NSAIDs and biologic therapy as the mainstay. Anti-IL12/23 and anti-IL17A are particularly effective in psoriatic arthritis with axial involvement and are licensed for first-line use alongside anti-tumour necrosis factor (TNF) treatment. Patients who fail to respond or who have contraindications to these may consider apremilast (anti-PDE4).
- All patients benefit from a multidisciplinary team approach.

Prognosis

The prognosis for psoriatic arthritis is generally good, with joint function being preserved in most cases. Chronic, destructive and deforming arthritis may occasionally develop.

REACTIVE ARTHRITIS

Clinical features

Reactive arthritis is an aseptic arthritis that occurs after an anatomically distant infection. It mainly affects young adults and the triggering infection is usually of the gastrointestinal or genitourinary tract. Occasionally the incidental infection is not found and other triggers such as drug treatment have been rarely found.

Symptoms start to develop a few days to weeks after the infection. The onset is sometimes acute, with stiffness, fatigue and occasionally fever.

RED FLAG

Remember that *Salmonella* and *Neisseria* can cause septic arthritis. Always ensure joint aspirate cultures are negative!

Musculoskeletal features

The arthritis is typically asymmetrical and oligoarticular. It targets the larger weight-bearing joints, fingers and toes. Dactylitis and enthesitis occur and some patients experience pain and stiffness in the sacroiliac region.

Conjunctivitis

This is sterile and can be unilateral or bilateral.

Urethritis

Sterile inflammation of the urogenital tract can cause symptoms of frequency, dysuria and urethral discharge. It is

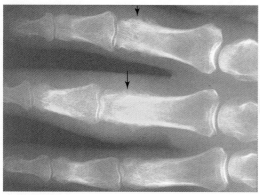

Fig. 13.8 Radiograph showing fluffy periosteal reaction and erosive changes (*arrows*) in the digits in a patient with psoriatic arthritis.

important patients are screened for sexually transmitted infections if at risk, as these can also trigger reactive arthritis.

Skin and mucosal lesions

Circinate balanitis can accompany uveitis. Some patients develop a sterile pustulosis on the palms of the hands and soles of the feet. This looks similar to pustular psoriasis and is called keratoderma blennorrhagia. Erythema nodosum is another recognized association.

Reiter syndrome

The triad of arthritis, conjunctivitis and uveitis following a bacterial infection is referred to as Reiter syndrome.

Investigations

- Full blood count, ESR and CRP show a similar picture to that of AS. CRP and ESR may be significantly elevated.
- Serological tests, including antibodies against *salmonella, campylobacter, chlamydia,* gonorrhoea and *Neisseria,* may help identify the causative organism.
- Synovial fluid from the affected joints should be examined for Gram stain and cultures performed. Cultures are negative in reactive arthritis, but it is important to exclude a septic arthritis or crystal arthropathy.
- A cervical/penile swab, midstream specimen of urine and stool sample should all be obtained for culture and to exclude ongoing infection. Partners should be offered advice where possible.
- X-ray images are initially normal. Later, fluffy periostitis may be seen in the calcaneus, digits or pelvis. Plantar spurs are common, but erosions are rare. Sacroiliitis and typical AS changes develop in some patients.
- HLA B27 is often associated with the risk of developing reactive arthritis and patients who are HLA B27 positive are more likely to have subsequent episodes.

Management

Reactive arthritis varies in severity from mild symptoms that do not require treatment, to relapsing inflammation requiring steroid/DMARD treatment. The course of treatment is generally as follows:

- Treat any underlying infection with antibiotics
- NSAIDs
- Corticosteroid joint injections +/- systemic steroids
- Rarely, DMARDs may be required

Prognosis

The vast majority of cases are mild and self-limiting. Relapses following a further infective trigger can occur. At least 60% of those affected will experience a further episode. Permanent joint damage can occur but is rare.

ENTEROPATHIC ARTHRITIS

Clinical features

Arthritis occurring with inflammatory bowel disease (IBD) is known as enteropathic arthritis. It occurs in approximately 10%–20% of patients with Crohn disease or ulcerative colitis.

Peripheral arthritis

A peripheral arthritis that is a mono- or oligoarthritis may develop. It worsens with flaring of the bowel disease and improves if the affected bowel is surgically removed.

Spondylitis and sacroiliitis

These are not related to the activity of the bowel disease and often predate the onset of Crohn disease or ulcerative colitis.

Enthesopathy

This can accompany peripheral or axial joint disease.

Investigations

Most X-ray images are normal. Spinal imaging may show changes similar to AS. In the case of active spinal inflammation, MRI is the imaging modality of choice. Blood tests are generally unhelpful, unless inflammatory markers correlate with active bowel disease activity. If inflammatory bowel disease is suspected, faecal calprotectin and inflammatory markers should be tested and the patient referred to a gastroenterologist.

Management

Treatment of the IBD is the priority and will help with active peripheral arthritis. Drugs, such as corticosteroids and sulfasalazine, should improve both bowel and joint disease. Anti-TNF biologics are licensed for IBD and are extremely effective in managing axial disease.

HINTS AND TIPS

Nonsteroidal antiinflammatory drugs often aggravate gastrointestinal symptoms in inflammatory bowel disease. They risk causing upper gastrointestinal (GI) bleeding, particularly in patients with Crohn disease, where inflammation/ulceration can occur at any point in the GI tract.

Chapter Summary

Spondyloarthropathies are a group of overlapping conditions associated with HLA B27.

- The general aetiology of spondyloarthritis is of inflammatory axial enthesitis with or without associated synovitis.
- Back pain is common; inflammatory back pain is recognized as being worse on rest and better on movement, often with associated stiffness.
- Ankylosing spondylitis is more common in men, typically does not involve the peripheral joints and is associated with the 'four-As': *a*cute anterior uveitis, *a*ortic incompetence, *a*pical lung fibrosis and *a*myloidosis.
- Psoriatic arthritis occurs in around 10% of patients with psoriasis, although it is more common in those with nail involvement. There are differing axial and peripheral patterns of disease.
- Reactive arthritis is commonly seen after a bacterial infection; always consider STIs in sexually active patients.
- Treatment for axial disease typically involves the use of biologic therapies: anti-TNF, anti-IL12/23 and anti-IL17.

FURTHER READING

van der Heijde, D., Ramiro, S., Landewé, R., et al., 2016. Update of the ASAS-EULAR management recommendations for axial spondyloarthritis. In: Annals of the Rheumatic Diseases. https://doi.org/10.1136/annrheumdis-2016-210770. Published online: 13 January 2017.

NICE, 2017. Spondyloarthritis in over 16s; diagnosis and management (NG65). Available online at: https://www.nice.org.uk/guidance/ng65.

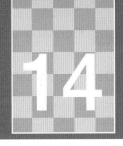
Connective tissue disease is a broad term used to describe conditions where the connective tissues of the body are targeted. There is no strict unifying definition, but generally these diseases are multisystem inflammatory disorders associated with immunological abnormalities. There are overlaps between many of the disorders, which share many clinical features.

SYSTEMIC LUPUS ERYTHEMATOSUS

Definition

Systemic lupus erythematosus (SLE) is an autoimmune inflammatory disease characterized by autoantibodies to nuclear material, which can involve almost any organ or system of the body.

Prevalence

SLE has an average worldwide prevalence of 10–50 per 100,000. However, this varies significantly according to ethnicity. It is more common in Indian and Afro-Caribbean people, than in Caucasians and affects women at least 10 times more frequently than men.

Aetiology

There are genetic, environmental and hormonal factors thought to be important to the aetiology. SLE can be induced by drugs, such as minocycline, hydralazine and the oral contraceptive pill. Oestrogen is thought to play a role in producing autoreactive B cells. Environmental triggers include viruses and ultraviolet B light. Drug-induced lupus tends to be mild and does not affect the kidneys.

Pathology

Immune function in SLE is abnormal, with T- and B-cell dysfunction causing B-cell hyperactivity and impaired immune complex clearance from tissues. Dysfunction of the complement system and aberrant programmed cell death means that intracellular material is not disposed of correctly, allowing autoantibody production to develop against nuclear material. A wide variety of autoantibodies have been described, some of which are directly pathogenic (anti-double-stranded DNA, anti-Ro). The coagulation system may be abnormal and vasculopathy is common, resulting from clotting cascade antibodies (anti-C).

Clinical features

SLE usually develops between the ages of 15 and 40 years. The clinical features are diverse and vary in severity over time. Initial symptoms may be mild and vague, but it is the exacerbations of SLE and resultant tissue damage that cause significant ill health. Severe lupus flares can result in life-threatening complications including renal failure and cerebral vasculitis. Factors that may trigger a flare of SLE are listed in the box.

FACTORS CAPABLE OF TRIGGERING FLARES OF SYSTEMIC LUPUS ERYTHEMATOSUS

- Overexposure to sunlight: ultraviolet light B > A
- Oestrogen-containing contraceptive therapy
- Drugs: hydralazine, minocycline, etc.
- Infection
- Stress

Constitutional features

Fatigue, malaise and weight loss are common features of SLE. Fatigue, in particular, can be extremely debilitating and difficult to manage.

HINTS AND TIPS

Hypothyroidism is more common in systemic lupus erythematosus than in the general population. It should be considered in patients with extreme lethargy.

Musculoskeletal features

Approximately 90% of patients with SLE experience arthralgia, usually polyarticular. Nonerosive arthritis occurs in approximately 25% of patients and symptoms are usually more dramatic than clinical signs. Deformity is due to tenosynovitis and fibrosis, rather than cartilage or bone erosions (Jaccoud arthropathy).

Myalgia is a common feature in SLE and myositis (inflamed muscle) can occur (see later section on myositis). Avascular necrosis of bone and osteoporosis are recognized but are usually a consequence of corticosteroid treatment or vasculopathy.

Dermatological features

There are many cutaneous manifestations of lupus. Photosensitivity is common (approximately 60%). The characteristic 'butterfly' malar rash develops over the nose and cheeks (Fig. 14.1). Discoid lupus (demarcated, pigmented or atrophic plaques) can develop with no systemic features (Fig. 14.2).

Hair loss reflects disease activity and patients may develop alopecia. Mucosal ulceration may affect the nose, mouth and vagina. Cutaneous vasculitis can present with urticarial lesions, livedo reticularis, palpable purpura and splinter haemorrhages.

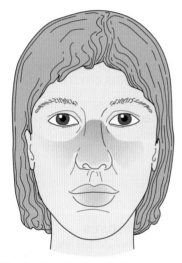

Fig. 14.1 The classic butterfly rash of systemic lupus erythematosus.

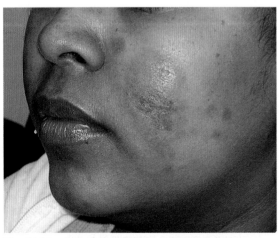

Fig. 14.2 Lesions of discoid lupus. With permission from Aranow C, Diamond B, Mackay M, Systemic Lupus Erythematosus. In: Rich RR et al (eds), Clinical Immunology: Principles and Practice, 5th ed., 2019, Elsevier.

Cardiovascular features

Serositis is common in SLE and pericarditis is the most common manifestation. It tends to cause a sharp pain in the chest, alleviated by sitting forward and associated with diffuse saddle-shaped ST-segment elevation on an electrocardiogram.

Myocarditis may accompany myositis and can present with arrhythmias or heart failure. Libman–Sacks endocarditis is due to noninfective vegetations and seldom causes clinical problems.

At least a third of patients with SLE suffer from Raynaud phenomenon (vasospasm, typically precipitated by the cold, causing peripheral ischaemia). This can be seen in the digits, tip of the nose, earlobes and occasionally the tongue, which become pale and numb before turning blue. The final phase is redness and flushing due to eventual vasodilation.

Vasculitis may present with digital infarcts, skin rashes or ulcers that can occasionally affect internal organs such as the lungs and brain.

Pulmonary features

Amongst the pulmonary features of SLE, pleurisy and pleural effusions are the most common. Acute pneumonitis can mimic pneumonia. Chronic pneumonitis causes fibrosis. Pulmonary hypertension is rare.

Renal features

Glomerulonephritis is the most common cause of lupus-related deaths in patients with SLE. Nephritis does not cause clinical symptoms until there is significant renal damage. It is important to monitor patients closely, checking their blood pressure and urine for blood and protein, so that renal disease can be acted upon early.

Neurological features

SLE can involve the central nervous system, cranial and peripheral nerves, producing a wide range of clinical features. These include headaches, neuropsychiatric problems, seizures, neuropathies and chorea.

Issues such as anxiety, depression and psychosis are well recognized effects of lupus.

Haematological features

Lymphopenia is very common in SLE but neutropenia is also found. When patients are taking immunosuppressants, it can be difficult to differentiate between drug effects and disease-related aetiology. Anaemia can be due to chronic inflammation or autoimmune haemolysis, which affects up to 5% of lupus sufferers. Antiphospholipid antibodies and coagulopathies are discussed later in this chapter.

Gastrointestinal features

Gastrointestinal (GI) features tend to be rarer than other systemic involvement. Aseptic peritonitis can present with abdominal pain and nausea, with or without ascites. Other manifestations include mild hepatosplenomegaly from haemolysis or vasculitis affecting the mesenteric vessels.

Investigations

Serological tests

SLE is characterized by the presence of serum autoantibodies against nuclear components (Table 14.1).

Other tests

- Urine should be tested with a dipstick to look for blood and protein. These are signs of nephritis.
- Full blood count should be performed regularly to look for anaemia, leukopenia and thrombocytopenia. Urea, creatinine and electrolyte levels should also be monitored.
- The erythrocyte sedimentation rate (ESR) will increase during a flare of SLE (see box) but may also be high even when the patient feels well. C-reactive protein tends to be normal or mildly elevated unless infection, synovitis or serositis is present.
- Complement levels (C3 and C4) can be lower in active SLE.
- Coombs test will be positive in patients with autoimmune haemolytic anaemia.

Table 14.1 Autoantibodies associated with systemic lupus erythematosus

Autoantibodies found in SLE	Comments
Antinuclear antibodies	Detected in >95% of patients
Anti-Ro and anti-La antibodies	Associated with secondary Sjögren syndrome and pulmonary fibrosis. Mothers are at risk of having babies with neonatal SLE and congenital heart block. Sensitivity = 25%
Anti-double-stranded DNA antibodies	Present in 50% of SLE patient. Very specific indicator of disease when present.
Antihistone antibodies	Often positive in drug-induced SLE; sensitivity = 90%
Antiphospholipid and anticardiollpin antibodies	May be positive in around 10%–20% of SLE patients

SLE, Systemic lupus erythematosus.

- Skin biopsy shows deposition of immunoglobulin G (IgG) and complement at the dermal–epidermal junction in patients with rashes (lupus band test).
- Renal biopsy is sometimes performed to aid diagnosis or to establish prognosis in patients with abnormal renal function.

Management

General measures

Education about SLE is essential. Patients are advised to avoid factors that can precipitate lupus flares (see earlier box). They should wear long-sleeved clothes and use complete sunblock in sunny weather. Infections should be treated promptly.

Pharmacological treatment

The choice of drug treatment depends on the severity of the disease and the organs involved.

Mild SLE

Patients with symptoms such as arthralgia, lethargy or a faint rash may respond to nonsteroidal anti-inflammatory drugs and/or antimalarials such as hydroxychloroquine.

Moderate SLE

Patients with more severe clinical features, such as serositis, severe arthritis, nephritis autoimmune haemolysis, thrombocytopenia and neurological or psychiatric disorders often require treatment with corticosteroids. Once disease remission is achieved, steroid-sparing agents such as azathioprine, methotrexate and mycophenolate mofetil are often used.

Severe SLE

An SLE flare may cause severe life-threatening complications such as acute renal failure, neurological or haematology problems and must be treated promptly with cytotoxic

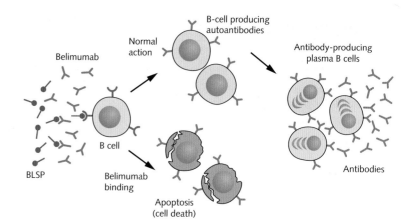

Fig. 14.3 B-lymphocyte stimulating protein is blocked by the monoclonal antibody, belimumab, thus inhibiting B-cells from producing pathogenic autoantibody.

medication and corticosteroids. Cyclophosphamide is very effective. Tacrolimus and mycophenolate are alternatives. Ciclosporin is often also used. Rituximab and belimumab are used in refractory lupus: belimumab blocks B-cell survival factor (see Fig. 14.3).

Adjunctive treatment

Hypertension due to nephritis should be managed aggressively. Intravenous immunoglobulin infusions may help thrombocytopenia or neutropenia. Antiplatelet medication or warfarin are required for patients with antiphospholipid syndrome (see later section). Anticonvulsants may be required for epilepsy associated with a disease of the central nervous system.

Prognosis

The outlook for patients with SLE is improving. Ten-year survival is over 90%. It is widely recognized that patients have a higher cardiovascular mortality and risks are managed aggressively. Malignancy and infection rates are higher.

THE ANTIPHOSPHOLIPID SYNDROME

Definition

The antiphospholipid syndrome (APS) is a systemic autoimmune condition characterized by arterial and venous thrombosis, fetal loss and thrombocytopenia associated with persistent levels of antiphospholipid antibodies.

Antiphospholipid antibodies often complicate other connective tissue diseases, such as lupus. In these cases, the patient is said to have secondary APS.

Incidence

Overall incidence of APS is unclear; it was first described in patients with SLE, but it has become apparent that it has its own clinical entity.

Pathology

The two main antiphospholipid antibodies are anticardiolipin and lupus anticoagulant. They have a procoagulant effect in susceptible individuals, associated impaired fibrinolysis and increased vascular tone, all contributing to clot formation and infarction.

Clinical features

The major features and additional clinical features of APS are shown in the boxes.

THE MAJOR FEATURES OF ANTIPHOSPHOLIPID SYNDROME	
Venous thrombosis	Deep vein thrombosis and pulmonary emboli are the most common Other veins can be affected (e.g., inferior vena cava, pelvic, renal, portal and hepatic veins)
Arterial thrombosis	Cerebral ischaemia (stroke, transient ischaemic attacks) Peripheral ischaemia
Fetal complications	Spontaneous abortion, premature births
Thrombocytopenia	Not severe enough to cause haemorrhage

Investigations

Diagnosis is based on the detection of anticardiolipin antibodies or a positive lupus anticoagulant assay on at least two occasions separated by at least a 12-week interval. The interval is necessary because the antibodies can sometimes develop transiently in relation to other events (such as infection) and exist harmlessly in the body.

Anticardiolipin antibodies bind to cardiolipin or β2-glycoprotein-1. The lupus anticoagulant assay measures the ability of antiphospholipid antibodies to prolong clotting tests such as the activated partial prothrombin time. Although the test is for an anticoagulant, the syndrome produces clotting and thrombosis. Thrombocytopenia may occur.

Management

General advice

The following steps are advisable:

- Avoidance of the oral contraceptive pill
- Avoidance of smoking
- Treatment of hypertension, diabetes and hyperlipidaemia

Asymptomatic patients

Current recommendations are that asymptomatic patients should be monitored closely, but those with no clinical features should not be treated. Those with high cardiovascular risk factors or with a concurrent separate autoimmune disease should receive low-dose aspirin prophylaxis. During high-risk periods, such as after elective surgery, patient should receive thrombosis prophylaxis with low-molecular weight heparin.

Venous or arterial thrombosis

Patients who experience thrombosis should be managed with conventional anticoagulation. However, anticoagulation should be lifelong, because there is an ongoing risk of repeated thrombosis. Warfarin is the typical anticoagulant used in patients with a confirmed arterial or venous

thrombus, with a target international normalized ratio (INR) of 2.5 (range 2–3).

Recurrent fetal loss

Warfarin should be stopped before conception, when attempting another pregnancy, because it is teratogenic. Subcutaneous heparin and aspirin should be given throughout pregnancy to reduce the risk of fetal loss.

SJÖRGEN SYNDROME

Definition

Sjörgen syndrome is a chronic autoimmune disease, characterized by inflammation of exocrine glands. The salivary and lacrimal glands are the most commonly involved, resulting in dryness of the mouth and eyes. Sjörgen syndrome can be primary or secondary (associated with another autoimmune disease). Causes of secondary Sjörgen syndrome are shown in the box.

Sicca syndrome is the presence of dry eyes or mouth as a result of nonautoimmune disease, such as smoking or drugs.

Prevalence

The prevalence is 1%–3%. It is nine times more common in women than in men.

Aetiology

The exact aetiology is unknown. The primary disease has a strong association with human leukocyte antigen (HLA class II DR and DQ) haplotypes and the signal transducer and activator of transcription 4 (STAT4) gene. It is thought that a viral infection might trigger an immune response in susceptible individuals.

Pathology

All organs affected by Sjörgen syndrome are infiltrated by lymphocytes. In the salivary glands, this results in duct dilatation, acinar atrophy and interstitial fibrosis. There is marked activation of B cells, resulting in increased immunoglobulin production. Sicca syndrome has no immune infiltrate when compared with Sjörgen syndrome.

Clinical features

Sjörgen syndrome predominantly affects people aged between 40 and 50 years. The main symptoms are ocular and oral.

Ocular symptoms

Reduced tear secretion results in the destruction of the corneal and conjunctival epithelium (keratoconjunctivitis sicca). Patients complain of dry, gritty, sore eyes that might be reddened. Bacterial conjunctivitis is common.

Oral symptoms

Xerostomia (dryness of the mouth) leads to difficulties in swallowing dry food or talking for long periods of time. On examination of the oral cavity, the mucosa is dry, there is very little saliva and the tongue may be fissured. Dental caries are more common and oral candidiasis often occurs. Intermittent parotid swelling affects at least half of patients with primary Sjörgen syndrome (Fig. 14.4) but is less common in secondary disease.

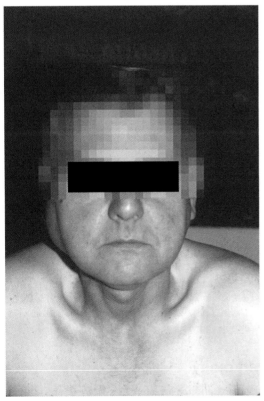

Fig. 14.4 Parotid swelling in Sjörgen syndrome.

Other symptoms of exocrine dysfunction

Secretions from other exocrine glands can also be affected. Patients may experience vaginal dryness and dyspareunia and lack of secretions in the GI tract can result in oesophagitis and gastritis.

Systemic features

Primary Sjörgen syndrome is a systemic disease and many patients develop extraglandular manifestations that mimic SLE:

- Constitutional features such as fatigue, weight loss and fever.
- Arthritis is episodic, nonerosive and very similar to the joint disease seen in SLE.
- Circulation: Raynaud phenomenon affects up to 50% of patients. Vasculitis affects approximately 5% of patients and usually causes cutaneous lesions, purpura and urticaria.
- Respiratory: interstitial lung disease is mild and often subclinical.
- Renal: interstitial nephritis can lead to renal tubular acidosis or nephrogenic diabetes insipidus.
- Neurological features vary widely. Peripheral neuropathies result from small vessel vasculitis. Cranial neuropathies, hemiparesis, seizures and movement disorders can also occur.
- Malignancy: lymphomas, usually B cell, are more common in patients with Sjörgen syndrome than in the general population. They develop in the salivary glands, reticuloendothelial system, GI tract, lungs or kidneys.

Investigations

Schirmer test

Schirmer test is used to demonstrate a reduction in tear production from the lacrimal glands. One end of a strip of filter paper is placed beneath the lower eyelid. Wetting the paper by less than 5 mm in 5 minutes suggests reduced tear secretion.

Labial gland biopsy and histology

Biopsy and histology of the buccal surface of the lower lip is very useful. Lymphocytic infiltration can be seen.

Blood tests

- ESR is usually elevated.
- Immunoglobulin levels can be very high.
- Anti-Ro/La antibodies are a diagnostic aid but rheumatoid factor and antinuclear antibodies (ANA) are often also found.

Management

Treatment of Sjörgen syndrome is mainly topical and symptomatic. Tear substitutes such as hypromellose eye drops can help to lubricate the eyes. Occlusion of the canaliculi can help block the drainage of tears and keep the conjunctiva moist.

Xerostomia can be treated with saliva substitutes. Pilocarpine tablets can help but might cause cholinergic side effects such as sweating, flushing and abdominal cramps. Careful attention to dental hygiene is essential.

Hydroxychloroquine can help the arthritis. Corticosteroids and other immunosuppressants are prescribed for serious complications such as vasculitis and renal disease.

POLYMYOSITIS AND DERMATOMYOSITIS

Definition

Polymyositis (PM) and dermatomyositis (DM) are autoimmune, inflammatory muscle diseases. DM also affects the skin.

Incidence

Both muscle diseases are rare, with a combined annual incidence of between 2 and 10 cases per million. There is a female predominance of 2:1.

Aetiology

The aetiology is unknown in both diseases. Family studies support a genetic predisposition. Associations with various HLA types have been reported but are weak.

Pathology

In both conditions, muscle fibres are infiltrated by inflammatory cells and there is subsequent degeneration, necrosis and phagocytosis. In PM, the main driver of damage is thought to be predominantly via cytotoxic T-cell damage. In DM, muscle damage is driven by complement-mediated damage of the intramuscular microvasculature. Skin biopsies in DM show the same histological features as in lupus.

Clinical features

Inflammatory muscle disease can affect people of any age, but the peak onset is between 40 and 60 years of age.

Myositis

PM and DM are characterized by an insidious, symmetrical and progressive proximal muscle weakness that develops over week and months. Patients describe difficulty in rising from a chair or walking up stairs. It can be difficult to reach things above head height.

Involvement of the intercostal muscles and diaphragm can affect ventilation and lead to a type 2 respiratory failure. Involvement of the muscles of the head, neck and oesophagus can result in dysphagia and regurgitation.

Patients may complain of muscle pain and tenderness. Muscle bulk and reflexes appear normal, except in advanced cases.

Cutaneous manifestations

The skin rashes of DM usually precede the weakness. Typical lesions are:

- Gottron papules: erythematous, scaly papules or plaques over the metacarpophalangeal and proximal interphalangeal joints and also over the extensor surfaces of the hands and elbows.
- A heliotrope rash develops over the eyelids; lilac discolouration is often accompanied by periorbital oedema.
- A macular erythematous rash may develop on the face, neck, chest, shoulders and hands.
- Cutaneous vasculitis can cause ulceration.
- Periungal telangiectasia may be seen and the cuticles are often thickened and irregular.

Extramuscular features of polymyositis and dermatomyositis

Constitutional features
Fatigue, malaise, fever and weight loss are common.

Skeletal features
Many patients develop polyarthralgia as well as myalgia.

Pulmonary features
Interstitial lung disease occurs in up to 30% of patients. Ventilatory failure can result from weakness of the intercostal muscles and diaphragm. Patients with dysphagia and regurgitation may develop aspiration pneumonia.

Cardiovascular features
Myocarditis can occur with heart failure and arrhythmias, but most cases are asymptomatic. Raynaud phenomenon and vasculitis can accompany myositis.

Gastrointestinal features

Vasculitis can result in intestinal haemorrhage or perforation. It is more common in juvenile DM.

Malignancy

Approximately 10%–15% of adults with inflammatory muscle disease have an underlying malignancy. The association is thought to be much stronger with DM than PM.

Investigations

Serum levels of muscle enzymes

Serum levels of muscle enzymes (such as creatine kinase) are elevated due to myositis.

Erythrocyte sedimentation rate

The ESR is usually raised but does not closely correlate with disease activity.

Autoantibodies

A positive autoantibody test is found in around 60% of patients with inflammatory myositis. Anti-Jo-1 antibodies are more common in patients with PM than those with DM and are associated with Raynaud phenomenon and interstitial lung disease (the antisynthetase syndrome). Anti-Mi-2 antibodies are specific for DM but are only found in around 25% of patients.

Muscle biopsy

This is the most definitive diagnostic test. Histology shows the typical inflammatory infiltrate pattern of PM or DM.

Electromyography and nerve conduction studies

Electromyography and nerve conduction studies can show that the weakness is due to a myopathic process but do not provide a specific diagnosis.

Magnetic resonance imaging

Magnetic resonance imaging (MRI) can identify areas of anatomical muscle oedema and then be used to target a biopsy.

Management

Although the muscle enzymes respond quickly to treatment, muscle strength is usually much slower to recover. Physiotherapy plays an important role in the rehabilitation of patients with inflammatory muscle disease.

Most patients with PM and DM require immunosuppressive therapy. Corticosteroids are used to control myositis. They are initially prescribed at high doses. Serum creatine kinase is monitored and, as it falls, the corticosteroid dose is gradually reduced. Methotrexate and azathioprine are used as steroid sparing agents. Cyclophosphamide

may be prescribed for patients with severe interstitial lung disease. If an underlying malignancy is found, it should be promptly treated.

HINTS AND TIPS

Steroid myopathy is a common complication of treatment. It may be difficult to distinguish from active myositis, but it should be considered in patients with normal creatine kinase levels whose muscle strength is deteriorating. Biopsy may help differentiate.

Prognosis

The 5-year survival for PM and DM has improved and is currently over 80%. Despite this, many patients are still left with persisting symptoms, or side effects due to their treatments.

SYSTEMIC SCLEROSIS

Definition

Scleroderma means hardening of the skin and describes a spectrum of disorders, which may be confined to the skin (cutaneous) or involve other organs (systemic sclerosis; see box). The systemic form is further subdivided into a limited and diffuse disease, the latter having more extensive skin involvement than the former.

CLASSIFICATION OF SYSTEMIC SCLEROSIS AND RELATED CONDITIONS

- Localized cutaneous scleroderma
- Morphoea linear scleroderma
- Systemic sclerosis
- Limited cutaneous systemic sclerosis
- Diffuse cutaneous systemic sclerosis
- Scleroderma sine scleroderma

Incidence and prevalence

These are rare conditions. The annual incidence of scleroderma is 0.6–1.9 per million. The UK prevalence is approximately 100 per million. Women are affected four times as often as men.

Aetiology

In most patients the aetiology is unknown.

Pathology

The two main pathological processes in systemic sclerosis are fibrosis and microvascular occlusion. Over-active fibroblasts produce excessive extracellular matrix in the dermis. Perivascular inflammatory infiltrates and intimal proliferation lead to narrowing of arteries and arterioles and obliteration of the capillary bed. There is immune activation and release of cytokines.

Clinical manifestations

Skin manifestations

Scleroderma begins with an inflammatory phase. The skin becomes puffy and tight and sometimes feels itchy. These symptoms typically affect the forearms, hands and feet initially. Over several months, skin thickening and induration develops. Common features found on examination are:

- sclerodactyly (Fig. 14.5)
- microstomia (Fig. 14.6)
- furrowing of the skin around the lips (Fig. 14.6)
- loss of normal skin creases
- tethering of skin to underlying structures
- skin hypo- and hyper-pigmentation
- flexion contractures at joints
- thinning and atrophy (late stage)

The skin changes can differ between the limited and diffuse forms of systemic sclerosis. They are outlined in Table 14.2.

The effects of systemic sclerosis on other body systems

In addition to causing disfiguring skin changes, systemic sclerosis can have profound effects on other organs. Limited disease is twice as common as diffuse disease and is sometimes referred to as CREST syndrome (CREST = *c*alcinosis,

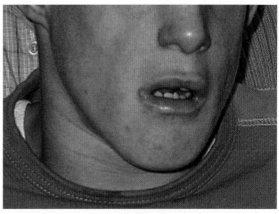

Fig. 14.6 Microstomia: note the tightness of the skin around the mouth. With permission from de Ravel TJ, Balikova I, Thiry P et al, Another patient with a de novo deletion further delineates the 2q33.1 microdeletion syndrome. European Journal of Medical Genetics, Volume 52, Issue 2, pp 120–122, 2009, Elsevier Masson SAS.

*R*aynaud phenomenon, o*e*sophageal disease, *s*clerodactyly and *t*elangiectasia). Symptoms develop most commonly between 40 and 50 years of age.

Involvement of internal organs is more frequent in diffuse than in limited disease.

Cardiovascular manifestations

Raynaud phenomenon

This occurs in nearly every patient with systemic sclerosis. Severe disease may cause ischaemic changes in the fingertips and possibly gangrene. Unlike in benign primary Raynaud phenomenon, there is destruction of the capillary structures at the peripheries, which can be seen using nailfold capillaroscopy techniques.

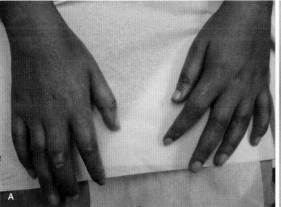
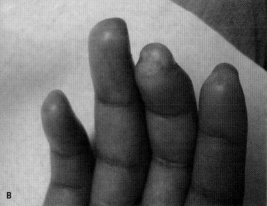

Fig. 14.5 (A) Sclerodactyly and (B) digital pitting and ulceration. With permission from Torok KS, Pediatric Scleroderma: Systemic or Localized Forms; Pediatric Clinics of North America, 2012-04-01, Volume 59, Issue 2, pp 381–405, 2012, Elsevier.

Table 14.2 A comparison of skin disease between limited and diffuse systemic sclerosis

	Limited systemic sclerosis	Diffuse systemic sclerosis
Distribution of skin fibrosis	Hands[a] and feet Over the face and neck	Limbs, face, neck and trunk
Skin tethering to underlying structures	Common	Less common
Inflammatory features	Mild	Swelling and pruritus prominent
Telangiectasia	Commonly occurs on the face and digits	Less common
Calcinosis	Cutaneous and subcutaneous Calcification common	Less common

[a] Scleroderma affecting the fingers is often referred to as sclerodactyly.

Cardiac disease

- Myocardial fibrosis can cause cardiac failure and arrhythmias.
- Pericarditis can be silent.

Pulmonary manifestations

Pulmonary disease is the most common cause of death in systemic sclerosis.

Interstitial lung disease

This affects around 25% of patients with limited disease and up to 40% of those with diffuse systemic sclerosis.

Pulmonary hypertension

This affects around 10%–15% of patients and now represents a major cause of death in scleroderma patients.

Primary pulmonary hypertension is more common in limited disease and is not associated with additional lung pathology. Secondary pulmonary hypertension is more common in diffuse disease and is caused by interstitial lung disease and fibrosis.

Renal manifestations

Scleroderma renal crisis

This is a cause of rapidly progressive renal failure associated with severe hypertension. It tends to occur in patients with diffuse cutaneous disease within 5 years of diagnosis and is often preceded by a deterioration in skin disease. Mortality is high and poor outcomes are common. Aggressive but cautious blood pressure control is the mainstay of treatment. Patients often present with headaches, blurred vision and sometimes seizures. Acute left ventricular failure can occur and death from renal failure is common without urgent intervention.

RED FLAG

Scleroderma renal crisis is a life-threatening medical emergency that requires urgent treatment.

Gastrointestinal manifestations

Scleroderma can affect any part of the GI tract but commonly involves the oesophagus. Reflux oesophagitis and dysmotility are common and are a significant source of distress and worry to patients. Hypomotility can lead to bacterial overgrowth, with constipation or diarrhoea. Many patients complain of worsening dysphagia to solids, which warrants a barium swallow study.

Musculoskeletal manifestations

Most patients suffer from a degree of arthralgia and joint stiffness, but overt synovitis is uncommon. Flexion contractors of the interphalangeal joints due to skin changes are common.

Neurological manifestations

Both central and peripheral neuropathies can develop and overlap myopathy/myositis is a recognized feature.

Investigations

The diagnostic criteria are based on clinical findings and serological status (see box). It is important to establish whether patients have limited or diffuse disease, as this impacts upon prognosis.

DIAGNOSTIC CRITERIA FOR SYSTEMIC SCLEROSIS

Item	Subitem	Score
Skin thickening of the fingers of both hands extending proximal to the MCP joints		9
Skin thickening of the fingers (only count the highest score)	Puffy fingers	2
	Sclerodactyly (distal to the MCP joints but proximal to the PIP joints	4

Item	Subitem	Score
Fingertip lesions (only count the highest score)	Digital tip ulcers	2
	Fingertip pitting scars	3
Telangiectasia		2
Abnormal nail-fold capillaries		2
Lung disease (max score is 2)	Pulmonary artery hypertension	2
	Interstitial lung disease	2
Raynaud phenomenon		3
Related antibodies (max score is 3)	Anticentromere	3
	Antitopoisomerase I (Scl-70)	
	Anti-RNA polymerase III	

The highest score for each criterion is counted.
Patients with a score of 9 or above are classified as having definite scleroderma (sensitivity 91%, specificity 92%).
MCP, Metacarpophalangeal; PIP, proximal interphalangeal.
Adapted from 2013 ACR/EULAR criteria for the classification of systemic sclerosis.

Table 14.3 Treatment of end-organ disease in systemic sclerosis

Complication	Intervention
Raynaud phenomenon	Hand warmers Vasodilators • Calcium-channel blockers • Angiontensin receptor blockers • Intravenous prostacyclin (iloprost) for severe ischaemia. Digital sympathectomy is useful for ischaemia of one or two digits
Pulmonary fibrosis	Prednisolone, with or without cyclophosphamide
Pulmonary hypertension	Anticoagulation Vasodilators • Calcium-channel blockers • Bosentan • Sildenafil • Prostacyclins Diuretics for right ventricular failure, if present
Gastrointestinal problems	Proton pump inhibitor for gastro-oesophageal reflux Antibiotics for small-bowel overgrowth Bulk-forming agents for constipation
Renal crisis	Antihypertensives (give immediately): • ACE inhibitors • Calcium-channel blockers • Temporary dialysis may be required
Cardiac problems	Diuretics and ACE inhibitors for cardiac failure Antiarrhythmics if necessary Corticosteroids for myocarditis

ACE, Angiotensin-converting enzyme.

Serological tests

ANA are found in most patients. The presence or absence of other autoantibodies can help predict complications and prognosis, for example:

- Anticentromere antibodies are associated with limited disease and a relatively good prognosis. They signify a risk of pulmonary hypertension, but not pulmonary fibrosis.
- Antitopoisomerase-I (Scl-70) antibodies are associated with diffuse disease, higher risk of pulmonary fibrosis, renal involvement and mortality.

Management

Treatment

To date, no definitive treatment exists. Symptoms and complications should be treated on an organ-by-organ basis (see Table 14.3).

Screening for complications

Monitoring pulmonary function tests, echocardiography, blood pressure and renal function help to detect complications early in systemic sclerosis.

Prognosis

The 5-year survival rate for scleroderma is about 85%, with 10-year survival less than 70%. Improving survival rates reflect better disease management, but many patients still suffer a significant burden of morbidity.

THE VASCULITIDES

Vasculitis is inflammation of blood vessels. It is a feature of many illnesses and can be primary or secondary. The primary vasculitides are uncommon diseases in which vasculitis is the predominant feature. Secondary vasculitis complicates other established diseases, such as rheumatoid arthritis and SLE.

In addition, vasculitis can be caused by infections, drugs and malignancy. Only primary vasculitis is dis-cussed below.

Pathology

Vasculitis is characterized by idiopathic autoimmune-driven inflammation caused by inflammatory cell infiltration of the blood vessel wall, resulting in fibrinoid necrosis. For this reason, the term necrotizing vasculitis is sometimes used. There is often associated granuloma formation. Vascular inflammation can have severe consequences:

- Vessel stenosis leading to occlusion and distal infarction.
- Aneurysm formation can lead to rupture of vessels and haemorrhage.

Antineutrophil cytoplasmic antibodies (ANCA) are particularly specific for vasculitis and helpful for diagnosis and classification. These antibodies bind to enzymes in the cytoplasm of neutrophils. There are two associated antigen/antibody subtypes:

- Proteinase-3 (PR3) is an enzyme found throughout the neutrophil cytoplasm and anti-PR3 antibodies are sometimes called c-ANCA (cytoplasm ANCA). This enzyme is found in patients with granulomatosis with polyangiitis (GPA, formerly Wegener granulomatosis) and is highly specific.
- Myeloperoxidase (MPO) is an enzyme found in a perinuclear distribution in neutrophils and anti-MPO antibodies are called perinuclear-ANCA (p-ANCA). This enzyme is found in eosinophilic granulomatosis with polyangiitis (EGPA, formerly Churg-Strauss syndrome), polyarteritis nodosum and microscopic polyangiitis.

Classification of primary vasculitis

The vasculitides are commonly classified by the size of the vessels they affect (see box).

CLASSIFICATION OF PRIMARY VASCULITIS

Large-vessel vasculitis

Giant cell (temporal) arteritis and polymyalgia rheumatica

Takayasu arteritis

Medium-vessel vasculitis

Polyarteritis nodosa

Kawasaki disease

Small-vessel vasculitis

Wegener granulomatosis[a]

Churg-Strauss syndrome[a]

Microscopic polyangiitis[a]

Henoch-Schönlein purpura

Essential cryoglobulinaemic vasculitis

[a] *Vasculitides are most commonly associated with antineutrophil cytoplasmic antibodies.*

Clinical features

Although vasculitis is rare, it can affect any system of the body and has the potential to be life threatening. It is important to be aware of the general effects it can cause (Table 14.4), but detailed knowledge of specific diseases is beyond the scope of this textbook.

Giant cell arteritis and polymyalgia rheumatic

Giant cell arteritis (GCA) is a large vessel vasculitis. It often coexists with polymyalgia rheumatic (PMR), a nonvasculitic illness, which is why they are discussed together here. They have an incidence of approximately 1–5 in 10,000. They both affect people over the age of 60 years and are twice as common in women than in men. About 50% of patients with GCA have symptoms of PMR and approximately 25%–50% of patients with PMR may experience GCA symptoms.

Giant cell arteritis

Most symptoms are due to inflammation of the carotid arteries and their branches, although any large artery can be involved. The onset of GCA can be insidious or abrupt with symptoms appearing overnight. Patients complain of:

- Severe unilateral headache and scalp tenderness from skin ischaemia.
- Pain on chewing food (jaw claudication from masseter muscle ischaemia).
- The temporal artery is thickened and beaded on palpation and may be pulseless.
- Visual change: optic artery ischaemia, which may be preceded by a temporary change such as amaurosis fugax.

Blindness can occur. This is due to ischaemia optic neuritis, caused by arteritis of the posterior cilliary artery and branches of the ophthalmic arteries. Patients may experience transient visual disturbance at first. A stroke is another serious complication.

Table 14.4 The effects vasculitis can have on specific body systems

Body system or organ	Manifestations of vasculitis
Constitutional	Fatigue, anorexia, weight loss, fever
Skin	Rashes Palpable purpura Ulceration Ischaemia (Fig. 14.7)
Joints	Arthralgia Arthritis
Kidneys	Glomerulonephritis
Gastrointestinal tract	Ischaemia
Nervous system	Neuropathies Stroke
Lungs	Pulmonary haemorrhage

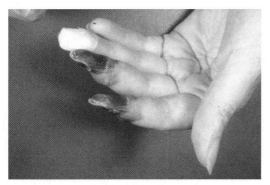

Fig. 14.7 Ischaemic changes in the fingers of a patient with vasculitis.

Polymyalgia rheumatica

Patients present with symmetrical pain and stiffness in the shoulder and pelvic girdle, often without synovitis. Proximal muscles are often tender. A medium-sized joint synovitis can occasionally occur. Constitutional features are common.

Investigations

The diagnosis of PMR is clinical. It is important to exclude mimics such as malignancy and other connective tissue diseases.

Temporal artery biopsy is the investigation of choice in GCA, but it does not always achieve a diagnosis. Arterial wall thickening may occur as skip lesions and the biopsy may fail to target one. Inflammatory cell infiltrates, giant cells and granulomas should be detected.

The ESR is typically raised in both conditions. However, a normal ESR does not exclude the diagnosis and if in doubt, other tests should be undertaken. There is a growing role for the use of colour Doppler ultrasound in the diagnosis of GCA. Anaemia is another common feature.

Management

Both GCA and PMR should be treated with corticosteroids. Prednisolone at a dose of 15–20 mg/day is usually prescribed for PMR. A higher dose of 1 mg/kg/day is used initially in GCA. Guidelines suggest blood tests should be monitored and clinical symptoms assessed regularly and when the patient has clinically improved, the steroid dose should be reduced.

There is usually a dramatic response to initiating steroids, provided an appropriate dose has been used. Failure to respond to steroids should challenge the diagnosis.

Most patients should be no longer receiving treatment after 2 years. Symptoms may occasionally flare at lower doses and if recurrent, a steroid sparing agent such as methotrexate or azathioprine should be prescribed to avoid longer-term high-dose steroid use. A small but significant number of patients remain on long-term low-dose steroids.

Takayasu arteritis

This is a rare disease that predominantly affects young women. The arteritis affects the aortic arch and its branches. Symptoms are due to vascular ischaemia and include claudication, visual disturbance, dizziness and stroke. Differences in blood pressure between limbs may occur, as well as subclavian bruits. Imaging with computed tomography (CT), MRI or positron emission tomography (PET) may help confirm the diagnosis. Steroids are the mainstay of treatment, but vascular complications are not uncommon and surgery, such as vascular bypass surgery, may be needed.

Polyarteritis nodosa

Polyarteritis nodosa is a necrotizing arteritis that leads to aneurysm formation. It affects men more commonly than women. Clinical features include skin ulceration and rashes (such as levido reticularis), peripheral neuropathy, renal disease and gut infarction, which presents as bleeding with abdominal pain. Angiography may show microaneurysms, which are usually found in the renal arteries and the coeliac axis. Renal, rectal and sural nerve biopsies can be helpful in achieving a diagnosis.

It is occasionally seen secondary to hepatitis B infection.

Treatment is with corticosteroids and, in severe cases, cyclophosphamide.

Kawasaki disease (mucocutaneous lymph node syndrome)

This vasculitis predominantly affects children under the age of 5 years but may rarely occur in adults. Features include desquamation of the skin of the hands and feet, conjunctival congestion, cervical lymphadenopathy, arteritis and coronary artery aneurysms, which can lead to myocardial infarction and heart failure. The characteristic finding in children is of a strawberry tongue. Treatment is with intravenous immunoglobulin and low dose aspirin.

Granulomatosis with polyangiitis

Granulomatosis with polyangiitis (GPA, formerly Wegener granulomatosis) is a granulomatous disorder associated with necrotizing vasculitis. It is strongly linked to the presence of PR3 ANCA. The peak age of onset is between 30 and 40 years of age. Many systems can be affected (Table 14.5), but it is the respiratory and renal complications that are often the most serious, including pulmonary haemorrhage and renal failure.

Survival in cases of GPA has improved significantly since the introduction of cyclophosphamide, which is given in conjunction with corticosteroids. Rituximab (B-cell depletion therapy) has been shown to have equivalence to cyclophosphamide and is licensed for treatment. Some patients with a more limited, non-life-threatening GPA are prescribed immunosuppressants such as mycophenolate, azathioprine and methotrexate.

Other forms of vasculitis

Eosinophilic granulomatosis with polyangiitis

Eosinophilic granulomatosis with polyangiitis (EGPA, formerly Churg-Strauss syndrome) usually has three stages.

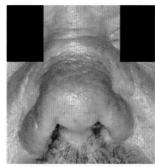
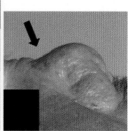

Fig. 14.8 Saddle nose deformity of granulomatosis with polyangiitis (late complication). With permission from Comarmond C, Cacoub P, Granulomatosis with polyangiitis (Wegener): Clinical aspects and treatment; Autoimmunity Reviews, 2014-11-01, Volume 13, Issue 11, pp 1121–1125, 2014, Elsevier B.V.

The atopic phase is characterized by atopy with allergic rhinitis and adult-onset asthma, often requiring frequent steroids. The eosinophilic stage is marked by abnormally high eosinophils in peripheral blood samples. Weight loss, night sweats, cough, diarrhoea and wheeze may be present due to the effects of eosinophils on the body's systems. The third phase, the vasculitis stage, is the hallmark of EGPA. Inflammation and damage to blood vessels results in rashes, a mononeuritis multiplex, renal failure and abdominal pains.

Treatment is as for GPA. MPO ANCA is commonly found in affected patients.

Microscopic polyarteritis

Microscopic polyarteritis (MPA) shares many features with GPA and presents with a rash, rapidly progressive glomerulonephritis and occasional alveolar haemorrhage.

Henoch-Schönlein purpura

Henoch-Schönlein purpura (HSP) typically presents with a palpable purpuric rash on the legs and buttocks in children and adolescents but it can occur at any age. GI involvement results in abdominal pains and there may be associated asymmetric arthritis. Around 40% of patients develop a glomerulonephritis, which is usually self-limiting. Treatment is usually supportive, but in rare cases immunosuppression may be required.

Behçet disease

This is a rare systemic inflammatory disorder that has features of vasculitis in a number of patients. The classical symptoms are of oral and genital ulceration, anterior and posterior uveitis or retinal vascular lesions, cutaneous lesions (erythema nodosum and cutaneous pustular vasculitis) and GI features of anorexia and diarrhoea.

Table 14.5 Clinical features of granulomatosis with polyangiitis

Body system or organ affected	Clinical features
Upper and lower respiratory tracts	Subglottic stenosis Lung nodules with or without cavitation Pulmonary haemorrhage Pulmonary infiltrates
Kidneys	Glomerulonephritis (often rapidly progressive)
Ear, nose and throat	Sensorineural deafness Nasal discharge, crusting and epistaxis • Saddling of the nose due to destruction of the septal cartilage (Fig. 14.8)
Joints	Arthralgia Arthritis
Skin	Rashes Palpable purpura Livedo reticularis
Nervous system	Cranial nerve palsies Peripheral neuropathy Granulomatous meningitis

Chapter Summary

- Connective tissue diseases (CTD) are a broad spectrum of inflammatory disorders affecting the connective tissues.
- SLE is a common CTD that presents with multisystemic symptoms. It is much more common in women than in men. Anti-dsDNA antibodies are commonly found.
- Antiphospholipid syndrome causes venous and arterial thrombosis and is associated with recurrent fetal loss. It may require lifelong treatment with anticoagulants.
- Sjörgen syndrome causes inflammation of the exocrine glands, resulting in dry eyes and a dry mouth.
- Inflammatory myositis (polymyositis and dermatomyositis) is rare but causes significant disability. Many patients require aggressive immunosuppression.
- Scleroderma/systemic sclerosis is a rare multisystem disorder characterized by fibrosis and vascular occlusion. Ulcerating Raynaud phenomenon is usually the presenting feature.
- Vasculitides cover a broad range of inflammatory conditions affecting the arteries. GCA and PMR are relatively common, with urgent high doses of steroids indicated in the former to reduce the risk of blindness.
- Table 14.6 contains a summary of the autoantibodies associated with various connective tissue diseases.

Table 14.6 Connective tissue diseases with corresponding associated autoantibody

Associated disease(s)	Autoantibody
Many connective tissue diseases	ANA
SLE	Anti-dsDNA
Drug-induced lupus	Anti-histone
Antiphospholipid syndrome & SLE	Antiphospholipid and anti-cardiolipin
Sjörgen syndrome	Anti-Ro/La
Polymyositis > dermatomyositis	Anti-Jo-1
Dermatomyositis	Anti-Mi-2
Systemic sclerosis - limited pattern	Anti-centromere
Systemic sclerosis - diffuse pattern	Antitopoisomerase-1 (Scl-70)
Granulomatosis with polyangiitis	c-ANCA (PR3)
Eosinophilic granulomatosis with polyangiitis	p-ANCA (MPO)

ANA, Antinuclear antibodies; ANCA, antineutrophil cytoplasmic antibodies; SLE, systemic lupus erythematosus.

FURTHER READING

Yates M, Watts R.A., Bajema I.M., et al. EULAR/ERA-EDTA recommendations for the management of ANCA-associated vasculitis. Annals of the Rheumatic Diseases. First published online: 23 June 2016. doi: 10.1136/annrheumdis-2016-209133.

Gordon, C., Amissah-Arthur, M.B., Gayed, M., et al., 2018. The British Society for Rheumatology guideline for the management of systemic lupus erythematosus in adults. Rheumatology 57 (1), e1–e45. 1 January.

Kowal-Bielecka O, Fransen J, Avouac J, et al. Update of EULAR recommendations for the treatment of systemic sclerosis. Annals of the Rheumatic Diseases. First published online: 09 November 2016. doi: 10.1136/annrheumdis-2016-209909.

Dasgupta, B., Borg, F.A., Hassan, N., et al., 1 August 2010. BSR and BHPR guidelines for the management of giant cell arteritis. Rheumatology 49(8), 1594–1597. https://doi.org/10.1093/rheumatology/keq039a.

Metabolic bone disease
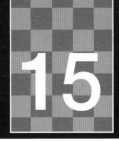

OSTEOPOROSIS

Because of the ageing population, fractures resulting from osteoporosis can put pressure on medical services incurring costs at both personal and societal levels.

Definition

Osteoporosis is a condition characterized by weakness of the bones, due to lower than normal bone mass or greater than normal bone loss. It results in increased bone fragility, which translates into an increased risk of fractures. Bone mineral density (BMD) is used to measure bone strength and is expressed as a T-score. This is the number of standard deviations by which the BMD varies in relation to the mean density of young adults. The World Health Organisation defines osteoporosis as a T-score of less than –2.5. Osteopenia is defined as a T-score of between –1 and –2.5. Normal bone density is expressed as a T-score greater than or equal to –1.

Aetiology and pathology

Peak bone mass is usually achieved around the age of 30 years and declines thereafter (Fig. 15.1). Bone loss is accelerated in osteoporosis by an imbalance between the rates of bone resorption and formation, which are governed by the activity of osteoclasts and osteoblasts respectively (Fig. 15.2). Risk factors for osteoporosis can be modifiable or nonmodifiable (see box: Risk factors for osteoporosis).

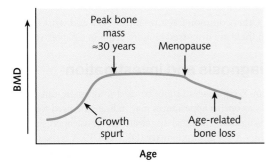

Fig. 15.1 Lifeline of bone mineral density.
BMD, Bone mineral density.

RISK FACTORS FOR OSTEOPOROSIS

Nonmodifiable	Modifiable
Age	Poor calcium and
Race (Caucasian, Asian)	vitamin D intake
Female sex	Lack of exercise
Early menopause	Smoking
Small size	Alcohol excess
Positive family history	

Osteoporosis is divided into primary (idiopathic and age related) and secondary (resulting from another disease process). The causes of secondary osteoporosis are shown in the box: Causes of secondary osteoporosis.

CAUSES OF SECONDARY OSTEOPOROSIS

- Hyperthyroidism
- Hyperparathyroidism
- Hypogonadism
- Cushing syndrome
- Rheumatoid arthritis
- Inflammatory bowel disease
- Coeliac disease and malabsorption states
- Renal failure
- Multiple myeloma
- Anorexia nervosa
- Medications:
  - corticosteroids
  - anticonvulsants
  - heparin

Clinical features

Patients present with pain, deformity and immobility due to fractures or they are detected by screening measurements

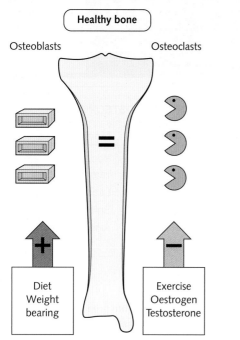

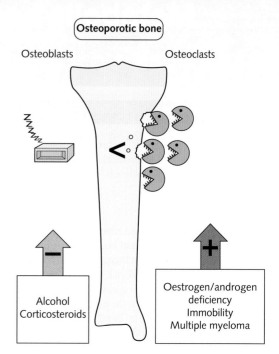

Fig. 15.2 Cell interactions in normal and osteoporotic bone.

of their BMD. Many areas now have automatic screening programmes for patients presenting with fragility fractures: these are fractures that occur during normal activities, such as a fall from standing height or less. The skeleton should be able to withstand this without injury.

The three typical fragility fractures are a Colles fracture of the wrist, a fractured neck of the femur and a vertebral body fracture.

COMMUNICATION

Osteoporosis is often asymptomatic and therefore the importance of treatment to prevent fractures must be emphasized to patients.

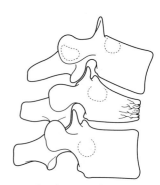

Fig. 15.3 Compression fracture of a thoracic vertebra.

Other common fractures include hip and wrist fractures and these are discussed in more detail in Chapter 18.

Vertebral fractures

Vertebral compression (or wedge) fractures (Fig. 15.3) usually present with thoracic or lumbar back pain after a minor fall. They are frequently multiple and result in a loss of height and kyphotic deformity of the spine. Some patients do not experience pain but complain that they are shrinking or becoming round-shouldered.

These fractures are stable and treatment is aimed at controlling symptoms with analgesia. Both vertebroplasty and kyphoplasty have been trialled. Trials involved the injection of cement into the fractured vertebra. Studies suggested the effect was no greater than with placebo treatment.

Diagnosis and investigation

Plain X-ray images cannot be used to diagnose osteoporosis, but osteopenia appearances may indicate the need for further investigation. The usual diagnostic test for osteoporosis is dual-energy X-ray absorptiometry (DEXA). DEXA is used in most departments to measure BMD at the lumbar spine and hip. Two photon beams are generated by the X-ray machine, which allows soft tissue and bone to be differentiated (Fig. 15.4).

A full history and examination should be performed when assessing a patient with low BMD. It is important to enquire about risk factors for osteoporosis as well as symptoms of potential secondary causes. Osteoporosis in men and young people is more likely to be due to a secondary cause.

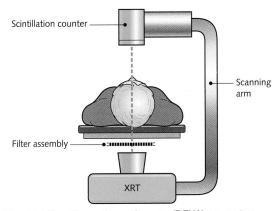

Fig. 15.4 Dual X-ray absorptiometry (DEXA) apparatus. The patient lies with the X-ray tube below. The filter allows two different beams to be produced, which are narrow to reduce scatter radiation. The beams are detected by the scintillation counter, which then generates an image. *XRT*, X-ray tube.

Investigations to exclude secondary causes will be necessary in some patients. Full blood count, alkaline phosphatase, renal function, serum electrophoresis, thyroid function, parathyroid hormone levels and vitamin D levels are commonly tested. Serum testosterone should be measured in men.

Management

The aim is to reduce the risk of fractures. This can be achieved by the following methods:

Modification of risk factors

Patients should try and change their modifiable risk factors (see box: Risk factors for osteoporosis), for example by stopping smoking or by increasing weight-bearing exercise.

Drug therapies to increase bone mass

Bisphosphonates

These are first line therapeutic drugs usually used in combination with calcium supplements and vitamin D. Bisphosphonates are antiresorptive and work by inhibiting osteoclast activity. Daily, weekly, monthly and yearly preparations are available and have good efficacy. Gastrointestinal intolerance is a problem for some patients.

Denosumab

This is a second line monoclonal antibody directed against RANK-L. RANK-L is a ligand produced by osteoblasts that upregulates osteoclast formation, activity and survival, which in turn causes loss of BMD. It is useful in patients who are intolerant to bisphosphonates.

Teriparatide

This is a parathyroid hormone analogue. It is very expensive but useful in patients intolerant to other treatments.

Intermittent parathyroid hormone exposure causes an increase in osteoblast activation (above that of osteoclasts) and therefore results in net BMD increases.

Other drugs

Raloxifene, a selective oestrogen receptor modulator, is sometimes used in postmenopausal women but its popularity has significantly decreased. Calcitonin is an antagonistic hormone to parathyroid hormone, reducing osteoclast activity and therefore increasing BMD.

Prevention of falls

As the majority of osteoporotic fractures are caused by falls, a significant amount of time and resources is spent on falls clinics to try to reduce the risk of falling. There are a number of factors that predispose patients to falls:

Intrinsic factors

- The ageing process: this leads to slower reaction times.
- Poor mobility: patients often have other conditions such as osteoarthritis and neurological issues.
- Poor eyesight.
- Medical comorbidities: syncope, cardiac arrhythmia, etc.

Extrinsic factors

- Lack of social support.
- Inadequate/unsafe housing environment.

Falls can be reduced through various interventions and often involve a multidisciplinary approach. Physiotherapists, occupational therapists, specialist nurses and social workers often have a key role to play.

HINTS AND TIPS

When looking at why patients fall, make sure to review a patient's drugs. Many drugs have mild sedative effects that might increase the risk of falling.

PAGET DISEASE

Definition

Paget disease is a disorder of bone metabolism characterized by focal increases in bone remodelling, resulting in abnormal bone production. This leads to mechanical weakness of the bone.

Incidence

The incidence varies greatly across the world. It is very rare in Asians, whereas the UK has the highest incidence in the world at approximately 2%–3% of people over the age of 40 years.

Aetiology

The cause of Paget disease is unknown. However, clustering in families has been observed suggesting a strong genetic contribution. Another hypothesis suggests that the disease process may be triggered by a virus.

Pathology

There is a dramatic focal increase in bone metabolism with increased bone resorption, mediated by large multinucleated osteoclasts. Osteoblasts then respond by producing weak, disorganized bone. Repeated cycles of this result in abnormal hypertrophied areas of bone with increased vascularity (Fig. 15.5).

Clinical features

Less than a third of patients are symptomatic and many patients are diagnosed incidentally due to abnormal blood test results (raised alkaline phosphatase) and X-ray examination findings.

Symptomatic patients present with bone pain, deformity and fractures. Bone pain is most common in the spine, pelvis, femurs, skull and tibia. Deformity may lead to compression of other structures, such as the 8th cranial nerve, resulting in unilateral deafness. Fractures, when they occur, are often atypical such as low-energy femoral shaft fractures.

Fig. 15.6 shows some possible complications from Paget disease.

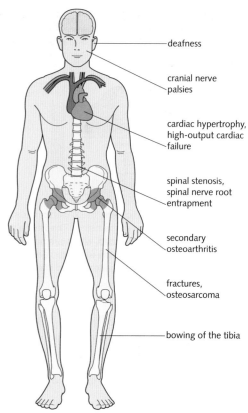

Fig. 15.6 Potential complications of Paget disease.

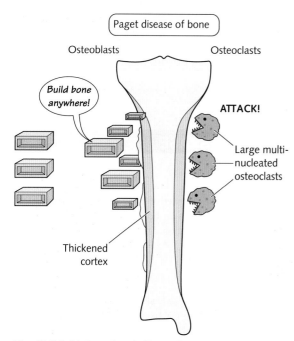

Fig. 15.5 Cell interactions in Paget disease of bone.

Diagnosis and investigation

- Serum alkaline phosphatase is elevated and correlated to the amount of skeletal involvement.
- Plain radiographs show areas of disorganized bone with areas of lysis and sclerosis. The cortex is usually thickened.
- Isotope bone scans often show multiple areas of focal increased uptake and are the most sensitive test for detecting pagetic lesions.

Treatment

Bisphosphonates are very effective in inhibiting bone resorption and reducing the symptoms of Paget disease. Calcitonin is sometimes also used but is less tolerated.

Asymptomatic disease may not require treatment and should simply be observed; the key is to determine whether lesions are active or inactive. Pain is often the main reason for commencing pharmacological therapies.

Surgical treatment is needed to manage complications:

- Fractures: need for surgical stabilization.
- Deformity: osteotomy is rarely performed.
- Osteosarcoma: this is a rare tumour seen in Paget disease. It is discussed further in Chapter 21.

RICKETS AND OSTEOMALACIA

Both of these conditions are the result of failure of mineralization of bone. Rickets affects the growing skeleton in children and is a disorder of effective mineralization of cartilage in the epiphyseal growth plates of children. Osteomalacia occurs in adults.

Aetiology

Vitamin D deficiency is the most common cause of both conditions. Hypophosphataemia is a much rarer cause. Fig. 15.7 illustrates the pathways of vitamin D metabolism. The causes of vitamin D deficiency are showing in the box.

CAUSES OF VITAMIN D DEFICIENCY

- Low dietary intake plus inadequate sunlight exposure
- Intestinal malabsorption (coeliac disease, gastric surgery)
- Liver disease
- Renal disease
- Drugs that affect vitamin D metabolism (anticonvulsants)

Pathology

Histological examination of bone biopsies in both conditions show increased amounts of osteoid with deficient mineralization.

Clinical features

The main features of rickets and osteomalacia are:

- bone pain
- skeletal deformity
- muscle weakness
- fracturing

Lethargy, tetany and convulsions due to hypocalcaemia can occur.

Rickets

Growth is impaired in children with rickets. The clinical manifestations depend on the age of the child. Those under 12 months of age may have softening and frontal bossing of the skull. There may be swelling of the epiphyses of the wrists and at the costochondral junctions (the rickety rosary). Older children develop bowing of the long bones and valgus or varus deformities of the knee.

The following radiological changes are seen in rickets:

- delayed opacification of the epiphyses
- widened growth plates
- thin cortices

Osteomalacia

Osteomalacia tends to present with vague bone pain, especially in the long bone and pelvis. Severe localized pain may be due to a fracture. Patients can develop proximal myopathy and often complain of lethargy.

Diagnosis and investigation

The following laboratory abnormalities are usually found:

- low or low/normal calcium
- low or low/normal phosphate

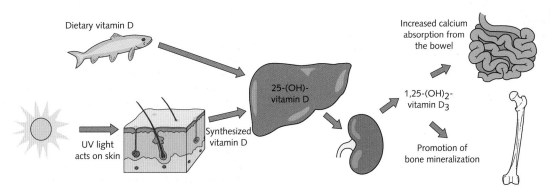

Fig. 15.7 Pathways of vitamin D metabolism.

- raised serum alkaline phosphatase
- low serum vitamin D
- raised parathyroid hormone levels
- low urinary calcium excretion

In osteomalacia, the characteristic appearance on X-ray images is Looser zones, which are spontaneous incomplete fractures.

Treatment

Both rickets and osteomalacia can be treated with vitamin D replacement. The underlying cause of the vitamin D deficiency should be addressed.

● Chapter Summary

- Osteoporosis results in increased risk of fractures in susceptible individuals.
- A DEXA scan is the diagnostic test of choice with a T-score of between −1 and −2.5 indicating osteopenia and a T-score less than −2.5 indicating osteoporosis.
- Treatment is with bisphosphonates, denosumab or teriparatide with calcium and vitamin D supplementation. Modifiable risk factors such as smoking should also be addressed.
- Paget disease is relatively common (2%–3% in the UK over 40 years of age), but many patients are asymptomatic. It causes abnormal bone metabolism resulting in areas of weakened and structurally abnormal bone.
- Vitamin D deficiency causes rickets in children and osteomalacia in adults. Treatment is with vitamin D replacement.

FURTHER READING

NICE, 2012. Osteoporosis: assessing the risk of fragility fracture (CG146). updated 2017. Available online, www.nice.org.uk/guidance/cg146.

Tuck, S.P., Layfield, R., Walker, J., et al., 1 December 2017. Adult Paget's disease of bone: a review. Rheumatology Volume 56 (Issue 12), 2050–2059. https://doi.org/10.1093/rheumatology/kew430.

National Osteoporosis Society, 2013. Vitamin D and bone health: a practical clinical guideline for patient management. National Osteoporosis Society. Available at www.nos.org.uk.

Gout and pseudogout | 16

GOUT

Definition

Gout is the consequence of high levels of hyperuricemia and uric acid crystal formation. Clinical features include:

- joint inflammation
- crystal deposition in soft tissues (tophi)
- renal disease
- uric acid renal stones

Prevalence

Gout affects 2.5% of people in the UK. It is more common in men, but the incidence in women is increasing.

Aetiology

Gout is caused by a sustained increase in serum uric acid levels. Uric acid is a breakdown product of purine bases, which are components of nucleic acids. Synthesis occurs mainly in the liver (Fig 16.1). Unlike many mammals, humans lack uricase, an enzyme that breaks down uric acid in a more readily excretable form, allantoin.

Many factors influence uric acid excretion by the kidneys; age, sex, body mass, diet and genetic factors all play a role.

Hyperuricemia is usually due to reduced renal excretion of uric acid, rather than increased production. A summary of risk factors for gout can be seen in the box.

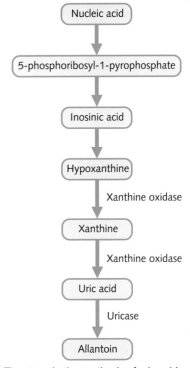

Fig. 16.1 The steps in the synthesis of uric acid.

RISK FACTORS FOR GOUT
- Alcohol: especially beer
- Diet: high protein, shellfish, red meats, high fructose content
- Obesity
- Diuretic use
- Male gender
- Hypertension and renal disease
- Cancer
- Psoriasis

Pathology

Prolonged hyperuricemia leads to the formation of monosodium urate crystals. These deposit in the synovium, connective tissues and kidneys. Joint inflammation is mediated by phagocytosis of the crystals by polymorphonuclear leucocytes. Uric acid crystal deposition in the kidneys can cause interstitial nephritis, renal stones and acute tubular damage.

Clinical features

Acute gout

Acute gout is extremely painful. Joint swelling develops suddenly and is often associated with shiny skin, skin redness, warmth and excruciating pain. It most commonly occurs as a monoarthropathy but might involve several joints at the same time in severe cases. The first metatarsophalangeal joint is the most commonly affected, but the ankles, knees, elbows, wrists and hands can also be involved. Attacks often subside spontaneously after days or weeks but often require treatment for symptom control.

The bursa can also be affected and gout is a common cause of acute olecranon bursitis.

Acute attacks usually resolve themselves, leaving the patients free of pain. Some people only suffer a single attack, although many have recurrent flares within a year. Without treatment, acute attacks become more frequent and bony erosive damage occurs.

Chronic gout

Chronic gout occurs in patients with longstanding hyperuricemia who have had many gouty flares. Within the skeleton and soft tissues, bony erosions form and tophi are deposited into the soft tissues; these can rupture, leading to discharge of chalky-white material, and can become infected. Progressive damage to bones, ligaments and tendons leads to deformity (Fig. 16.2).

Within the kidneys, longstanding urate deposition may lead to progressive nephropathy. Uric acid stones may also form in the urinary tract.

Investigations

Synovial fluid analysis

This is the most important test for suspected gout. Synovial fluid should be obtained by needle aspiration from symptomatic joints and examined with a microscope under polarized light. Monosodium urate crystals are needle-shaped and show strong negative birefringence (Fig. 16.3). This means crystals parallel to the plane of light appear yellow and those perpendicular appear blue. Material aspirated from tophi can be examined in a similar way. Fluid should be examined soon after aspiration to increase the chance of seeing crystals.

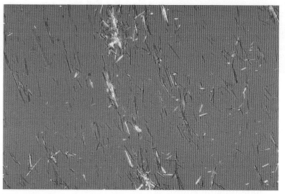

Fig. 16.3 Monosodium urate crystals under polarized light. With permission from Klatt, EC, Bones, Joints, and Soft-Tissue Tumors; Robbins and Cotran Atlas of Pathology, 3rd ed, Saunders 2015, Elsevier.

RED FLAG

Septic arthritis is another common cause of an acute monoarthropathy. Gram stain and culture should be performed on samples to exclude infection. Look for other features of systemic upset or shock in keeping with sepsis (high temperature, tachycardia, a high respiratory rate and low blood pressure). If in doubt, treat the patient with antibiotics. Septic arthritis can be life threatening!

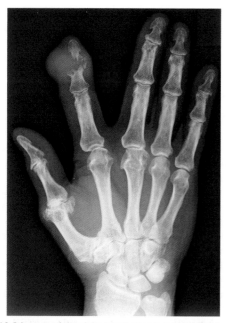

Fig. 16.2 Image of the right hand showing extensive bone erosive destruction of the 2nd digit with soft tissue calcified tophi on X-ray.

Blood tests

Serum uric acid is usually elevated, but one-third of patients have normal serum uric acids during an acute flare. Erythrocyte sedimentation rate (ESR) and C-reactive protein (CRP) are often elevated in an acute flare, as is white blood cell count.

Radiology

Radiological appearances are not normally visible until years of recurrent gouty flares have occurred. X-ray images show erosions in the juxta-articular regions with surrounded sclerosis of the bone, which helps differentiate between gouty erosions and erosions from inflammatory joint disease such as rheumatoid arthritis (RA).

Management

Acute Gout

Acute gout treatment should be initiated promptly after diagnosis during an acute flare

- Nonsteroidal antiinflammatory drugs (NSAIDS) are most commonly used first. They should be continued until pain and inflammation subside.

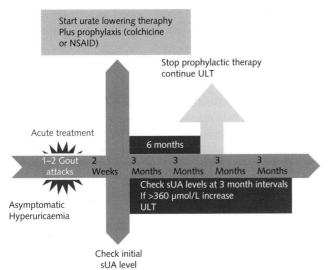

Fig. 16.4 Proposed treatment pathway for managing gout.
NSAID, Nonsteroidal antiinflammatory drugs; *sUA,* serum uric acid; *ULT,* urate-lowering therapy.

- Colchicine is a suitable alternative in those with contraindications to s (asthma, previous peptic ulcers, etc.). A dose of 500 μg two to three times daily is commonly used because higher doses cause diarrhoea.
- Corticosteroids are useful in patients who are unable to tolerate NSAIDs or colchicine. They are not suitable for long-term use. Steroid injections into affected joints are very successful in relieving symptoms.

Prophylactic therapy

Drugs that lower serum uric acid levels can be used to prevent gout attacks. A suggested treatment and monitoring regime is suggested in Fig. 16.4.

Allopurinol should be used first. It reduces uric acid production by inhibiting the enzyme xanthine oxidase. The dose should be increased until the patient's uric acid level is <360 μg/mL. Caution is needed in the elderly and those with renal disease.

Febuxostat is another xanthine oxidase inhibitor that can be used as an alternative to allopurinol. Newer uricosuric drugs such as lesinurad, which encourage renal excretion of uric acid, will soon be available. Polyethylene glycol (PEG) uricase and rasburicase have a value in treating severe tophaceous gout. Anti-tumour necrosis factor (TNF) drugs have shown some promise in reducing inflammation in extremely difficult cases.

HINTS AND TIPS

Changes in serum uric acid levels can precipitate acute flares. Urate lowering drugs should not be prescribed until an acute flare has completely settled. Sometimes coprescription of NSAIDs/colchicine is needed.

Lifestyle factors

Identify and reduce the patient's alterable risk factors, encourage good dietary practices and a reduction in alcohol intake.

COMMUNICATION

It is important to take a detailed drug and alcohol history from patients.

HINTS AND TIPS

Do not stop allopurinol in acute flares unless indicated for another reason, i.e., acute renal impairment.

CALCIUM PYROPHOSPHATE DIHYDRATE DISEASE

Definition

Calcium pyrophosphate dihydrate (CPPD) disease is an arthropathy associated with the deposition of CPPD crystals.

Prevalence

CPPD disease is much less common than gout, but much more common in the elderly. There is a slight female preponderance to the condition.

Aetiology

The absolute cause is unknown but the condition is associated with osteoarthritis and other metabolic bone diseases. Attacks are often preceded by intercurrent illness, episodes of physical stress and dehydration.

METABOLIC DISEASES THAT PREDISPOSE TO CALCIUM PYROPHOSPHATE DIHYDRATE DISEASE

- Hypothyroidism
- Hyperparathyroidism
- Haemochromatosis
- Acromegaly
- Gout

Clinical features

There are two main clinical presentations of CPPD disease:

1. Acute synovitis (pseudogout): This is the most common cause of acute monoarthritis in the elderly. Wrists and knees are most commonly affected. Patients experience pain, swelling, stiffness and occasionally fever. The clinical appearance of affected joints is very similar to gout.
2. Chronic pyrophosphate arthropathy: This is very similar to osteoarthritis with a gradual onset of pain, swelling and loss of joint function. Again, the knees and wrists are most commonly affected, along with the hips, shoulders, elbows and metacarpophalangeal joints. Some patients experience acute attacks of synovitis. Examination reveals changes in keeping with osteoarthritis.

Investigations

Synovial fluid examination

Synovial fluid examination with polarized light microscopy is key to the diagnosis. The CPPD crystals are small rhomboid or rod-shaped crystals that show weak positive birefringence. As with gout, fluid examination should include Gram stain and culture to exclude infection.

Radiology

CPPD causes changes in osteoarthritis that are visible on radiographs, with associated chondrocalcinosis. This calcification is often seen in the menisci of the knee, triangular cartilage of the wrist and symphysis pubis.

Other investigations

Serum calcium should be checked in younger patients. CPPD is very unusual in those <50 years old and if found, prompt screening should be performed for other metabolic diseases.

Management

Attacks of pseudogout are treated with analgesia. Joint aspiration, joint injection with steroids and the use of colchicine can also help. Unlike gout, there is no prophylactic medication that can be given. Other lifestyle factors include losing weight, physiotherapy, pain control and occasionally joint replacement.

● **Chapter Summary**

- Gout is one of the most common causes of an acute monoarthropathy.
- Clinical features of acute gout include a hot, extremely tender, swollen joint, often with red shiny skin over it. The 1st metatarsal-phalangeal joint is often the first site affected.
- In chronic gout, erosive changes appear on X-ray images, the joints affected may be deformed and there are often hard, chalky deposits (tophi) within the soft tissues.
- Acute gout is managed with nonsteroidal antiinflammatory drugs, colchicine and occasionally corticosteroids. Urate-lowering therapies, such as allopurinol, help prevent against future attacks.
- Newer drugs are available for those intolerant or for whom these medications are contraindicated.
- Calcium pyrophosphate dihydrate disease (pseudogout) is another crystal-arthropathy more common in the elderly and is associated with osteoarthritis and other metabolic bone diseases. It predominantly affects different joints from those affected by gout (wrists and knees). Acute flares of pseudogout are managed similarly to gout attacks.
- Joint aspiration and fluid microscopy is the gold standard test to differentiate between the two conditions.

FURTHER READING

Perry, M., 2017. Gout: Risk Factors, Prevalence and Impact on Health, first ed. Nova, New York.

Hui, M., Carr, A., Cameron, S., et al., 1 July 2017. The British Society for Rheumatology Guideline for the Management of Gout. Rheumatology Volume 56 (Issue 7), e1–e20. https://doi.org/10.1093/rheumatology/kex156.

NORMAL VARIANTS

The majority of referrals to paediatric orthopaedic surgeons are for normal variations in growth of a healthy child noticed by anxious parents. The single most reassuring feature is the symmetrical appearance of the limbs. If the child has only one side affected, the condition is much more likely to be pathological.

Examples of normal conditions commonly referred include the following.

Flat feet

This condition is usually physiological, painless and may be associated with laxity of ligaments. Simple advice should be given as even the use of insoles is questionable and most children develop normally regardless. Pain or fixed deformity suggests an underlying pathological condition.

Toe walkers

Children often take their first steps on tiptoes. Usually the child grows out of this, but examination is required to exclude a tight Achilles tendon or an underlying condition such as cerebral palsy.

In-toeing gait

Causes of in-toeing are at three levels: the hip, the tibia and the foot.

Persistent femoral torsion leaves the patient with an excessive internal rotation and the child often sits in a W position rather than cross-legged (Fig. 17.1). This condition usually resolves spontaneously as the child grows, but a small number require femoral osteotomy.

Internal tibial torsion also results in in-toeing but almost always resolves with no treatment.

In the foot, metatarsus adductus (inwardly pointing forefoot) is the cause of in-toeing and again this usually resolves over time.

Bow legs (genu varum)

It is normal for toddlers to have bow legs and they almost always grow out of this. Very rarely, pathological conditions such as rickets can cause bowing, but the child is usually older and the disease is on one side only.

Knock knees (genu valgum)

Older children (3–8 years old) gradually become more valgus as they grow and the majority straighten spontaneously.

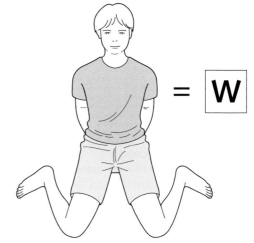

Fig. 17.1 Child sitting in the W position in excessive femoral anteversion.

Pathological genu valgum is rare, usually asymmetrical, severe and progressive.

PAEDIATRIC HIP DISORDERS

Of all the joint disorders affecting children, the most important to the orthopaedic surgeon are those affecting the hip. Many children with these disorders will require hip replacement surgery in adult life, with the most severely affected having such surgery aged in their 20s or 30s and even in teenage years.

Developmental dysplasia of the hip

Introduction
Previously called congenital dislocation of the hip (CDH), developmental dysplasia of the hip (DDH) is due to the failure of normal development of the acetabulum resulting in abnormal hip anatomy. This disorder encompasses the spectrum of disease from a frankly dislocated hip to acetabular dysplasia (in which the angle of slope of the acetabular roof is too steep).

Incidence
The UK incidence is approximately 1–2 per 1000 live births; however, the majority of these settle, stabilize and develop normally without treatment.

Fig. 17.2 Anatomy of the hip showing (A) normal and (B) pathological hip development. *DDH,* Developmental dysplasia of the hip.

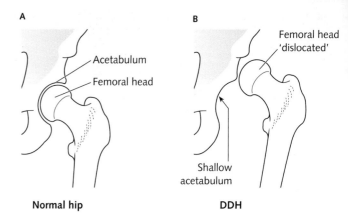

Normal hip   DDH

Aetiology and pathology

The condition is four times more common in females. It is also more common in certain races (northern Italy and North American indigenous population).

DDH is associated with:

- breech presentation
- family history
- other congenital and packaging deformities.

The left side is more commonly affected but the condition is bilateral in 20% of cases.

The acetabulum relies on the presence of the femoral head for normal development. In DDH there is excessive laxity of the joint with a shallow acetabulum (Fig. 17.2). This allows the femoral head to develop out of the socket, in severe cases forming a false acetabulum (located above the normal one).

Clinical features

The majority are picked up on routine baby checks and referred appropriately.

Late-presenting DDH can occur as the child begins to walk. The child will have a limp and shortness of one leg (if unilateral).

The clinical findings of DDH include:

- loss of abduction
- leg length discrepancy
- asymmetrical posterior skin crease

The special tests for dysplastic hips are called Barlow and Ortolani tests.

Barlow test

This is an attempt to dislocate a reduced hip.

The examiner holds the child's thigh so that the thumb is on the medial aspect of the thigh with the middle finger on the trochanter. Then with the child's hip and knee flexed to 90 degrees, the hip is slightly adducted and a gentle downward force applied to try to dislocate the hip. A clunk is felt if positive (Fig. 17.3).

Ortolani test

This is an attempt to reduce a dislocated hip.

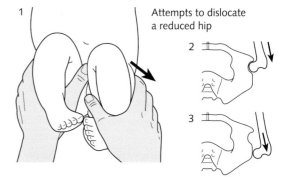

Fig. 17.3 Barlow test: attempts to dislocate a reduced hip.

Both hips are examined together. The hand is placed in a similar position and the hip is flexed to 90 degrees and then gently abducted. The test is positive if the hip reduces with a clunk.

Diagnosis and investigation

All babies are screened clinically by examination at birth but unfortunately this is unreliable. At-risk babies with the factors listed above are screened with ultrasound. If there is doubt, this investigation can be repeated.

Once the femoral head has ossified, older children should be investigated using X-ray images, which should clearly show if there is a dislocation (Fig. 17.4).

Management

This depends on whether the hip is dislocated and, if so, whether the hip is easily reducible.

Conservative

An abduction splint is used to hold the hip in an abducted and stable position, keeping the hip in the joint. The Pavlik harness is an example of such splintage (Fig. 17.5).

Surgical

If the hip is not reduced, closed or open, reduction is performed.

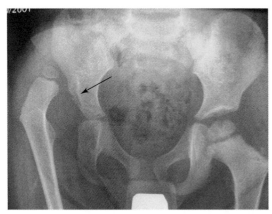

Fig. 17.4 X-ray image showing developmental dysplasia of the hip (*arrow*).

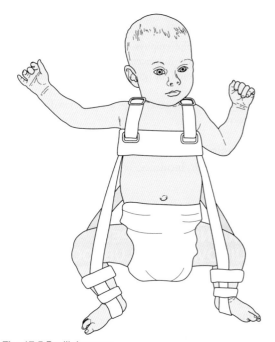

Fig. 17.5 Pavlik harness.

A variety of surgical osteotomies to the pelvis or femur can be used to correct anatomy and maintain reduction.

Prognosis

The outcome depends upon the degree of dysplasia, duration of dislocation and whether or not complications such as osteonecrosis develop. Secondary osteoarthritis is common in this group of patients.

Perthes disease

Introduction

This is a rare disease of unknown aetiology, in which blood supply to the femoral head is interrupted, causing segmental avascular necrosis and collapse of the femoral head. It is often referred to as Legg-Calvé-Perthes disease.

Epidemiology

Approximately 5–12 in 100,000 are affected. Perthes disease is four times more common in boys and is bilateral in 12%. It usually presents between the ages of 4 and 8 years but can affect children from the age of 2 years to 12 years. It is more common in Caucasians than other ethnic groups.

The condition is associated with:

- family history
- lower socioeconomic groups
- low birth weight children
- delayed bone age
- northerly latitude regardless of race

Variable amounts of the femoral head are involved and this affects the outcome. In severe cases of collapse, the femoral head migrates out of the joint (subluxation).

Clinical features

The child (usually a boy) presents with a gradual history of hip or knee pain associated with a limp or Trendelenburg gait. Clinical features will show loss of hip motion, particularly abduction and internal rotation, and there may be fixed deformity. Complete loss of abduction is a worrying sign and may signify subluxation of the hip.

Diagnosis and investigation

Acute Perthes disease in a child could be confused with septic arthritis and therefore inflammatory markers should be checked. These markers are normal in Perthes disease.

A plain X-ray image (Fig. 17.6) is the mainstay of diagnosis. The features of Perthes on X-ray images are:

- medial joint space widening (earliest)
- loss of epiphyseal height
- increased density of the femoral epiphysis
- subchondral fracture, partial collapse and fragmentation of the head.
- abnormal shape and size of femoral head
- subluxation

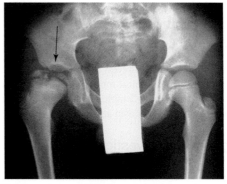

Fig. 17.6 X-ray image of Perthes disease (*arrow*).

Magnetic resonance imaging (MRI) is very sensitive for diagnosis and staging.

Treatment

This depends upon the age of the patient and the extent of the disease.

Conservative

Overall, 75% of children require no treatment and will have a good long-term outcome. Young patients with less than 50% involvement of the femoral head have a good prognosis.

Surgical

Older patients and female patients (closer to skeletal maturity) and patients with greater than 50% involvement of the epiphysis have a poor prognosis and significant early osteoarthritis is likely. These children may require containment of the femoral head with surgery, e.g., a pelvic or femoral osteotomy.

Slipped upper femoral epiphysis (or slipped capital femoral epiphysis)

This condition is a disorder in which there is structural failure through the growth plate of an immature hip.

Incidence

Approximately 10 per 100,000 children are affected.

It is more common in boys than in girls, usually occurring during the early adolescence growth spurt between 11 and 14 years of age. Approximately 17%–50% of cases are bilateral.

Aetiology and pathology

Two groups are affected: athletic children of either sex or overweight boys with delayed puberty.

The exact cause is not known but may relate to failure of the epiphyseal cartilage to mature as the child grows. Obesity is the single greatest risk factor, along with position of femoral head and previous radiation to femoral head. Some hormonal conditions are associated, e.g., hypothyroidism and diabetes mellitus.

The slip results in the epiphysis lying posterior and inferior to the femoral neck.

Clinical features

The child presents with groin or knee pain (or both) and a limp. The history can be acute or gradual.

Examination findings reveal an external rotation deformity with limitation of most movements. There might be a slight discrepancy in leg length. Check for evidence of hypogonadism, hypopituitarism and hypothyroidism.

Diagnosis and investigation

Diagnosis is based on changes seen in X-ray images. An anteroposterior (AP) X-ray image is taken, but the frog lateral view demonstrates the pathology most clearly (Fig. 17.7).

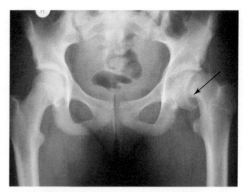

Fig. 17.7 X-ray image of slipped upper femoral epiphysis (*arrow*).

Management

Surgical

Once diagnosed, the epiphysis should be pinned in situ to prevent further displacement as soon as possible. Consideration should be given to fixing the other hip prophylactically.

Attempts to reduce severe slips are associated with avascular necrosis.

Prognosis

There is a high incidence of secondary degenerative osteoarthritis.

CONGENITAL TALIPES EQUINOVARUS (CLUBFOOT)

Congenital talipes equinovarus encompasses a deformity of the lower limb with calf wasting and the classic inwardly pointing foot.

Incidence

The incidence is approximately 1 per 1000 live births. Boys are affected twice as often as girls and half of cases are bilateral.

Aetiology and pathology

The exact aetiology is not known, but arrest of normal limb bud development in utero may be the cause. Genetic factors play a role, with family history being important.

The basic pathology is at the level of the subtalar joint with a cavus deformity (high arch) and metatarsus adductus (Fig. 17.8). The Achilles tendon is also tight, resulting in an equinus deformity.

Associated soft-tissue contractures occur on the medial side.

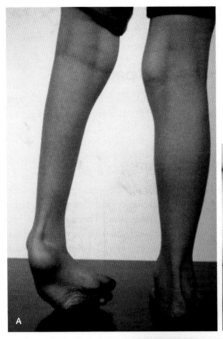
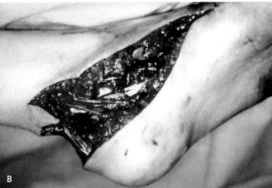
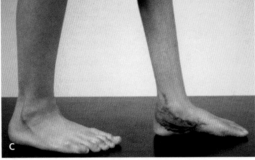

Fig. 17.8 (A) Untreated talipes equinovarus showing inversion contracture. (B) Intraoperative view showing release of soft tissues. (C) Postoperative image showing corrected deformity and soft tissue coverage. With permission from Zuker RM, Bains RD. Gracilis Flap. In: Wei FC, Mardini S (eds), Flaps and Reconstructive Surgery, 2nd ed, 2017 Elsevier.

Clinical features

The condition is easily noted at birth as a fixed varus and equinus deformity of the foot. The calf is underdeveloped when compared with the normal side.

The baby should be examined for associated syndromes or conditions (such as spina bifida or DDH).

Diagnosis and investigation

The diagnosis is a clinical one and X-ray images are usually taken after initial treatment or surgery.

Management

Conservative
Initial treatment is with serial manipulation and casting changed weekly for up to 3 months, achieving a 90% success rate.

Surgical
Surgery is reserved for those cases that fail to correct fully or for later recurrence.

Prognosis

The foot and limb will never be normal in terms of appearance but most patients lead a normal life.

OSTEOGENESIS IMPERFECTA

Also known as brittle bone disease, osteogenesis imperfecta (OI) is a type 1 collagen disorder predisposed to multiple fractures.

Incidence

The condition is rare.

Aetiology and pathology

There are four different types of OI. The primary abnormality is a defect in the synthesis of type 1 collagen, leading to either abnormal collagen or decreased quantities.

OI is usually inherited as an autosomal dominant condition (types 1 and 4), although sporadic and recessive cases can occur (types 2 and 3). 90% of cases have an identifiable genetic mutation.

Clinical features

The child may present with a low-energy fracture and the diagnosis is made subsequently, following examination and investigation.

Blue sclerae are pathognomonic and present in types 1 and 2 OI. Children are usually small with bony deformities (including scoliosis) and joint abnormalities. Associated features include deafness, joint laxity, altered dentition (brownish teeth), dysmorphic facies and valvular defects.

Diagnosis and investigation

X-ray images may show:

- multiple fractures (can lead to saber shin appearance of tibia)
- deformity
- thin-looking cortex

Treatment

Conservative

Gentle handling is needed to prevent fractures.

Bisphosphonates such as pamidronate can be given intravenously to try to improve bone strength.

Surgical

Intramedullary telescoping rods are the mainstay of treatment for the prevention of deformity and further fracture.

Established deformity is treated with osteotomy.

Prognosis

The outcome depends on the type of OI: some types, such as type 2, are lethal.

CEREBRAL PALSY

Definition

This is a nonprogressive upper motor neurone, neuromuscular disorder that results from injury to an immature brain.

Incidence

Incidence is 2 per 1000 births.

Aetiology and pathology

The cause is often unknown but can include prematurity, perinatal anoxia, perinatal infection, including meningitis and kernicterus.

Clinical features

There is a mixture of muscle weakness and spasticity. This can lead to characteristic joint deformities, contractures, fractures and hip subluxation. There may be athetosis and ataxia. This can be associated with varying degrees of cognitive impairment and emotional disturbance. Children may also develop seizures.

CLINICAL NOTES

Characteristic joint deformities associated with cerebral palsy

Flexion at elbows and wrists with clasped fingers

Adductor spasticity of the hips, resulting in a scissors stance

Flexion at the hips and knees

Equinus deformity of the feet

Diagnosis and investigation

Cerebral palsy is a clinical diagnosis based on a thorough birth and developmental history and is normally apparent within the first 2 years of life. MRI of the brain may show periventricular leukomalacia.

Management

Conservative

Depending on the severity of the disease, children will benefit from physiotherapy, occupational therapy, speech and language therapy and other forms of special needs care.

Surgical

In children who have not developed fixed contractures, intramuscular botulinum injections can temporarily reduce spasticity. For fixed deformity, soft-tissue release or tendon lengthening is required to improve function. Severe muscle imbalance can result in bone deformity, sometimes requiring corrective osteotomy.

NONACCIDENTAL INJURY

Nonaccidental injury (NAI) is becoming increasingly recognized and is often diagnosed late. A diagnosis is important because the child may die if undiagnosed.

Clinical features

The history is often vague, inappropriate or changes each time it is told. In young children (<2 years), it is rare for accidental fractures to occur, particularly in long bones. Delayed presentation is often a feature of NAI.

The child may have external features of abuse such as bruising in other areas of the body away from the fracture. The child may be withdrawn, particularly when the parents are present.

Diagnosis and investigation

In suspected cases, a skeletal survey or bone scan is performed to look for occult fractures. Certain fractures such as of the rib or tibial metaphysis are typical of NAI.

Conditions such as OI can be confused with NAI.

Management

The child should be admitted for protection if NAI is strongly suspected and the fracture should be treated in the usual way.

Paediatricians and social workers should be involved early on.

Prognosis

A child left in an abusive environment has a 5% risk of death.

PAEDIATRIC KNEE CONDITIONS

Osgood-Schlatter disease

Definition
Osgood-Schlatter disease is traction apophysitis of the tibial tuberosity.

Incidence
The condition is very common, usually in adolescent boys.

Aetiology and pathology
It occurs during a period of rapid growth and is related to the pulling force of the patellar ligament on the tibial tuberosity (Fig. 17.9).

It is more common in athletic individuals.

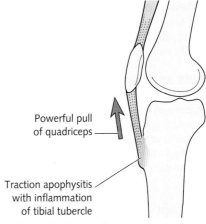

Powerful pull of quadriceps

Traction apophysitis with inflammation of tibial tubercle

Fig. 17.9 Osgood-Schlatter disease.

Clinical features
The patient complains of localized pain over the tubercle. The pain is usually made worse by activity and relieved by rest.

Clinically, a tender swollen tuberosity is found.

Diagnosis and investigation
Fragmentation and sclerosis of the tibial tuberosity are present. Sometimes a visible ossicle remains.

Management

Conservative
Treatment is rest if the knee is very inflamed, with simple analgesia and modification of activities. Parents are usually very worried and need reassurance. The child may choose to put up with the pain and continue sporting activities and this has no detrimental effect and will not prolong the natural history of the disease process.

Surgical
Surgery is used only for a painful ossicle.

Prognosis
The natural history is complete resolution of symptoms after 2 years.

Osteochondritis dissecans

Definition
Osteochondritis dissecans is a small area of avascular bone on an articular surface, usually in the knee.

Incidence
The incidence is 4 per 1000. Presentation is between 10 and 15 years of age and is more common in boys.

Aetiology and pathology
The condition is most common in the knee (medial femoral condyle) but can affect other joints. It is thought to be due to repeated trauma in a susceptible patient.

Clinical features

The patient has intermittent ache, swelling and catching in the knee. The patient may complain of the knee giving way owing to acute sharp episodes of pain.

Diagnosis and investigation

X-ray images show a variably sized lesion on the medial femoral condyle, which is fragmented in the child, but in mature adults the lesion shows as a clear, demarcated sclerotic zone. The lesion can be attached or may be a loose body.

An MRI scan will help define the lesion. An isotope bone scan confirms the presence of activity and hence healing potential.

Management

Conservative

Activity modification with avoidance of sporting activity is adequate to allow small well-fixed lesions to heal. Younger age correlates with better prognosis.

Surgical

Lesions that become detached or give significant persistent symptoms require surgical stabilization. If the fragment becomes a loose body, removal may be the only option.

JUVENILE IDIOPATHIC ARTHRITIS

Definition

Juvenile idiopathic arthritis (JIA) is a chronic inflammatory condition in children primarily involving synovial joints. It does not include specific diseases such as systemic lupus erythematosus or arthritis of inflammatory bowel disease.

JIA is a persistent autoimmune inflammatory arthritis lasting > 6 weeks in patients younger than 16 years of age. It is a diagnosis of exclusion.

JIA has been classified into seven subtypes. This classification is based partly on the number of joints involved 3 months into the disease process. It is useful as a guide to prognosis.

CLINICAL NOTES

THE SUBTYPES OF JUVENILE IDIOPATHIC ARTHRITIS

- Oligoarticular disease
- Extended oligoarticular disease
- Polyarticular disease: rheumatoid factor-negative
- Polyarticular disease: rheumatoid factor-positive
- Systemic-onset disease
- Enthesitis-related arthritis
- Psoriatic arthritis

Incidence and prevalence

Incidence is approximately 1 per 10,000 and prevalence is 10 per 10,000 children.

Clinical features

Joint disease

Children develop symptoms and signs of joint inflammation similar to those in adults, including joint pain, stiffness and swelling. Presentation depends on the joints affected and the age of the child. A 12-year-old with knee synovitis will complain of pain, whereas a 2-year-old may just be irritable and reluctant to mobilize. Paediatric Gait Arms Legs Spine (p-GALS) is a useful screening tool when examining children.

Joints from most frequently affected to least affected: knee > hand/wrist > ankle > hip > cervical spine.

Eye disease

Some forms of JIA can be associated with anterior uveitis. Acute anterior uveitis presents with pain and redness of the eye. Chronic anterior uveitis, however, is more insidious and can cause significant visual loss. All children with JIA need regular eye checks.

Constitutional symptoms

Fatigue, malaise and other systemic symptoms affect JIA patients, in particular those with systemic-onset disease. Growth retardation is an important consequence of prolonged inflammation in childhood.

Juvenile idiopathic arthritis subtypes

Oligoarticular disease

Between one and four joints are affected, commonly in the lower limb. The prognosis is good and many children grow out of it. This group of patients has the greatest risk of developing chronic anterior uveitis.

Extended oligoarticular disease

Initially, fewer than four joints are involved, but these patients gradually develop polyarthritis after the first 3 months. The outcome is often poor.

Polyarticular disease

More than four joints are affected from an early stage. There are two types. Rheumatoid factor–negative arthritis targets small and large joints and tends to persist into adult life. Rheumatoid factor–positive arthritis is the equivalent of adult rheumatoid arthritis. It is seen mainly in teenage girls and frequently has a poor outcome.

Systemic-onset disease

This arthritis is characterized by prominent systemic symptoms. It was previously known as Still disease. Patients present with a swinging fever, plus any of the following features:

- evanescent rash
- hepatomegaly
- splenomegaly
- anaemia
- lymphadenopathy
- serositis, especially pericarditis

The differential diagnosis includes infection and malignancy. Joint involvement may initially be mild or absent.

Enthesitis-related arthritis

Inflammation of entheses, e.g., Achilles tendonitis, is a prominent feature. Enthesitis-related arthritis encompasses juvenile ankylosing spondylitis. A positive family history of ankylosing spondylitis or related diseases is common and patients are often HLA B27-positive.

Psoriatic arthritis

This is usually oligoarticular and often involves weight-bearing joints. A personal or family history of psoriasis is common.

Investigations

The diagnosis of JIA is clinical. X-ray images are helpful in excluding other causes of joint pain, such as malignancy, but are usually normal in early JIA.

Blood tests are useful, but not diagnostic. Full blood count may reveal anaemia or thrombocytosis and the erythrocyte sedimentation rate and C-reactive protein are usually elevated. Serum rheumatoid factor should be measured. It is also important to know whether the patient has positive antinuclear antibodies, as they are associated with an increased risk of uveitis.

HINTS AND TIPS

All children with juvenile idiopathic arthritis should be seen by a rheumatologist.

Management

Physiotherapy

This is vital to maintain mobility and function. Hydrotherapy is commonly used and is popular with children. Splinting is sometimes required to prevent deformity.

Drug treatment

Initial treatment is with nonsteroidal antiinflammatory drugs and corticosteroid joint injections. Disease-modifying therapy with drugs such as methotrexate is used. Corticosteroids may be necessary in severe or systemic-onset disease. Biological agents, such as the anti-tumour necrosis factor drugs, are indicated for children with persistent major synovitis or unresolving systemic features.

Eye screening

Children should have their eyes examined regularly by an ophthalmologist.

HINTS AND TIPS

Eye screening is particularly important in young children with juvenile idiopathic arthritis, as they do not reliably report visual disturbance to their parents.

CLINICAL NOTES

Still disease
Acute onset juvenile rheumatoid arthritis presenting in children aged 5–10 years.
- multiple joint involvement
- fever
- rash
- splenomegaly
Infection must be ruled out.

Chapter Summary

This chapter discusses conditions that are important to consider when dealing with a painful joint.

- There are many normal variations of gait that do not need intervention. However, there are several conditions that require investigation and intervention.
- Developmental dysplasia of the hip should be picked up on examination after birth, but this is not always the case. An abduction brace such as a Pavlik harness can often treat it.
- Perthes disease is avascular necrosis (AVN) of the femoral head and can cause significant osteoarthritis at a young age and can require pelvic osteotomy.
- Slipped upper femoral epiphysis should be picked up on X-ray examination and is most common between 11 and 14 years of age. The most common position of the leg is in fixed external rotation. It is also likely to happen on the other side. It often requires fixation in situ rather than reduction due to the AVN risk.
- Clubfoot or talipes equinovarus is often treatable in a cast and only rarely requires surgery.
- There are four different types of osteogenesis imperfecta and they can lead to multiple fractures due to weak bones. It should not be confused with nonaccidental injury.
- Knee pain is common in children and can be caused by hip problems. Osgood-Schlatter disease and osteochondritis dissecans can also cause knee pain.
- Cerebral palsy can have orthopaedic manifestations with a mixture of weakness and spasticity causing contractures.
- Juvenile idiopathic arthritis has several subtypes and is a chronic inflammatory condition involving synovial joints.

FURTHER READING

Orthobullets website http://www.orthobullets.co.uk

Cassidy, J.T., Petty, R.E., 2001. Textbook of Pediatric Rheumatology. Saunders, Philadelphia.

Prakken, B., Albani, S., Martini, A., 2011. Juvenile idiopathic arthritis. Lancet 377, 2138–2149.

Prince, F.N., Otten, M.H., van Suijlekom-Smit, L.W., 2010. Diagnosis and management of juvenile idiopathic arthritis. Br. Med. J. 341, 6434.

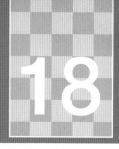
In this chapter we will discuss the principles of managing basic fractures particularly of the wrist, hip and ankle. Advanced trauma life support and the management of a multiply injured patient are covered in Chapter 19.

INCIDENCE

Fractures are very common and most of us will have at least one during a lifetime. They occur in peaks during childhood, young adult life and again in the elderly when osteoporosis has weakened bony structures (see Chapter 15).

DEFINITIONS

The following are the terms used to describe fractures (Fig. 18.1):

- Fracture: loss of continuity of the cortex of a bone.
- Pathological fracture: a fracture through bone weakened by a preexisting pathological process.
- Simple: a bone fractured into two pieces.
- Comminuted: a bone in three or more pieces.
- Segmental: fractures at two levels of the same bone.
- Closed: a fracture with intact skin overlying it.
- Open: a fracture with a skin breach over it (formerly known as a compound fracture).
- Extraarticular: a fracture that leaves the adjacent joint entirely undamaged.
- Intraarticular: a fracture that involves a joint.
- Undisplaced: a fractured bone with its anatomy entirely unchanged.
- Displaced: a fracture whose components are no longer in their original anatomical position. Displacement describes the position of the distal fragment in relation to the proximal fragment. A displaced fracture may involve translation, angulation, rotation or distraction/compression.
- Fracture pattern: may be transverse, oblique or spiral.

The causes of pathological fractures are shown in the box.

UNDERLYING CAUSES IN PATHOLOGICAL FRACTURES

Tumours
- Benign
- Malignant:
  - Metastasis (most common)
  - Primary

Paget disease

Metabolic bone disease
- Osteomalacia/rickets
- Hyperparathyroidism
- Osteogenesis imperfect

Other malignancy
- Lymphoma
- Myeloma

Rheumatoid arthritis

Infection

In children, the fracture may occur through the growth plate (physis) and these injuries are classified as shown in Fig. 18.2.

When concentrating on the bone, it is easy to forget the soft tissues surrounding the bone. Soft-tissue integrity is vital, as it is the soft tissues that will eventually provide a healing environment to the injured bone. However, soft tissues are unable to heal without bony stability underneath. A fracture should be thought of as a soft-tissue injury with a broken bone inside; both must be carefully considered before healing can occur.

CLINICAL FEATURES

The patient almost always gives a clear history of an injury. Difficulties can arise if the patient cannot give a history, e.g., because of dementia in the elderly, intoxication or coma in major trauma (see Chapter 19). In cases where the history cannot be directly elicited, information must be obtained from a third person such as a carer, witness to the accident or ambulance personnel.

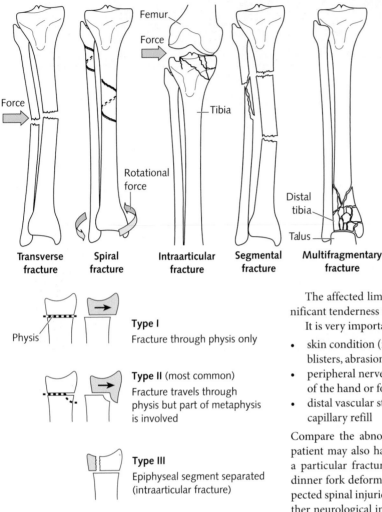

Fig. 18.1 Fracture patterns.

Transverse fracture — Force

Spiral fracture — Rotational force

Intraarticular fracture — Femur, Force, Tibia

Segmental fracture

Multifragmentary fracture — Distal tibia, Talus

Physis

Type I
Fracture through physis only

Type II (most common)
Fracture travels through physis but part of metaphysis is involved

Type III
Epiphyseal segment separated (intraarticular fracture)

Type IV
Fracture crosses physis and involves joint interface
Requires accurate reduction to prevent growth problems leading to deformity

Type V
Crush injury
Difficult to diagnose initially becomes obvious later when growth arrest occurs

Fig. 18.2 The Salter-Harris classification of fractures of the growth plate (physeal fractures).

Patients will complain of pain. They may have noticed a deformity (e.g., my ankle pointed the wrong way, doctor).

The patient should be examined as a whole for associated injuries and then the injured limb.

The affected limb will be swollen and bruised with significant tenderness to palpation.

It is very important to note and to document:

- skin condition (i.e. open or closed, but also note blisters, abrasions and swelling)
- peripheral nerve function: any weakness or numbness of the hand or foot
- distal vascular status: assess peripheral pulse and capillary refill

Compare the abnormal limb with the normal limb. The patient may also have a clinical deformity associated with a particular fracture, such as angulation, shortening or a dinner fork deformity in Colles fracture. Patients with suspected spinal injuries need to be log-rolled to avoid any further neurological injury when performing a full peripheral nervous system examination.

DIAGNOSIS AND INVESTIGATION

X-ray images should be taken in two orthogonal planes (90 degrees to each other), usually anteroposterior (AP) and lateral, and include both ends of the injured bone. The anatomical area in question should be in the centre of the X-ray image (Fig. 18.3). Special views are required for certain fractures (e.g., scaphoid views).

Computed tomography (CT) scans are helpful to diagnose and categorize complex fractures and to plan surgery.

Magnetic resonance imaging (MRI) or isotope bone scans are occasionally used to diagnose a fracture where doubt exists or to assess associated soft-tissue injuries.

Describing X-ray images

This is something that requires a systematic approach and practice.

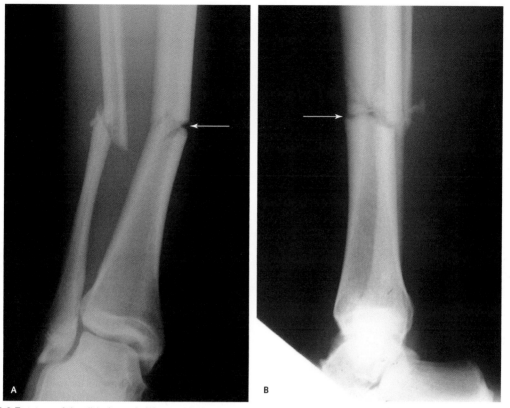

Fig. 18.3 Fracture of the tibia (*arrow*): (A) anteroposterior view showing angulation; (B) lateral view.

When asked to comment on an X-ray image, state:

- name and age of patient and date of X-ray examination.
- which anatomical region is shown, e.g., AP X-ray examination of pelvis, lateral X-ray examination of a wrist.

Remember ABC:

- A is for *a*dequacy and *a*lignment (is the film rotated? of acceptable quality, i.e., too light or too dark?).
- B is for *b*one:
  - state which bone is fractured, e.g., tibia
  - state where in the bone the fracture is, i.e., metaphysis/diaphysis/epiphysis
  - state whether the fracture is simple or comminuted
  - fracture pattern: transverse, oblique, spiral, segmental
  - displacement of the fracture (Fig. 18.4).
  - Joint: intraarticular, dislocation
- C is for *c*overing soft tissues: look for air (may indicate an open fracture), foreign material, swelling or joint fluid (haemarthrosis or lipohaemarthrosis).

MANAGEMENT

Initial management

Ensure the patient's general condition is optimized: airway, breathing, circulation, fluid management and oxygenation. Then:

- Control any external bleeding by direct pressure.
- For open fractures, cover any wounds with sterile dressings. Ensure antibiotic cover and tetanus prophylaxis. (See Chapter 19 and BOAST guideline 4).
- Immobilize the fractured bone: plaster, splint, brace, sling.

Fig. 18.4 Deformity associated with fractures.

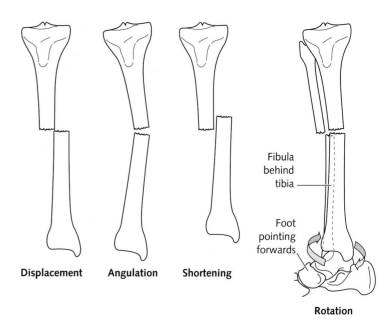

Displacement   Angulation   Shortening

Fibula behind tibia

Foot pointing forwards

Rotation

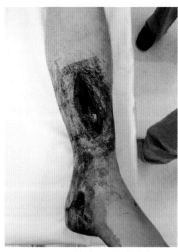

Fig. 18.5 An open tibial fracture. With permission from Jones CB, and Wenke JC, Open Fractures, in: Browner, B, Jupiter JBM Krettek C, Anderson P (eds); Skeletal Trauma: Basic Science, Management, and Reconstruction; Fifth Edition, 2015, Saunders, Elsevier.

- Give adequate and appropriate analgesia: this will often require intravenous opiates.
- Arrange imaging and further investigations.

Definitive management

The basic principles for the treatment of any fracture are:

- reduction of any deformity (displacement, angulation, rotation), i.e., put the bones back into the correct place
- stabilization (maintain reduction until healing occurs)
- rehabilitation (rehabilitate the limb and the patient)

Reduction

Reduction can be performed in either a closed or open manner.

- Closed reduction is performed by manipulating the fracture into position. This can be done under sedation or a general anaesthetic.
- Open reduction is performed in the operating theatre and involves a surgical procedure to open the fracture site and to reduce the bones accurately under direct vision. It is usually accompanied by operative stabilization.

Intraarticular fractures are usually treated with open reduction so that the joint can be accurately reduced, minimizing the risk of secondary osteoarthritis.

Stabilization

This can be achieved by external splintage, e.g., plaster cast, without an operation. Intraoperative fixation can be with percutaneous pinning with wires, plates and screws, intramedullary nail for long-bone fractures or external frame fixation (Fig. 18.6).

Rehabilitation

Following healing, or if the fracture is stable, the limb can be mobilized and range-of-movement exercises begun. One of the principles of operative stabilization is to allow early mobilization. The physiotherapist may need to instruct the patient in the use of crutches for restricted weight bearing.

Rehabilitation of the limb may often take as much time as the fracture took to heal.

Following a hip fracture, elderly patients require intensive input from physiotherapy, occupational therapy and social workers in order to become self-caring and safe prior to discharge.

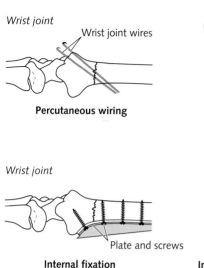

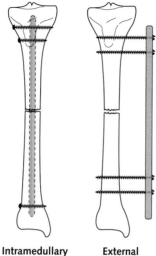

Fig. 18.6 Methods of surgical stabilization of fractures.

Wrist joint — Wrist joint wires

Percutaneous wiring

Wrist joint

Plate and screws

Internal fixation

Intramedullary nail

External fixation

COMPLICATIONS OF FRACTURES

Any complication can be local or general and immediate, early or late.

Immediate

Local

Initial displacement can cause the skin to tear, resulting in an open fracture. Fracture fragments may press on nerves, producing a nerve palsy (common in the humerus, resulting in radial nerve palsy), or on blood vessels, producing ischaemia (e.g., femur: popliteal vessels).

Very occasionally, nerves and blood vessels are completely torn and repair is needed.

General

Haemorrhage from fractures can be excessive, especially from femoral, pelvis, open or multiple fractures. Hypovolaemic shock may result (see Chapter 19).

Early

Local

Compartment syndrome

Compartment syndrome is a true emergency in orthopaedics. It results from excessive pressure developing in a closed fascial muscle compartment; the forearm and lower leg are the most common sites. Whilst uncommon, if left untreated, the condition can be limb- or even life-threatening. Following an injury (within a few hours usually), swelling can cause the blood supply to the muscle to be impaired, causing muscle ischaemia. This occurs at the level of small vessels and peripheral pulses are usually still present. The patient will complain of extreme pain (much more than normal) and increased pain on passive stretching of the muscles in the compartment. Paraesthesia and lack of pulse are late signs; in such cases irreparable damage has already occurred. The diagnosis is clinical (it is possible to confirm it with pressure monitoring). Any circumferential bandage or splint should be removed immediately and analgesia given. If the pain does not settle within 15 minutes, surgical decompression (fasciotomy) is required at once.

> **RED FLAG**
>
> **COMPARTMENT SYNDROME**
>
> An emergency not to be missed:
> - Pain exceeding the expected level, particularly on passive stretch through affected compartment. This is the first sign and the most important. If the symptoms progress to areas below the injury, the damage may already have occurred.
> - No pulse
> - Paraesthesia

Infection

This can occur early or late, following operative stabilization or open fracture. See Chapter 20.

Complex regional pain syndrome

This unusual condition can occur after any injury or operation. The exact cause is not known but is thought to relate to the sympathetic nervous system.

Usually the upper limb or foot and ankle are affected. The patient might have red, swollen, shiny fingers with excessive joint stiffness. Atypical pain is a feature. Referral to a multidisciplinary pain management team is indicated.

General

Thromboembolism

Deep vein thrombosis can occur after any lower-limb injury. Prevention in the form of mechanical (foot pumps, graduated compression stockings) or chemical agents is routinely used.

The limb will be swollen and may be painful because of the injury. If in doubt, obtain a duplex scan or venogram. Patients are treated prophylactically with anticoagulation with lower-limb fractures unless contraindicated. Pulmonary embolism is a rare, but potentially fatal, complication.

CLINICAL NOTES

DEEP VEIN THROMBOSIS PROPHYLAXIS

Used in all cases where prolonged immobility is likely and no contraindications. Local guidelines will vary. See NICE clinical guidance CG92 for further information.

Mechanical: Anti embolism stockings, pneumatic compression devices

Pharmacological: low molecular weight subcutaneous heparin injection. Used for 28–35 days after hip fracture surgery

---

Fat embolus

This condition may occur after long-bone fractures (particularly of the femur) and occurs due to fat entering the circulation and embolizing to the lungs. The condition occurs because the medullary canal of long bones contains fat. Early stabilization of fractures reduces the risk.

The patient presents with shortness of breath, petechial haemorrhages and sometimes confusion from low circulating oxygen levels (pO2) usually 2–3 days after injury.

This condition is potentially very serious and may lead to acute adult respiratory distress syndrome, which can be fatal.

Treatment is supportive with oxygen and fluids. Transfer to a high-dependency unit is advised.

Late

Delayed union/nonunion

Some fractures are slow to unite or fail to do so despite adequate treatment. Certain fractures (e.g., of the tibia) are more prone to this and it is more likely if the initial injury was high-energy or complicated by compartment syndrome. Further surgery and insertion of grafted vascular bone may be required to encourage the bone to heal.

Malunion

The fracture heals but in an abnormal position. This can be due to inadequate reduction or stabilization of the fracture. The resulting deformity may reduce movement in an associated joint and predisposes to late arthritis.

Osteoarthritis

Osteoarthritis, which is discussed in Chapter 11, is more common after intraarticular fractures.

Stiffness

Prolonged immobilization can result in severe joint stiffness. The joint may be held in a flexed position from ligament and capsular contracture.

Growth disturbance

Fractures occurring through the growth plate in children can stop growth. Growth arrest can be partial (i.e., one side of the limb grows, the other does not), leading to deformity, or complete, leading to shortness of the limb. Growth arrest can also be caused by placing wires/screws across growth plates but should be kept to a bare minimum. Treatment of such problems is complex.

COMMON FRACTURES

Any bone can be fractured and the patterns and treatment options are extensive. It is beyond the realms of this book to cover all of them. We have selected the three most common fractures: distal radial, hip and ankle.

Distal radial fractures

These are common at all stages of life, from greenstick fractures in children to osteoporotic fractures in the elderly. They are usually the result of a fall on to an outstretched hand.

Clinical features

The patient will present with a grossly swollen and frequently deformed wrist (the deformity will depend upon the type of fracture). Pain will be the main complaint. The patient will have a markedly reduced range of motion at the wrist. The patient may complain of altered sensation in the hand due to compression of the median nerve. The most common fracture is dorsally translated and dorsally and radially angulated. This is a Colles fracture. A distal radius fracture that is volarly translated and angulated is a Smith fracture (Fig. 18.7).

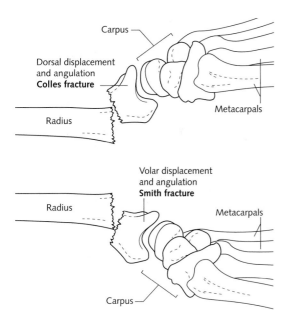

Carpus

Dorsal displacement
and angulation
Colles fracture

Radius

Metacarpals

Volar displacement
and angulation
Smith fracture

Radius

Metacarpals

Carpus

Fig. 18.7 Common distal radial fractures (lateral view).

Investigations

Wrist fractures are diagnosed by plain X-ray examinations. Heavily comminuted or intraarticular fractures may require a CT scan, for planning prior to theatre.

Treatment

The fracture pattern and the age, comorbidity and function of the patient will influence treatment.

Undisplaced fractures of the wrist, minimally angulated fractures and angulated fractures in the elderly may require immobilization in a cast for 4–6 weeks or simply splintage if they are comfortable. Very comminuted and intraarticular fractures and angulated fractures in higher demand, or more active, patients will require open reduction and internal fixation.

Whichever treatment option is used, the wrist will often be stiff afterwards and require physiotherapy to restore movement.

Hip fractures

Hip fractures (femoral neck fractures) are very common. They particularly occur in elderly patients with osteoporosis. Femoral neck fractures can also occur as pathological fractures related to metastatic malignancy. They are rare in young patients when they occur after high- energy trauma and are subject to different considerations. Hip fractures in the elderly place a huge impact on health resources, as well as having major implications for the patient with regard to mortality, disability and loss of independence. Approximately one-third of patients with a hip fracture will die within a year of injury.

Hip fractures can be broadly divided (Fig. 18.8) into:

- intracapsular fractures
- extracapsular fractures (intertrochanteric, subtrochanteric)

The blood supply to the femoral head originates predominantly from the medial femoral circumflex artery via the ascending cervical arteries. These travel from the capsular attachment along the intertrochanteric line to the femoral head and are closely attached to the posterior femoral neck. Consequently:

- In an intracapsular fracture (Fig. 18.9A), the fracture line is between the blood supply and the femoral head, potentially severing the blood supply to the head. This leads to a risk of avascular necrosis and nonunion.
- In an extracapsular fracture (Fig. 18.9B), the femoral head is in continuity with its blood supply and therefore there is no risk of avascular necrosis.

Aetiology

Most hip fractures are the result of a simple fall from standing height.

Clinical features

The patient will complain of severe pain around the affected hip or in the groin. This pain will be exacerbated by any attempt to move the leg. The patient will usually be unable to bear any weight.

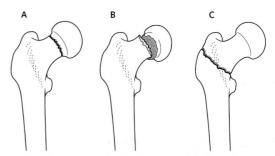

A   B   C

Fig. 18.8 Fractures of the femoral neck. (A) Undisplaced intracapsular fracture; (B) Displaced intracapsular fracture; (C) Extracapsular trochanteric fracture.

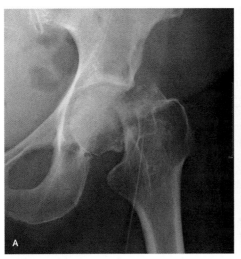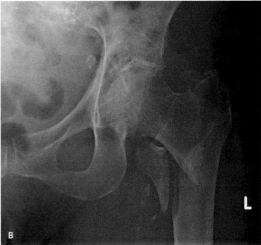

Fig. 18.9 (A) Intracapsular fracture with the fracture line potentially severing the blood supply to the head; (B) extracapsular fracture with blood supply intact.

Classically, patients will have a shortened and externally rotated leg on the affected side. They will be unable to raise the leg straight because of pain in the hip or groin. The patient might demonstrate tenderness on palpation over the greater trochanter or in the groin.

Diagnosis

Femoral neck fractures are usually diagnosed with plain film X-ray images (AP pelvis and lateral hip views). However, occult fractures might not show up on X-ray examination and further imaging such as MRI may be required.

Treatment

Nonoperative treatment with immobilization has high mortality and morbidity. In the vast majority of cases, femoral neck fractures are treated surgically. Postoperative patients are mobilized early to minimize these complications. Even when faced with a bed-bound nursing home resident, surgeons usually operate to provide pain relief.

Intracapsular fractures can be divided into undisplaced and displaced.

- Undisplaced fractures have a low chance of disruption to their blood supply and can be treated with internal fixation (Fig. 18.8A). However, a third will develop avascular necrosis or a nonunion and must be followed closely.
- Displaced fractures (Fig. 18.10) are normally treated with hemiarthroplasty; the femoral head is removed, leaving the artificial head articulating with the normal acetabulum. A total hip replacement may be more appropriate in young or active patients.

Extracapsular fractures are trochanteric or subtrochanteric and are treated with internal fixation with either a dynamic hip screw or an intramedullary nail.

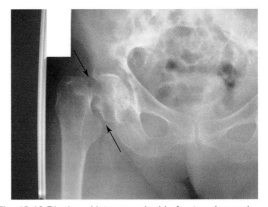

Fig. 18.10 Displaced intracapsular hip fracture (*arrows*).

CLINICAL NOTES

The subtrochanteric region is a common place for metastatic deposits. Be suspicious of a fracture in this region and consider getting preoperative imaging ± biopsy.

Ankle fractures

The tibia and fibula form a mortice in which the talar dome sits, supported by ligaments. Damage to the bones or ligaments can lead to instability.

Clinical features

The patient will describe pain and swelling around the ankle and might be unable to bear weight. The ankle might be obviously deformed. There will be tenderness over fracture

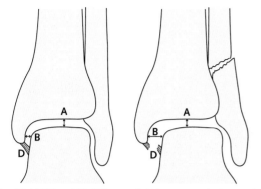

Fig. 18.11 Talar shift. If the medial clear space between the talus and tibia (*B*) is significantly greater than than the joint space (*A*), talar shift is present. Talar shift is suggestive of disruption of the medial ligaments (*D*) and indicates the fracture is likely to be an unstable pattern requiring fixation. *A*, Tibio-talar joint space; *B*, medial clear space; *D*, medial (deltoid) ligament.

or ligaments. The fibula can fracture anywhere along its length: palpate for tenderness along its entire length. A high fibular fracture results in an unstable ankle (a Maisonneuve fracture). It is important to check the neurological and vascular status of the foot.

Diagnosis

Diagnosis is made by X-ray examination. However, you should not wait for an X-ray examination before you reduce an obviously deformed ankle. If no fracture can be seen at the ankle in cases of significant ankle injury or if there is proximal fibular tenderness, a full-length tibia and fibula X-ray image is required.

Management

Fracture patterns thought to be stable can be managed conservatively with external splintage. Unstable ankle fractures—usually injuries that involve both the medial and lateral sides of the ankle—require surgical stabilization.

Chapter Summary

- Fractures can be pathological with an underlying cause or due to trauma. Differentiating these is important for fixation technique and prognosis.
- Open fractures must be recognized and treated appropriately with antibiotics in the Emergency Department as per guidelines.
- Fractures should be seen clearly on X-ray images including angulation, displacement, pattern of fracture including comminuted and simple, as well as whether they are intraarticular.
- Recognize the specific problems of certain broken bones such as the hip. Understand that there are very few situations where this fracture will be left to heal without an operation due to the challenge and pain of walking with a broken hip.
- Casting is often a good immobilization technique for fractures and can treat a vast majority of undisplaced fractures.
- Operative fixation is often indicated in unstable or very displaced fractures. These methods include open reduction and internal fixation, external fixation and intramedullary nailing.
- If a patient needs to undergo surgical fixation of a fracture, they are at risk of perioperative complications, the worst of which can be death, limb loss and compartment syndrome.
- A Colles fracture is a dorsally angulated, dorsally displaced fracture of the distal radius, a Smith fracture is the opposite.
- Femoral neck fractures are divided, based around the blood supply to the femoral head, into intracapsular and extracapsular fractures. These are managed differently, different ages and fitness ranges requiring different procedures.
- Ankle fractures can be treated operatively or nonoperatively, based on whether the fracture pattern is stable or unstable.

FURTHER READING

Charnley, J., 1999. The closed treatment of common fractures, new Golden Jubilee edition. Colt Books, Cambridge. (gives an excellent practical account of plaster and traction techniques).

McRae, R., 2008. Practical Fracture Treatment. Churchill Livingstone.
Orthobullets website. Available at http://www.orthobullets.com
BOAST guidelines https://www.boa.ac.uk/publications/boa-standards-trauma-boasts

DEFINITION

Trauma can refer to any injury but, in the context of surgery, normally refers to a patient with major isolated or multiple injuries. Major changes have occurred in how trauma treatment is delivered, with focus on rapid delivery of standardized care in major trauma centres from dedicated trauma teams.

INCIDENCE

Trauma is the leading cause of death for those aged 1–44 years.

CLINICAL FEATURES

Advanced trauma life support

Advanced trauma life support (ATLS) is a system developed in the USA for managing and assessing trauma in a uniform and timely fashion. It prioritizes examination and intervention by system so that most immediate threats to life are addressed. This primary survey forms the basis for the ATLS system and whilst its structure is rigid it is designed to prevent the inexperienced or anxious minds from missing reversible, life-threatening pathology. The following box

PRIORITIES FOR ADVANCED TRAUMA LIFE SUPPORT

A: Airway with cervical spine control	Cervical spine immobilized (blocks + tape/manual) Assess airway • Talking in full sentences • Obstruction: facial/neck trauma. Stridor • Reduced conscious state: GCS < 8 = immediate intubation • Aspiration: suction should be used but cautiously to avoid pushing vomitus further • Oedema: burns, heat/chemical/smoke inhalation High flow oxygen for all patients initially
B: Breathing	Assess breathing • Respiratory effort • Symmetrical chest wall movements • Respiratory rate • Visible wounds • Oxygen saturation • Auscultation • Percussion: dull in haemothorax, hyperresonant in pneumothorax • Tracheal position: deviated away from pneumothorax • Neck vein distension: in cardiac tamponade/tension pneumothorax • Crepitus/tenderness: rib fracture
C: Circulation with haemorrhagic control	Assess circulation • Pulse: rate, character • Blood pressure • Capillary refill time: centrally at sternum or peripheral at nail bed • Pallor • Urine output: excellent guide to volume status • Obvious external bleeding sources: initially treat with pressure but tourniquet use if unsuccessful, urgent theatre if ongoing bleeding • Abdomen/pelvis as source of bleeding: palpate abdomen but use caution with palpation of pelvis unless experienced.
D: Disability/neurological	Assess neurological status • GCS/ AVPU • Check blood sugar • Head wounds

summarizes the primary survey process that should be remembered as ABCDE.

The first step is a quick initial assessment and A, B, C and D can be achieved by asking the patient's name and what happened. Appropriate responses suggest intact airway and breathing adequate to generate speech and no major reduction in level of consciousness. Failure to respond appropriately mandates immediate assessment of A, B and C.

A- Airway

Lack of oxygenated blood delivered to the brain and other major organs causes rapid death in the injured patient. A protected, unobstructed airway is a priority in order to avoid hypoxia. A definitive airway can be achieved either through intubation or surgical techniques. A patient's airway can be compromised with:

- a decreased level of consciousness Glasgow Coma Scale (GCS) < 8 (head injury, hypoxia, hypovolaemia, drugs).
- facial trauma
- neck trauma
- aspiration of vomit or teeth
- swelling of subcutaneous tissues associated with burns or smoke inhalation

Assessment of airway patency should be rapid (earlier box). All trauma patients should receive oxygen initially.

Cervical spine control

All trauma patients should be assumed to have unstable neck injuries until proven otherwise, especially in those with an altered level of consciousness or with injuries above the level of the clavicle. The cervical spine is not considered immobilized unless held manually or with an appropriately sized hard collar, sandbags and tape across the patient's forehead. The patient should remain immobilized until the cervical spine can be cleared both clinically and radiologically.

B- Breathing

Adequate ventilation is required to oxygenate blood and therefore major organs such as the brain. Causes of ventilatory compromise include:

- Central nervous system depression (head injury, alcohol, drugs, cervical spine injury).
- Tension pneumothorax (needs immediate decompression with cannula in second intercostal space midclavicular line, followed by formal chest drain).
- Open/simple pneumothorax requiring chest drain (see Table 19.1).
- Rib fractures/flail chest (a condition where fractures at both ends of a rib leave it floating and severely affect the ability of lung to create negative pressure and inhale.
- Haemothorax

C- Circulation

Shock is defined as inadequate organ perfusion and tissue oxygenation. The most common cause of this in the trauma patient is hypovolaemia secondary to haemorrhage.

It is important to recognize hypovolaemic shock so that treatment is not delayed. The patient should have pulse rate, blood pressure, capillary refill, urinary output and level of

Table 19.1 Common causes of respiratory compromise in trauma

	Tension pneumothorax	Cardiac tamponade	Open pneumothorax	Haemothorax
Features	Tachycardia Tracheal Deviation Air hunger/Respiratory distress Neck vein distension Hyper resonance Absent breath sounds Cyanosis: late sign Hypotension	Tachycardia Neck vein distension Hypotension Cyanosis	Tachycardia Air hunger/ Respiratory distress Hyper resonance: unilateral Absent breath sounds: unilateral Cyanosis Hypotension Search for open wound	Tachycardia Air hunger/Respiratory distress Dullness to percussion Hypotension Cyanosis
Treatment	Large bore needle decompression to 2nd intercostal space midclavicular line	Needle pericardiocentesis: urgent discussion with cardiothoracic team	Occlusive dressing secured on three sides to create flutter type valve	Chest drain: 5th intercostal space just anterior to midaxillary line

Table 19.2 Physiologic response to haemorrhage				
	1	2	3	4
Blood loss (mL)	<750	750–1500	1500–2000	>2000
Blood loss (%)	<15	15–30	30–40	>40
Pulse rate (beats/min)	<100	100–120	120–140	>140
Blood pressure	Normal	Decreased	Decreased	Decreased
Respiratory rate (breaths/min)	14–20	20–30	30–40	>35
Urine output (mL/h)	>30	20–30	5–15	Negligible
CNS symptoms	Normal	Anxious	Confused	Lethargic

(Adapted from Committee on Trauma: Advanced Trauma Life Support Manual. Chicago: American College of Surgeons, 9th edition, 2012)

consciousness closely monitored. Clinical findings allow the doctor to estimate the circulating blood volume (approximately 5 L in adults). Blood pressure can be normal with up to 30% blood loss, but, as the patient decompensates, there is tachycardia, hypotension and confusion as shown in Table 19.2.

There are five areas to consider to identify potential blood loss: chest, abdomen, pelvis, long bones and on the floor (at the scene of the accident as well as in hospital). Intravenous access should be gained as soon as possible and fluid resuscitation commenced. In the case of haemorrhage, this means IV blood transfusion to be given as soon as possible and major haemorrhage protocols are present in all hospitals in the UK.

It is also important not to forget neurogenic or spinal shock in cases of head or spinal injuries respectively.

D- Disability/neurological status

This is based on the GCS and ranges from 3 to 15. This should be monitored regularly to observe for deterioration in the patient's condition. A simpler method to determine level of consciousness is AVPU (see box).

NEUROLOGICAL ASSESSMENT USING AVPU

A	Alert
V	Responds to *v*erbal stimuli
P	Responds to *p*ain
U	*U*nresponsive

E- Exposure and secondary survey

Look from head to toe for other injuries. This includes log-rolling the patient (with cervical spine control) to assess for trauma to the back and spine. A rectal examination should be carried out at this point.

The secondary survey involves a full history and examination of all systems. It is important that the secondary survey does not begin until the primary survey is complete and initial management has begun.

It is very common at secondary survey to find injuries missed in the primary survey. The examination should be from top to bottom and palpate all bony portions, as well as revisiting all the areas previously covered in the primary survey. Injuries commonly missed are those in the wrist and hands, with scaphoid fractures particularly hard to detect with distracting injuries.

COMMUNICATION

When taking a history from a multiply injured patient, the assessment should be rapid to avoid delays in diagnosing life-threatening conditions. Specifically ask about allergies, drug history, medical history, the last time the patient ate or drank and the events surrounding the injury. Seek a collateral history from others such as paramedics or people at the scene for clues about the mechanism (e.g., damage to the car) and to gain an idea of the patient's initial condition.

INVESTIGATIONS

A trauma series of X-ray images (taken in the resuscitation area) should include at least chest and pelvis films and, if indicated, cervical spine films. Major trauma will now often be directed rapidly to a CT scan for imaging as soon as safe. Blood tests include full blood count, urea and creatinine and clotting. Blood group should be identified and blood stored in case the patient needs blood transfusion.

TREATMENT

Treatment is guided initially by ATLS principles and early imaging has changed the way trauma is managed. Rapid access to blood and rapid transfer to the dedicated operating theatres have reduced mortality. The concept of damage control surgery is now used in trauma and revolves around the principle that trauma patients die from coagulopathy, hypothermia and metabolic acidosis, not from imperfect fixation of their fractures. Temporizing measures such as external fixators are used to stabilize adequately the patient physiologically for the definitive procedure.

OPEN FRACTURES

Definition

An open fracture is when there is an external wound leading to the fracture site, potentially allowing contamination with bacteria (see Fig. 18.6). They were formerly called compound fractures.

Incidence

Incidence of open fracture is approximately 23 per 100,000 patients per year.

Aetiology and pathology

Most open fractures are the result of high-energy trauma and are associated with significant damage to soft tissues. They can also occur when the fracture is grossly angulated or displaced and the sharp fracture end exits through the skin. The greatest risk to the bone is infection and the development of chronic osteomyelitis.

Clinical features

Check ABCDE. Assess the fractured limb for deformity and neurovascular status. Any wound around the fracture site should be assumed to communicate with the bone. Also look for evidence of compartment syndrome (still possible in open fractures).

Management

The wound should be photographed then irrigated and dressed with saline-soaked swabs. Splint the limb and start intravenous antibiotics as soon as possible. Give tetanus prophylaxis if immunizations are not up-to-date. The wound should be aggressively debrided in theatre as soon as possible (without putting the patient's health at risk) to minimize bacterial infection of the fracture. The fracture can then be stabilized with a suitable method of internal or external fixation.

CLINICAL NOTES

OPEN FRACTURES

Treat as per BOAST 4 guideline:

- Assess neurological status carefully: urgent surgery if compromised or wound heavily contaminated.
- Intravenous antibiotics within 3 hours
- Washout in Emergency Department and cover with soaked swabs
- Photography
- Definitive stabilization and debridement in normal working hours unless vascular compromise or contamination

SPINAL INJURIES

Definition

Spinal injuries include fractures and subluxations/dislocations of vertebrae. They also include damage to the spinal cord, even in the absence of a fracture.

Incidence

This is a common injury in trauma patients. Overall, 10%–20% of patients with a spinal fracture will have a second spinal fracture at another level. Patients with significant trauma to lower limbs are at risk of spinal fractures, for example 10% of calcaneal fractures will have a concurrent vertebral fracture.

Aetiology and pathology

Spinal injuries often occur after road traffic accidents. Other examples include neck injuries from diving into a shallow pool, thoracic injuries from hyperflexion and lumbar injuries, which commonly occur from falls from a height. Thoracolumbar injuries often occur as a result of wearing a lap belt in a road traffic accident. In elderly patients with osteoporosis, low-energy trauma can result in simple wedge fractures (see Chapter 15).

The stability of the spine depends on the bony structures and the integrity of strong ligaments. The spine can be thought of as three columns (Fig. 19.1). Fractures involving one column only, such as anterior wedge fractures, are usually stable (see Fig. 15.5) and can be treated conservatively. Fractures involving two or three columns, such as a high-energy burst fracture (Fig. 19.2), are often unstable. Injuries may involve the bony structures only, both ligaments and bones or purely ligaments. This means that even if the X-ray

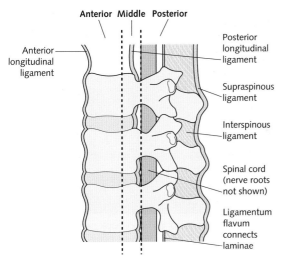

Anterior　Middle　Posterior

Posterior longitudinal ligament

Anterior longitudinal ligament

Supraspinous ligament

Interspinous ligament

Spinal cord (nerve roots not shown)

Ligamentum flavum connects laminae

Fig. 19.1 Anatomy of the spine divided into its three columns.

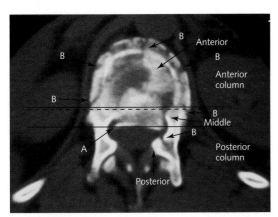

B　Anterior

B

B

Anterior column

B

B
Middle

B

A

Posterior column

Posterior

Fig. 19.2 Axial computed tomography scan showing an unstable two-column burst fracture (*arrows B*) with retropulsion of a bone fragment (*arrow A*) into the spinal canal.

examination is normal, you cannot assume the spine is stable as *all* the ligaments may be torn. However, this is type of injury is extremely rare. If there is doubt, magnetic resonance imaging (MRI) will show the soft tissues.

CLINICAL NOTES

Be careful with spinal injuries. It is very distressing for the patient and staff if fractures are missed. To exclude injury, you need good X-ray images (and/or computed tomography) and a fully conscious patient. If in doubt, get senior help.

Clinical features

Check ABCDE. A conscious patient will complain of pain at the level of injury (beware in patients with a decreased level of consciousness).

HINTS AND TIPS

Patients with facial or head injuries should be presumed to have a significant neck injury until proven otherwise.

Clinical examination may reveal tenderness, a boggy swelling or bony step. The patient should be log-rolled with cervical spine control in order to examine the thoracic and lumbar spine. Check limbs for abnormal neurology. A full neurological examination should include a rectal examination for anal tone and sensation (sacral nerves). Knowledge of dermatomes and myotomes will guide the doctor to the level of spinal cord injury if present.

Remember that spinal injury might cause bradycardia and hypotension (spinal shock). These patients should receive intravenous fluids cautiously.

Diagnosis and investigation

Neck: anteroposterior, lateral (to at least T1) and odontoid peg views.

Thoracic and lumbar spine: anteroposterior and lateral views if indicated.

X-ray images can be normal, even with spinal cord trauma.

Further imaging may be required: computed tomography (CT) scan in the case of equivocal or inadequate X-ray images; MRI to look for ligament and spinal cord damage.

Treatment

Treatment depends on the stability of the fracture.

Stable fractures can be mobilized.

Unstable fractures require immobilization (e.g., halo vest), bracing or possibly internal fixation.

Prognosis

Patients with spinal cord damage and neurological symptoms have a poor prognosis and often require extensive rehabilitation on a spinal unit.

PELVIC FRACTURES

Pelvic fractures are high-energy injuries commonly associated with massive bleeding, urethral, bladder and abdominal injuries.

Incidence

Pelvic fractures are rare injuries and careful assessment of the polytraumatized patient is necessary to avoid missing them.

Aetiology

The pelvis can be thought of as a stable ring formed by the sacrum, ilium and pubis bones held together by strong ligaments. The basic mechanisms of injury are anteroposterior compression (blow from the front: Fig. 19.3), lateral compression (side impact), vertical shear forces (usually fall from height) or a combination of all three.

Clinical features

Once again check ABCDE. The patient will have pain and may be shocked due to blood loss.

Clinical examination may reveal asymmetry to the pelvis or lower limbs and bruising and swelling around the pelvis itself. There may be blood at the urethral meatus (urethral tear) and bruising in the scrotal region. Rectal examination may reveal blood or a boggy, high-riding prostate (urethral tear). Bone fragments may be palpable. Do not assess pelvic stability by bimanual compression of the iliac wings (springing the pelvis) as this may displace a clot and cause renewed bleeding.

Diagnosis and investigation

An anteroposterior X-ray image of the pelvis should be checked for fractures, symmetry and normal contours. Once stable, a CT scan will enable a more accurate identification of the fracture.

Emergency treatment

The patient should be managed according to ATLS protocol and resuscitated with intravenous fluids. Patients who either transiently respond or do not respond are likely to

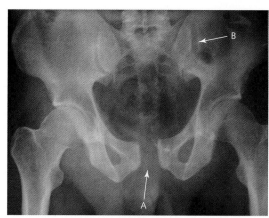

Fig. 19.3 X-ray image of an open-book pelvic fracture. There is widening at the symphysis pubis (*arrow A*) and the left sacroiliac joint (*arrow B*).

have ongoing bleeding. There might be haemorrhage from bones, the pelvic venous plexus and, rarely, arteries.

Bleeding can be reduced by stabilizing the pelvis. This can be done immediately by tying a bed sheet around the pelvis (at the level of the greater trochanters) or applying a pelvic binder to close the pelvic ring and reduce its volume. If this fails, angiography and embolization of bleeding vessels or laparotomy may be required. A pelvic external fixator can also be of use in certain specific situations. However, a well placed binder is usually sufficient for immediate purposes.

Stable fractures require pain relief and mobilization.

Unstable fracture patterns require surgical fixation.

Prognosis

Mortality can be high, especially when the patient has associated head, chest or abdominal injuries. Complications such as urethral tears, sciatic nerve damage or persistent sacroiliac pain can affect the quality of life in the long term.

Chapter Summary

- The most important step in managing any trauma is the ABCDE approach: this should be your first step.
- Spinal fractures should be assessed as either stable or unstable using the three-column rule. Any neurological deficit should be carefully documented and will influence operative decisions.
- Open fractures should be treated with early antibiotics and photographs of wound. External fixation or plastic surgery might be required to close the wound.
- Pelvic fractures can be life-threatening injuries and should be addressed as part of the primary survey.
- Managing major trauma requires a team approach and should be practised and updated on a regular basis. Courses such as the Advanced Trauma Life Support (ATLS) are attended by doctors treating trauma.

FURTHER READING

Committee on Trauma, American College of Surgeons, 2012. Advanced Trauma Life Support for Doctors, 9th ed. American College of Surgeons, Chicago, IL.
www.orthobullets.com.

Introduction

Bone and joint infection has become much less common in western society over the last century. This is explained by the increasing use of antibiotics and the general improvement in nutrition and health of the population as a whole.

Infection still occurs and needs to be recognized and treated promptly to avoid potentially fatal complications.

In this chapter we will discuss osteomyelitis (infection in bone) and septic arthritis (infection in a joint).

OSTEOMYELITIS

Infection of bone can be caused by direct inoculation (exogenous) or blood-borne bacteria (haematogenous).

In childhood or adolescence, osteomyelitis is usually caused by the haematogenous spread of bacteria. In adults, the source is more likely to be exogenous, most commonly due to infection developing after surgery or after a penetrating injury (particularly in the case of an open fracture).

Incidence

Osteomyelitis is now uncommon.

Aetiology and pathology

In children, there is often a history of preceding trauma, which may predispose the limb to infection. The most common infecting organism overall is *Staphylococcus aureus*; other pathogens are shown in Table 20.1. If unusual organisms are present, consider specific predisposing factors, as listed in the box; for example, patients with acquired immunodeficiency syndrome (AIDS) can get fungal infections.

Table 20.1 Common pathogens in osteomyelitis

Patient's age	Common organisms
Newborns (younger than 6 months)	*Staphylococcus aureus*, *Streptococcus* (group A and B), *Enterobacter*
Children (6 months to adult)	*Staphylococcus aureus*, *Haemophilus influenzae*, *Streptococcus*, *Enterobacter*
Adult	*Staphylococcus aureus*, *Streptococcus*, *Enterobacter*
Immunocompromised	*Pseudomonas*, *Mycobacterium tuberculosis*, fungal infection

---

CLINICAL NOTES

CONDITIONS ASSOCIATED WITH OSTEOMYELITIS

Congenital	Acquired
Sickle cell disease	Diabetes
Haemophilia	Renal failure
	Intravenous drug use
	Malnutrition
	Immunosuppression
	HIV/AIDS

AIDS, Acquired immunodeficiency syndrome; HIV, human immunodeficiency virus.

The three most common causes of osteomyelitis are:

1. Posttrauma osteomyelitis
2. Postsurgery osteomyelitis
3. Acute haematogenous osteomyelitis

Posttrauma osteomyelitis

An open fracture means the skin is broken, allowing bacteria direct access to the bony surfaces. Large dirty wounds associated with high-energy injuries are more likely to result in posttrauma osteomyelitis. Urgent surgical debridement and lavage are required to remove contaminated material and dead bone and to reduce the risk of subsequent osteomyelitis. Inadequate or delayed surgery will lead to osteomyelitis due to bacteria being harboured within dead bone. In these circumstances, the fracture will often fail to heal: an infected nonunion.

Postsurgery osteomyelitis

Many surgical procedures in orthopaedics involve using implants such as joint prostheses or plates and screws. These foreign bodies can harbour infection if bacteria are introduced at the time of surgery. Due to the lack of blood supply to the implants, eradication is almost impossible without surgery. For this reason, orthopaedic surgeons are fastidious about aseptic techniques in the operating theatre and routinely use antibiotics as prophylaxis. Despite this, infection still occurs and might spread around the implant, devitalizing bone.

Acute haematogenous osteomyelitis

This form of osteomyelitis is usually seen in children and may develop spontaneously, but frequently may be precipitated by trauma. Blood supply to bone is from the endosteum and periosteum.

The pathogenesis of acute haematogenous osteomyelitis is as follows (Fig. 20.1):

1. Bacteraemia that settles in the metaphysis of a long bone.
2. Inflammation and pus formation within the bone.
3. Pus escapes through the haversian canals to form a subperiosteal abscess.
4. Pus is now present on both sides of the bone, causing this part of the bone to die.
5. Dead bone, called sequestrum, harbours infection.
6. Periosteal new bone, called involucrum, forms around the sequestrum as the body tries to fight the infection.

Acute osteomyelitis can easily become chronic if the sequestrum is neglected or not completely excised at surgery.

Other conditions associated with osteomyelitis

The above three causes of osteomyelitis are the most common, but it also occurs in the other conditions listed in the earlier box.

Bone and joint infection are common among intravenous drug users. These patients are often malnourished and immunosuppressed (possibly human immunodeficiency virus (HIV)-positive). They frequently inject themselves deeply with dirty needles, often neglecting small abscesses, leaving these patients at risk of opportunistic infections.

Clinical features

Acute osteomyelitis causes pain, fever and loss of function (often a limp if the lower limb is involved).

It is more common in the tibia and femur. The limb will be tender to palpate, erythematous and possibly swollen.

At the extremes of age (neonate, infant or elderly), the symptoms and signs are often nonspecific (such as general malaise). These patients can be seriously ill and it can be extremely difficult to pinpoint the exact site of the problem.

Occasionally, a patient presents with multiple sites affected or there may be another focus of infection that has spread from or to bone, for example infective endocarditis. This is called seeding of infection.

In postsurgery and posttrauma osteomyelitis, the wound will be painful, red and inflamed. Normally, once postoperative pain has settled, patients are comfortable and can mobilize without pain. If pain persists or increases, infection is a possible cause. Wounds will continue to leak and eventually break down or there will be dehiscence. If left untreated, a sinus will result.

A limb with chronic osteomyelitis will be swollen and have thickened, woody skin. Here the focus of infection remains within the bone as sequestrum and the infection can remain quiescent for a period of time (maybe many years) and then flare up unexpectedly, often producing an abscess. A chronic discharging sinus can result.

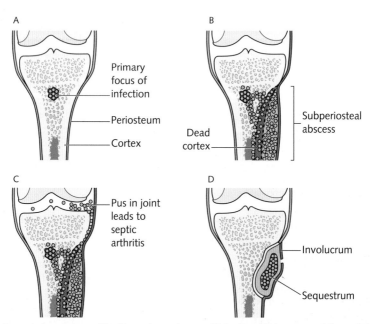

Fig. 20.1 Sequence of events in osteomyelitis. The primary focus of infection (A) has spread through bone, causing the death of cortical bone and formation of a subperiosteal abscess (B). Infection can spread into the joint (C), causing septic arthritis. Death of a segment of bone (sequestrum) occurs (D), and the area is surrounded by new subperiosteal bone (involucrum).

Diagnosis and investigation

The diagnosis may be obvious on clinical features, particularly if the history reveals a clear predisposing factor.

A raised white cell count (WCC), erythrocyte sedimentation rate (ESR) and C-reactive protein (CRP) will be present on blood tests.

Initially X-ray images will be normal, but after 10 days, features of lysis, periosteal elevation and new bone formation are seen. Later, sequestrum may be seen as a sclerotic area. A Brodie abscess may be seen in the metaphysis of long bones (Fig. 20.2).

Early osteomyelitis can be detected before it can be seen on X-ray images by using a bone scan or white cell-labelled scan (shows increased uptake) or magnetic resonance imaging (MRI).

It is very important to take microbiology specimens such as blood cultures prior to starting antibiotics.

Management

Conservative

The patient needs adequate analgesia, splintage of the affected limb and appropriate antibiotics. Most hospitals or health boards will have an antibiotic policy; however, consultation with the microbiologist is advisable.

As the majority of infections are with *Staphylococcus aureus*, flucloxacillin is the first-line antibiotic, usually in combination with fusidic acid or rifampacin. The course is initially given intravenously for 6 weeks, with additional oral antibiotics if necessary.

Antibiotic-resistant strains such as meticillin-resistant *Staphylococcus aureus* (MRSA) are becoming more prevalent and, if suspected, then vancomycin or teicoplanin can be used instead after consultation with a microbiologist.

Antibiotics will suffice provided the patient does not have an abscess or dead bone is not present.

Surgical

If an abscess is present, this should be drained surgically. Dead bone (sequestrum) needs to be removed, otherwise eradication is impossible.

In a chronic case, if the patient and surgeon decide to attempt to cure the infection, extensive surgery is required to remove all infected bone and implants if present. Techniques for doing this vary depending on the extent of involvement and the site.

It is possible simply to treat the flare-ups and suppress the infection with antibiotics when required, particularly in patients not fit for major surgery.

Complications

Complications occur if:

- Osteomyelitis persists.
- The physis is damaged, leading to growth disturbance and deformity.
- The infection spreads to the joint, causing septic arthritis.

Prognosis

In cases of acute osteomyelitis, the outcome is good and the majority make a full recovery provided none of the above complications occur. In chronic cases following surgery or trauma, many surgical procedures are often required and amputation is not an uncommon outcome.

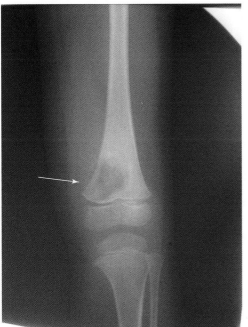

Fig. 20.2 Brodie abscess (*arrow*).

HINTS AND TIPS

Chronic osteomyelitis is very difficult to treat. It may remain dormant for many years and then flare up intermittently, causing pain and loss of function. These flare-ups are often managed with antibiotics. Some people cannot tolerate long-term loss of function of the limb, in which case amputation may be indicated.

COMMON PITFALLS

Patients with amputation can still go on to develop osteomyelitis and careful assessment with MRI and counselling is required.

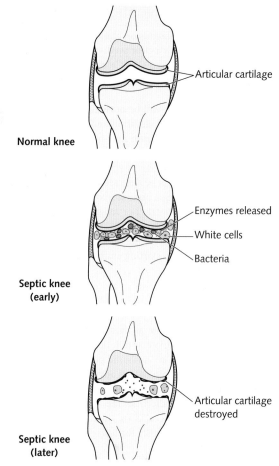

Fig. 20.3 Sequence of events in septic arthritis.

SEPTIC ARTHRITIS

Septic arthritis is infection within a synovial joint.

Incidence

The condition is uncommon but is seen more often in children, young adults and the elderly. It is more common in the developing world and in patients with a predisposing factor. In children, it is less common than osteomyelitis.

Aetiology and pathology

Infection reaches a joint via the haematogenous route, direct spread from the metaphysis or penetrating trauma/surgery. Associated conditions are similar to those for acute osteomyelitis (see box: Clinical notes, Conditions associated with osteomyelitis), with the addition of rheumatoid arthritis and crystal arthropathy. In all groups, *Staphylococcus aureus* is the most common causative pathogen; however, certain organisms are more common at different ages. *Haemophilus influenzae* used to be the most common infecting organism in infants prior to the introduction of the vaccination programme. In young sexually active adults, the *Neisseria gonorrhoeae* is more common.

In haematogenous septic arthritis, the bacterium settles in the synovium, which may be inflamed due to trauma or disease. Proliferation of bacteria causes an inflammatory response by the host with numerous leukocytes migrating into the joint. The variety of enzymes and breakdown products produced damages the delicate articular cartilage very quickly (within hours) and, if left unchecked, permanent damage will ensue (Fig. 20.3).

Clinical features

The patient will have an acutely hot swollen joint with a fever and be systemically unwell (see Chapter 6). An infant or young child will be distressed, unwell and difficult to assess. There may be a history of recent systemic infection such as otitis media.

Septic arthritis is more common in the hip and knee but can present in any synovial joint.

Any movement at all causes intense pain and weight-bearing will not be tolerated. If the joint is superficial, an effusion is palpable.

In neonates and infants, the diagnosis may be less obvious, particularly if the joint is deeply situated, such as the hip. These patients may be seriously unwell, and systemically compromised.

Diagnosis and investigation

- WCC, CRP and ESR will be elevated.
- X-ray images will be normal initially and show joint destruction late.

- If available, ultrasound scanning is useful to see if there is a joint effusion when the hip is the suspicious joint.
- Any joint suspected of infection must be aspirated and the fluid sent for urgent Gram stain, culture and examination for crystals.

Management

Relieve pain by giving analgesia and splinting the limb. Aspiration should be performed at the earliest opportunity, preferably before the commencement of antibiotics. Give appropriate antibiotics as directed by the microbiologist, depending on the age of the patient and any predisposing illness. Treatment can be either medical with serial aspiration or surgical with arthroscopy/arthrotomy, both in conjunction with antibiotics. If infection is serious, whether the patient is young or old, the chances of full recovery are slim once the articular cartilage is destroyed. Further procedures, often in the form of arthroplasty, may be needed in the future to return to normal function.

Complications

- Seeding of infection can occur to the spine or other organs.
- Recurrence of infection.
- Joint destruction with long-term arthritis or even ankylosis (bony fusion across the joint).
- Avascular necrosis (particularly in the hip).

Prognosis

If treated promptly, prognosis is good, but if joint destruction occurs, prognosis is very poor. Septic arthritis, if missed or left untreated, can be fatal.

TUBERCULOSIS

Incidence

Tuberculosis (TB) is common in global terms and causes significant morbidity and mortality in Africa and Asia.

TB has made a comeback in the UK, with over 10,000 cases per year, most of which are in the Asian community or immunocompromised patients but it is increasingly seen in all communities.

Aetiology and pathology

TB is due to *Mycobacterium tuberculosis* or *M. bovis* infection.

Histologically, the classic appearance is of granulating caseating necrosis.

Musculoskeletal TB results when primary TB (lung) becomes widespread or when later reactivation or reinfection occurs (immunosuppressed patients).

Clinical features

Patients have general symptoms of ill health, such as malaise, weight loss, cough and loss of appetite. The most common musculoskeletal sites affected by TB are the spine, hip and knee.

Unlike other orthopaedic infections, TB presents with gradual symptoms of pain and may be initially diagnosed as osteoarthritis or inflammatory arthritis.

Diagnosis and investigation

The two most common tests for TB exposure are the Mantoux and Heaf tests, which are skin hypersensitivity tests.

For confirmation, large samples of bone or synovial fluid are required, which need to be cultured (Löwenstein-Jensen medium) for a prolonged period (6 weeks).

If mycobacterial infection is suspected, samples should be submitted to a Ziehl-Neelsen stain to look for acid/alcohol-fast bacilli. Remember to ask for this specifically when requesting a Gram stain.

X-ray images show variable amounts of joint destruction with periarticular osteopenia.

In the spine, vertebra plana may be found with almost complete collapse of the vertebral body (see Fig. 9.9).

Treatment

Drugs commonly used are rifampicin, isoniazid and ethambutol and multidrug therapy is required.

A spinal abscess may need drainage with stabilization of the spine.

Ankylosed joints from previously treated TB can be replaced (usually the hip).

● Chapter Summary

- The most common causative organism for septic arthritis in all ages is *Staphylococcus aureus*. Aspiration of the joint will give fluid for culture.
- Osteomyelitis can develop either posttraumatically or from haematogenous spread. Sequestrum and involucrum are terms relating to the effect of infection on bone and its response.
- The clinical features of septic arthritis in children and adults are redness, swelling, pain, difficulty moving the joint, difficulty bearing weight and systemic upset and in some cases sepsis can be caused by joint infection.
- Septic arthritis should be investigated and treated aggressively. An aspiration should be done to confirm the diagnosis and to obtain samples for culture and antibiotic treatment should be started. Arthroscopic washout of a large joint or open washout of smaller joints may be indicated to save cartilage.
- For the diagnosis of bone and joint sepsis, inflammatory markers, X-ray imaging and aspiration should be used as diagnostic methods.
- Tuberculosis differs from other infections in orthopaedics in that it can lie dormant for a number of ears before reactivating and can cause significant collapse of the spine.

FURTHER READING

www.orthobullets.com.

Solomon, L., Warwick, D., Nayagan, D. (Eds.), 2001. Apley's System of Orthopaedics and Fractures. 8th ed. Hodder Arnold, London.

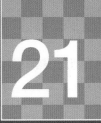
This chapter covers bone tumours (benign and malignant; primary and secondary) and other malignant conditions presenting as a musculoskeletal disorder. Tumours may be discovered incidentally as a lesion on X-ray examination, when the X-ray image was taken for another reason or as the primary symptom requiring further investigation to locate the primary pathology. Examples include a chest X-ray image taken for respiratory disease showing a lesion in the clavicle or a pelvic X-ray image taken for hip disease showing metastatic prostate carcinoma.

Benign lesions are quite common. Thankfully, primary bone malignancy is extremely rare. Secondary bone tumours are common in the elderly. It is important to remember that infection and metabolic bone disease can present as a bone lesion.

BENIGN TUMOURS/DISORDERS

- osteochondroma
- osteoid osteoma
- enchondroma
- bone cysts
- fibrous dysplasia

MALIGNANT TUMOURS

- Primary:
  - osteosarcoma
  - Ewing sarcoma
  - chondrosarcoma
- Secondary (metastatic):
  - breast
  - lung
  - prostate
  - renal
  - thyroid
  - bowel
- Haemopoietic diseases:
  - myeloma
  - leukaemia
  - lymphoma

INFECTION

- Osteomyelitis

METABOLIC BONE DISEASE

- Paget disease

While the clinical features, treatment and prognosis will depend upon the specific pathology, the way a bone tumour is approached remains the same. We will address the general approach to the history, examination and investigation to bone tumours and discuss the individual pathologies separately.

HISTORY

The following points must be elicited in the history, looking for clues as to the diagnosis.

Age of patient

Certain lesions such as bone cysts are more common in children and other benign bone lesions such as enchondroma usually occur in young adults.

Overall, primary malignant tumours are rare and metastatic bone disease is a disease of the elderly.

Pain

Pain that is severe and does not respond to simple analgesia, particularly if night pain is a feature, suggests a malignant process. Pain that worsens and is not related to any trauma is suspicious.

Swelling

Benign lesions are more likely to present with swelling, particularly osteochondroma, a lesion commonly found around the knee.

Malignant tumours may have pain and swelling, but it is rare for a bone tumour to present with swelling only.

General health

General features of ill health such as tiredness, weight loss, poor appetite and fever suggest a systemic illness such as malignancy, haemopoietic disorders or infection.

Primary bone malignancy is unlikely to present with widespread features of malignancy as patients will usually present with pain and swelling before these general features have developed.

It is important to ask about any other areas of pain in the musculoskeletal system, particularly if considering widespread metastatic disease.

Medical history

A history of cancer is extremely important when dealing with such a patient. The lesion should be treated as a metastatic lesion until proven otherwise.

Breast malignancy can be dormant for many years prior to representing with metastases.

EXAMINATION

Site

Different lesions are more common in certain locations, for example enchondromas are more common in the hand.

Secondary bone metastases tend to be found in the central skeleton and proximal limbs (hips and shoulders).

Limb examination

On initial examination, the affected limb will usually appear normal.

Tenderness, redness and swelling would be present in:

- impending or actual fracture associated with a bone metastasis
- osteomyelitis
- osteoid osteoma
- malignant primary bone tumour

Malignant secondaries or bone lesions from haemopoietic diseases rarely show any external features.

Generalized

In secondary malignancy with unknown primary, it is important to examine:

- breast (for carcinoma)
- chest (for lung tumours)
- abdomen (for renal or bowel tumours and evidence of haemopoietic disease such as liver and spleen enlargement)
- per rectum (PR; prostate)
- thyroid (for carcinoma).

INVESTIGATION

The X-ray examination

It is important to obtain two views taken at 90 degrees (orthogonal) to one another and to obtain full-length views of the entire bone (to ensure there are no further lesions along the same bone).

Most benign lesions need no further investigation and repeat X-ray examinations after 6 months are useful to ensure the bone lesion does not change in appearance and develop any sinister features.

COMMUNICATION

Practice describing bone defects and lesions whenever possible. The following should be covered when describing a lesion.

1. Name and age of patient.
2. Site, i.e., which bone and where in the bone
   - The lesion can be in the diaphysis (shaft), metaphysis (cancellous bone between the growth plate and shaft) or epiphysis (between the growth plate and the joint).
   - The lesion can primarily affect either the cortex or medulla of the bone.
3. Appearance
   - The lesion can be lytic (e.g., breast metastasis; Fig. 21.1), sclerotic (e.g., prostate metastasis), mixed or calcified (enchondroma).
   - Ground glass (fibrous dysplasia; Fig. 21.2).
   - Abnormal bony architecture, e.g., postosteomyelitis.
4. Zone of transition
   - A well-defined border between the lesion and the normal bone suggests a benign slow-growing lesion (it is clearly demarcated).
   - A broad, irregular or indistinct zone of transition where the change from abnormal to normal is poorly defined suggests a malignant process (Fig. 21.3).
5. What is the bone doing in response?
   - A significant periosteal reaction, with Codman triangle (elevation of periosteum; see Fig. 21.7B), onion skinning (Fig. 21.4A) and sunray spicules (Fig. 21.4B), is a feature of malignancy.
   - Infection can also cause a periosteal reaction.
6. What is the lesion doing to the bone?
   - Cortical destruction is typical of a malignant process.
   - Cortical thinning does occur in benign disease due to expansion.

Further investigation

Further investigation is necessary if there is any doubt about the diagnosis or to confirm or to exclude malignancy.

COMMUNICATION

It is not uncommon for patients to present with a lesion on X-ray examination to find they have metastatic disease from an unknown primary. Make sure this news is broken in the right way, preferably once all the information is available, a plan has been made and with relatives and nursing staff present.

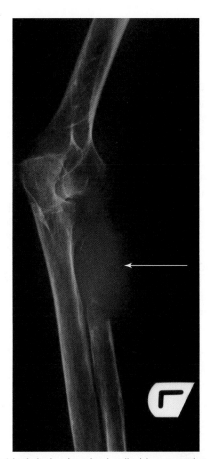

Fig. 21.1 Lytic lesion (proximal radius) is suggestive of malignancy (*arrow*).

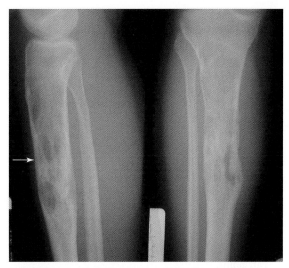

Fig. 21.3 A poorly defined zone of transition (*arrow*) suggests malignancy.

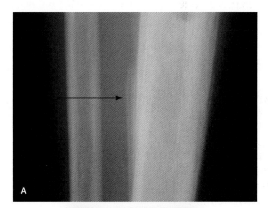

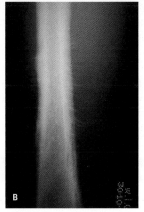

Fig. 21.4 Primary bone tumour showing: (A) onion skinning (*arrow*) and (B) sunray spicules.

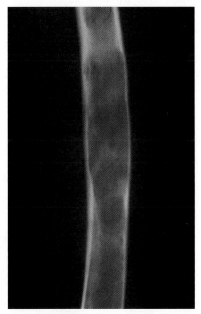

Fig. 21.2 Fibrous dysplasia. (Reproduced with permission from Hochberg, MC, Silman, AJ, Smolen, JS et al. (eds) 2011. Rheumatology, 5th ed. London: Mosby).

Blood tests

- A full blood count may show anaemia of chronic disease.
- Liver function tests could be deranged if liver metastases are present.
- The calcium profile is often elevated in generalized malignancy and alkaline phosphatase is elevated in Paget disease.
- C-reactive protein (CRP) and erythrocyte sedimentation rate (ESR) are elevated in infection or malignancy.
- A very high ESR suggests myeloma. It is confirmed with serum electrophoresis and urinary Bence Jones proteins.
- Prostate-specific antigen (PSA) is elevated in prostate malignancy.
- Carcinoembryonic antigen (CEA) is elevated in bowel carcinoma.

Isotope bone scan

This is a very useful tool to detect further lesions in malignancy or to establish whether a lesion is active (i.e., hot on bone scan). Infection will show up hot, as will malignant lesions.

Of the benign lesions, only osteoid osteoma will show increased uptake.

Computed tomography

Computed tomography (CT) is used to confirm osteoid osteoma.

Magnetic resonance imaging

Magnetic resonance imaging (MRI) can detect early metastatic lesions before features are apparent on X-ray images.

It is also used to define the extent of malignant bone tumours and can help to distinguish between benign and malignant lesions.

Biopsy

It can be very difficult to be certain of the diagnosis in some cases. A biopsy will prove whether the tumour is benign or malignant and exclude infection as the cause.

PRIMARY BONE TUMOURS

Primary tumours of bone can be benign or malignant.

Benign bone tumours

Enchondroma

An enchondroma is a benign bone lesion of cartilaginous origin.

Incidence

Enchondromas are quite common, occurring usually in adulthood.

Aetiology and pathology

Enchondromas develop from aberrant cartilage (chondroma) left within bone ('en'). They are usually found in the metaphysis of long bones (femur or humerus) but are also common in the hand (Fig. 21.5).

Clinical features

An enchondroma is usually asymptomatic and may be found incidentally. Large lesions causing cortical erosion can be painful and the patient may notice a swelling, particularly in the hand.

Diagnosis and investigation

Typical features on X-ray examination show a well-demarcated calcifying lesion in the metaphysis of the bone. Serial X-ray images may be obtained to make sure the lesion is not growing rapidly.

Treatment

Usually no treatment is required, but if the lesion is significantly painful or associated with fracture, excision or curettage may be performed.

Osteochondroma

Incidence

This is the most common benign bone lesion, presenting from childhood through to adult life.

Aetiology and pathology

The lesion develops from aberrant cartilage remaining on the surface of the cortex. It is usually found around the knee, most commonly on the distal femur (see Fig. 21.5).

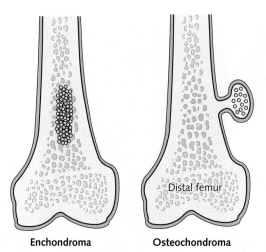

Enchondroma   Osteochondroma

Fig. 21.5 Benign cartilage tumours.

The pathological appearance is of a bone lesion continuous with the cortex of the bone, capped with hyaline cartilage. It can be sessile or pedunculated (see Fig. 21.5).

Clinical features
The majority are asymptomatic, presenting incidentally or as a swelling. Rarely, pain or pressure effects on nerves or vessels occur.

Diagnosis and investigation
The typical appearance of a pedunculated lesion in continuity with the cortex clinches the diagnosis. If there is doubt, CT or MRI may reassure.

Treatment
Usually no treatment is needed; rarely, excision is carried out, if symptomatic.

Prognosis
It is extremely rare for either osteochondroma or enchondroma to undergo malignant change.

Osteoid osteoma

Osteoid osteoma is a painful, self-limiting benign bone lesion.

Incidence
The lesion is uncommon, usually presenting between 5 and 30 years of age.

Aetiology and pathology
It is caused by a nidus of osteoblasts located in the cortex of bone and is usually found in the tibia, spine or femur.

Clinical features
Patients have intense pain, particularly at night. Tenderness over the lesion is usual. In the spine, scoliosis may be present.

Diagnosis and investigation
X-ray images show a radiolucent nidus surrounded by a dense area of reactive bone (Fig 21.6A). CT scans confirm and accurately locate the lesion (Fig. 21.6B).

Treatment
Pain is typically relieved by nonsteroidal antiinflammatory drugs. CT-guided ablation is now preferred over surgical excision.

Prognosis
The tumour is eventually self-limiting.

Fibrous dysplasia

This is not strictly a bone tumour.

Incidence
Fibrous dysplasia is relatively common, usually presenting by the age of 30 years.

Aetiology and pathology
It is most commonly found in the tibia, femur and ribs and is caused by developmental abnormality of bone with numerous fibrous proliferations.

Clinical features
The condition is usually asymptomatic, discovered as an incidental finding, but can present with pain, swelling, deformity or fracture.

Diagnosis and investigation
A typical ground-glass appearance is diagnostic (Fig. 21.2).

Treatment
No treatment is usually required, but if the dysplasia is significant, curettage and bone grafting can be performed.

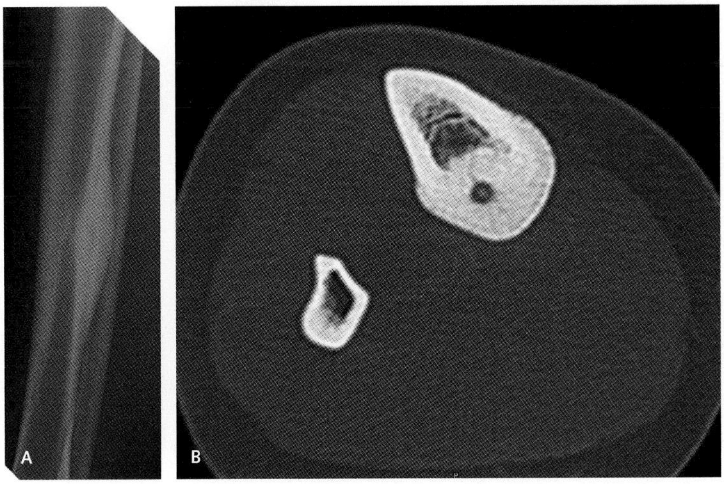

Fig. 21.6 (A) X-ray image showing an osteoid osteoma. (B) Computed tomography scan will confirm.

Malignant primary bone tumours

Primary malignant bone tumours are very rare indeed. We will discuss two of those most likely to be encountered.

Osteosarcoma

Incidence
There are approximately 1 or 2 cases per million of population. Presentation is in adolescence and young adulthood or in the elderly where they develop in pagetic bones.

Aetiology and pathology
Paget disease or radiation can predispose, but most cases occur sporadically. The tumour is highly malignant and secretes osteoid. Local spread occurs quickly, destroying the cortex, but it may also metastasize.

The most common location is around the knee; other sites include the proximal humerus and femur.

Clinical features
The patient presents with pain and sometimes swelling. Clinically, there is usually warmth over the affected area and there may be a palpable mass. 10%–20% of patients present with pulmonary metastases.

Diagnosis and investigation
X-ray images (Fig. 21.7) may show:

- an ill-defined lesion with an indistinct zone of transition (Fig. 21.7A)
- sclerotic or lytic areas within the lesion
- cortical destruction
- Codman triangle (elevation of periosteum; Fig. 21.7B)
- sunray spicules (calcification within the tumour but outside the bone)

Biopsy might be necessary to confirm the diagnosis. Further investigations such as CT and MRI are required to stage the lesion.

Treatment
A combined multidisciplinary team approach is adopted.

Preoperative chemotherapy followed by limb salvage surgery is performed if possible. Amputation is occasionally required.

Prognosis
Five-year survival is 60%.

Chondrosarcoma

Incidence
Chondrosarcomas are more prevalent with age, with most tumours arising after the age of 40 years. The peak incidence is approximately eight cases per million at the age of 80 years. Men are more commonly affected than women.

Aetiology and pathology
A chondrosarcoma can be either a primary lesion or a secondary conversion of a benign cartilaginous tumour such as osteochondroma or chondroma. A chondrosarcoma can be separated into low-grade and high-grade. Little difference can be seen histologically between a low-grade chondrosarcoma and a benign cartilaginous lesion. High-grade chondrosarcomas demonstrate a more abnormal cell structure and are consequently more aggressive. The most common areas of growth are in the pelvis and around the hip.

Clinical features
Similar to osteosarcoma, the main clinical features are that of pain and localized swelling. On examination, there might be a bony mass palpable.

Diagnosis and investigation
X-ray images usually show a lytic lesion with cortical destruction and central calcification. Low-grade lesions may resemble benign cartilaginous lesion. CT or MRI may be required to investigate the lesion further.

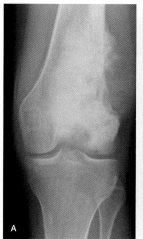
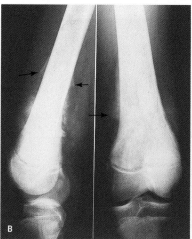

Fig. 21.7 X-ray images of osteosarcoma. (A) Ill-defined lesion. (B) Codman triangles (*arrows*).

Treatment

A multidisciplinary approach is once again adopted. Chemotherapy and radiotherapy are less effective. Wide excision of the lesion is sometimes possible, as chondrosarcomas are slow-growing and metastasize late in the disease. However, amputation may be the only viable option.

Prognosis

Prognosis is grade-dependent: 5-year survival for low-grade lesions is 90%, whereas for high-grade lesions it is 5%.

Ewing sarcoma

Incidence

Ewing sarcoma is extremely rare (less common than osteosarcoma), occurring between 5 and 25 years of age.

Aetiology and pathology

Histologically, this is a small-cell sarcoma. It occurs as frequently in flat bones as in long bones, being most common in the femur or tibia (long bone), pelvis or vertebra (flat bones).

These tumours are highly malignant and often large at presentation.

Clinical features

Patients present with pain and may be unwell with a fever. Clinically, the area is warm and swelling may be present.

Diagnosis and investigation

Diagnosis is usually made from X-ray examination (Fig. 21.8). It usually appears as a lytic lesion with a laminated periosteal reaction (onion skinning). CT and MRI help to stage the lesion. Biopsy may be necessary.

Treatment

A combined multidisciplinary team approach is adopted.

Preoperative chemotherapy and radiotherapy followed by limb salvage surgery are performed if possible.

Prognosis

Five-year survival is 60%.

SECONDARY BONE TUMOURS

Incidence

Secondary bone tumours are the most common bone-destroying lesions in the older patient.

Aetiology and pathology

The tumours most likely to metastasize to bone are:

- breast
- lung
- prostate
- renal
- thyroid
- bowel

Metastatic lesions are most commonly found in the spine, pelvis, ribs and proximal long bones. The mechanism of metastasis is shown in Fig. 21.9. Bone is destroyed by metastatic disease and weakened, predisposing to fracture. A majority of metastases appear osteolytic, but those from prostate cancer appear sclerotic.

Clinical features

Patients with a known primary

The patient has a clear history of previous malignancy, which in the case of breast carcinoma may have been many years previously. Unrelenting bone pain in the axial skeleton then makes the patient seek medical help. Night pain is often a feature that does not respond to simple analgesia. There may be constitutional symptoms such as weight loss and malaise.

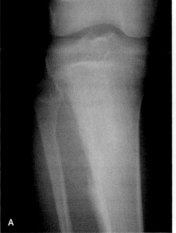
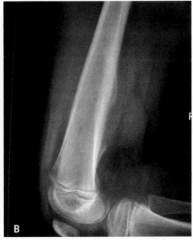

Fig. 21.8 X-ray images of Ewing sarcoma. (A) demonstrating lysis and periosteal reaction in a proximal tibial lesion. (B) demonstrating periosteal reaction in a distal femoral lesion.

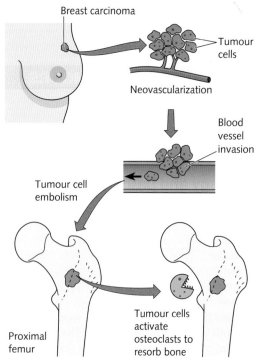

Fig. 21.9 Mechanism of long-bone metastasis.

Patients with no known primary

The patient presents with bone pain as described above but with no history of previous malignancy. In this case it is important to ask about symptoms suggestive of malignancy such as cough and haemoptysis (lung), urinary symptoms (prostate) or change in bowel habit (bowel). Patients often do not have any symptoms of the primary. Clinical examination should concentrate on likely sources of primary tumours. Therefore the following should be examined:

- breast
- chest
- prostate (per rectum)
- thyroid
- abdomen (kidney and bowel)

Fracture

The patient usually has a history of bone pain preceding the event (usually minor trauma) that caused the fracture. The patient is then either admitted or seen in a fracture clinic.

HINTS AND TIPS

Patients who present with significant fractures after a very minor injury (e.g., after lifting a suitcase) may have a malignancy.

Spinal cord compression

Patients with malignancy can appear to be 'off their legs' with weakness and/or altered sensation at a demonstrable spinal level (change in neurological signs corresponding to the specific vertebral level affected). There may be a history of preceding spinal bony pain and then weakness, numbness and loss of bladder and bowel control (cauda equina syndrome). An MRI scan is urgently needed to assess the spinal cord and radiotherapy may shrink the tumour, preserving spinal cord function.

CLINICAL NOTES

METASTATIC CORD COMPRESSION

Clinical suspicions of cord compression caused by metastases should be investigated urgently with MRI scanning. It can be a very difficult decision whether or not to operate on a patient with spinal cord compression in the presence of malignancy. Surgery has significant risks, but most spinal surgeons will try to stabilize the spine if at all possible to preserve the patient's mobility and dignity. Patients will know they are terminally ill but will not want to spend the last few months of life immobile and incontinent.

Diagnosis and investigation

Any bone-destroying lesion could be due to infection or malignancy. The following should be investigated:

- Check the white cell count and inflammatory markers (CRP and ESR). These are elevated in infection but may also be elevated in malignancy (myeloma).
- Further blood tests may identify the primary such as CEA or PSA.
- Plain X-ray images may show an osteolytic, sclerotic or mixed lesion.
- If strong clinical suspicion exists then an MRI scan is more sensitive.
- Cortical thinning suggests impending fracture.
- A bone scan will be hot and is useful to exclude further distant lesions.
- In an unknown primary, further investigation to find the primary is warranted (Fig. 21.10).

Treatment

Treatment depends on the primary and on the life expectancy of the patient. A multidisciplinary approach is required involving oncologists.

Conservative
- Adequate analgesia and splintage.
- Radiotherapy is used frequently for bony metastatic pain.

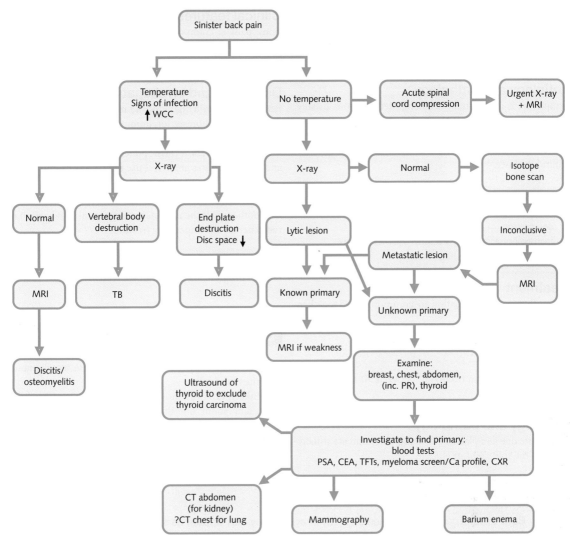

Fig. 21.10 Algorithm for the investigation of sinister back pain.
Ca, Calcium; *CEA*, carcinoembryonic antigen; *CT*, computed tomography; *CXR*, chest X-ray examination; *MRI*, magnetic resonance imaging; *PR*, per rectum; *PSA*, prostate-specific antigen; *TB*, tuberculosis; *TFTs*, thyroid function tests; *WCC*, white cell count.

- Chemotherapy may have a role in certain tumours.
- Hormonal therapy is useful in breast disease.
- Intravenous bisphosphonates are now being used to inhibit osteoclastic resorption of bone.

Surgical

- Intramedullary fixation of long bones is performed for fracture or impending fracture. This should be discussed carefully with the patient, but even in palliative care it can be a pain-relieving procedure to keep mobility in a patient's final months of life.
- Joint arthroplasty is sometimes used around the hip and shoulder.
- Spinal decompression and stabilization for acute cord compression.

Prognosis

The prognosis depends on the primary.

HINTS AND TIPS

Patients with renal tumours and a solitary metastasis may be cured by resection of both.

HAEMOPOIETIC DISEASES

Lymphoma and myeloma can present with bone destruction.

Lymphoma

Incidence
Lymphoma is rare but can occur at any age.

Aetiology and pathology
Lymphoma is a malignant haematopoietic tumour usually occurring secondarily but rarely primarily in bone. Primary bone lymphoma has a better prognosis. It can occur in any bone, most commonly the pelvis, spine and ribs, but also around the knee.

Diagnosis and investigation
- X-ray images show a long lesion with mottled bony destruction.
- Isotope bone scanning excludes further lesions.
- Biopsy confirms the diagnosis.

Treatment
Chemotherapy and irradiation are commonly used together.

Myeloma

Incidence
This is a rare tumour, occurring between 50 and 80 years of age.

Aetiology and pathology
Lesions are due to a plasma cell malignancy and are usually found in the spine, ribs or clavicle.

Clinical features
Bony pain is common and there may be a pathological fracture. Systemic symptoms of fatigue and fever are very common.

Diagnosis and investigation
Patients will have a high ESR and may have hypercalcaemia. Serum electrophoresis for immunoglobulins and urinary analysis for Bence Jones proteins confirm the diagnosis.

X-ray images show classic punched-out lytic lesions. MRI and CT procedures are of less use than X-ray examinations.

Treatment
Chemotherapy is the mainstay with surgical stabilization or radiotherapy for impending fracture.

Prognosis
Overall prognosis is poor, with survival averaging 2 years.

LEUKAEMIA

The last malignancy to mention is leukaemia: a malignancy of white blood cells.

Leukaemia is the most common malignancy of child-hood and about one-third of patients have bone pain. Leukaemia can also present with an acutely hot, swollen joint very similar to septic arthritis.

Chapter Summary

- Bone lesions can often be seen on X-ray images. They may appear as subtle lucencies or obvious deformities.
- Where X-ray examinations are concerned, features for malignancy are involvement of the cortex, periosteal reaction (Codman Triangle) and indistinct transition zone.
- Investigation for a patient with an incidental bone lesion visible on X-ray examination will often take the form of an MRI scan, but primary malignancy causing bony metastases should always be considered.
- Primary bone tumours should be classified into benign and malignant.
- Tumours that commonly metastasize to bone are breast, lung, prostate, thyroid and renal.
- Bone metastasis may present as pathological fractures or simply as regional pain.
- Available treatments for primary and secondary bone tumours may involve primary excision, a wide local excision, amputation, radiotherapy and chemotherapy.
- Haemopoietic diseases such as myeloma can present with bone destruction.
- Spinal cord compression is possible if metastases are present. If suspected, it should be investigated with MRI scanning. Treatment is usually with radiotherapy.

FURTHER READING

Canale, S.T., 2006. Campbell's Operative Orthopaedics, 11th ed, vols. 1–4. St Louis, Mosby. vols. 1–4.

Orthobullets website: http://www.orthobullets.com

Solomon, L., Warwick, D., Nayagan, D. (Eds.), 2001. Apley's System of Orthopaedics and Fractures. 8th ed. Hodder Arnold, London.

Sports injuries 22

KNEE INJURIES

Introduction

The knee is commonly damaged in sports involving twisting injuries. This chapter will discuss injuries to the menisci, ligamentous injuries of the knee and patellar dislocation.

Meniscal injuries

The menisci are two semicircular fibrocartilage structures that lie between the femoral and tibial articular surfaces (Fig. 22.1). They act as shock absorbers and are prone to injuries caused by the large forces crossing the knee.

Incidence

Meniscal injuries are common, usually occurring in young adult patients who participate in sports.

Pathology and aetiology

The medial meniscus is more commonly injured because it is fixed, in comparison to the more mobile lateral meniscus.

Meniscal tears can be traumatic or degenerative:

- Traumatic tears. The meniscus is normal and injury usually occurs after landing or twisting with the knee flexed. This can be associated with a ligamentous injury, such as an anterior cruciate ligament (ACL) tear. A chronically unstable knee is prone to further tears.
- Degenerative tears. These occur in an older population through abnormal cartilage. They may occur with little or no injury.

Types of meniscal tears (Fig. 22.2)

1. Bucket handle. The tear extends over a distance, remaining attached at the anterior and posterior horns. A locked knee results when a large bucket-handle tear flips over and becomes trapped in the joint, resulting in loss of complete extension.
2. Radial.
3. Horizontal cleavage.
4. Flap/parrot beak.

It is clinically important to establish how peripheral the tear is. Very peripheral tears occur through vascular tissue and are amenable to repair, as these tears can heal. Meniscal tears further away from the blood supply (i.e., further into the knee) cannot heal.

Meniscal cysts result from synovial fluid being pumped into the meniscal tear. A valve effect means the fluid in the cyst cannot drain back into the knee (see Fig. 22.2).

CLINICAL FEATURES

Patients usually incur this injury while playing sport, with the incident occurring during a tackle or when twisting or changing direction.

A patient may present immediately after injury with a painful locked knee or with a gradual chronic nagging pain with associated swelling over months or years following minor injury. In the chronic setting, the symptoms are often intermittent in character.

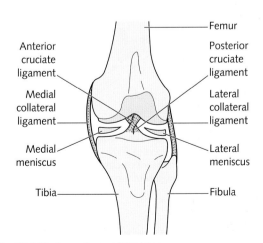

Fig. 22.1 Basic anatomy of the knee.

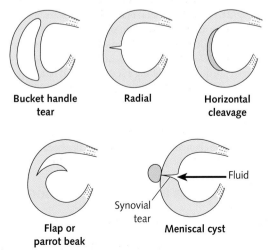

Fig. 22.2 Meniscal lesions.

Mechanical symptoms such as locking and giving way suggest meniscal pathology. A clicking joint does not necessarily mean there is pathology.

A more major injury with acute swelling and instability suggests associated ligamentous injury.

Examination may reveal:

- A locked knee.
- An effusion:
- A large acute effusion can be caused by a very peripheral tear but should raise suspicion of another cause such as ligament injury or fracture.
- A small chronic effusion is common.
- Joint line tenderness: this is an important part of the examination and is usually positive in a patient with a torn meniscus.
- A meniscal cyst, which may be palpable over the lateral joint line.

A variety of special tests are described for meniscal tears (such as McMurray test) and none are very reliable. A good history is often the best tool in diagnosing meniscal pathology.

Diagnosis and investigation

In most cases, the diagnosis is made solely on the basis of history and examination.

X-ray images are usually normal and are performed to exclude fracture or osteoarthritis or other rare causes of knee pain.

Magnetic resonance imaging (MRI) is used to confirm the presence of torn menisci, but the most accurate way to confirm the diagnosis is with arthroscopy of the knee.

Management

Conservative

Initially rest, ice, compression, elevation (RICE) is used for an acutely swollen knee. Early physiotherapy is essential to encourage movement.

Surgical

Surgery is now performed using arthroscopic techniques (see Fig. 24.1). For peripheral bucket-handle tears, meniscal repair has the advantage of retaining the meniscus.

For tears not amenable to repair, meniscal resection is commonly performed. Partial meniscectomy removes the damaged portion only, leaving a stable rim and reducing the risk of osteoarthritis in the future.

Prognosis

Removal of a significant portion of a meniscus can lead to osteoarthritic changes developing in the knee because of increased load on the articular surface.

Ligamentous injuries of the knee

Anterior cruciate ligament

Incidence

One per 3000 of the population per year is affected.

Aetiology and pathology

The ACL is the primary restraint to anterior tibial translation and a restraint to rotation. The mechanism of injury is usually a twisting or valgus strain pattern of injury commonly occurring in soccer or skiing (Fig. 22.3).

The knee is usually extended or slightly flexed with the foot fixed. Associated injuries to the medial collateral ligament (MCL) and either meniscus are common (the unhappy triad). The patient often hears a pop or feels something go inside the knee.

ACL-deficient knees are susceptible to further meniscal tears.

Clinical features

With an acute ACL rupture, the patient will be unable to play on and may have to be carried from the field. Many patients present a long time after injury with symptoms of instability.

Swelling typically occurs within the timeframe of minutes to hours, unlike meniscal tears, which swell over 24 hours, because the ACL is more vascular than the menisci.

Once initial symptoms have settled, the patient may complain of giving way of the knee. This occurs when the patient tries to turn rapidly. Patients will frequently report being able to run in a straight line but not being able to twist and turn. This giving way or instability is pain free.

Clinically, patients have a tense effusion after an acute injury.

The anterior drawer test (see Chapter 2), Lachman test are positive.

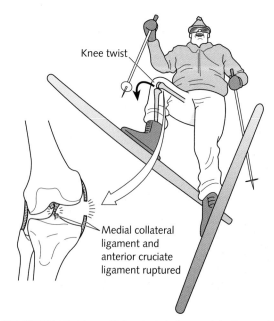

Knee twist

Medial collateral ligament and anterior cruciate ligament ruptured

Fig. 22.3 Mechanism of injury in anterior cruciate ligament rupture.

Diagnosis and investigation

The majority can be diagnosed clinically. In some patients, it is difficult to achieve positive examination findings and in those patients an MRI scan is used to confirm the diagnosis. Arthroscopy is the most reliable diagnostic tool and findings do not always match the MRI. X-ray images will usually be normal.

Management

Conservative—Initial treatment is with RICE and physiotherapy. In the absence of instability, the majority of patients can modify their activities and manage with a hamstring rehabilitation programme only.

Surgical—ACL reconstruction is indicated for functional instability of the knee. This can be performed either through open or arthroscopic surgery using a hamstring tendon or patellar tendon graft. Meniscal tears can also be addressed at the time of surgery.

Posterior cruciate ligament

The PCL is the primary restraint to posterior movement of the tibia on the femur.

Incidence

PCL injuries are rare.

Aetiology and pathology

PCL injuries require a significant force occur either in sporting activities or from road traffic accidents (dashboard injury; Fig. 22.4). It is an injury often sustained by goalkeepers in football, the mechanism of injury being the knee combining with an onrushing attacking player forcing the tibia backwards. The PCL can also rupture when the knee is forcibly hyperextended. The majority of PCL tears occur in combination with other ligamentous injuries and, rarely, injuries to the popliteal artery. It is important to check the distal vasculature in suspected cases of PCL rupture as the knee may have been dislocated (see box: Clinical notes, Knee dislocation).

CLINICAL NOTES

KNEE DISLOCATION

This is a rare injury but carries significant morbidity. It should not be confused with a patellar dislocation. It is usually the result of high-energy trauma and can result in devastating neurological and vascular injury with a 50% vascular injury rate in anterior and posterior dislocations. The knee will need to be reduced urgently and reconstructed after an interval. It is rare to recover preinjury function after a dislocated knee.

Clinical features

The patient will have a substantial injury to the knee and will usually be unable to bear weight. Swelling is usually less obvious than with an ACL injury. Patients complain less of instability than with ACL injuries. Clinically, patients will have a posterior sag and positive posterior drawer test. Careful assessment is needed to look for associated injuries such as lateral collateral ligament (LCL) injuries.

Diagnosis and investigation

All patients with suspected PCL injury should undergo an MRI scan.

Treatment

Conservative—Almost all isolated PCL injuries can be treated with rehabilitation alone.

Surgical—Patients with combined injuries or symptomatic instability require reconstruction.

Collateral ligament injuries

Incidence

MCL injuries are common injuries in isolation or combined with ACL injury, whilst LCL injuries are rare injuries.

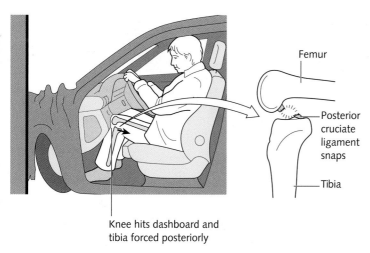

Fig. 22.4 Mechanism of injury in posterior cruciate ligament injuries.

Femur

Posterior cruciate ligament snaps

Tibia

Knee hits dashboard and tibia forced posteriorly

Aetiology and pathology

In the case of MCL injuries, there is a valgus strain pattern of injury. The injury can be complete or partial and is frequently associated with ACL injury. Isolated LCL injuries occur when a varus strain is placed on the knee (i.e., a hit from the medial side; Fig. 22.5).

Clinical features

Collateral ligament injuries are usually sporting injuries; the patient may feel something go but an effusion is not a feature of an isolated collateral ligament tear (they are extraarticular structures). The patient will complain of pain and possibly instability.

When the MCL is injured, there will be tenderness over the broad attachment of the MCL and opening up of the joint on valgus stress. In the normal knee, the LCL is easily palpable as a cord-like structure. When the LCL is ruptured, the area is tender and indistinct. Opening up of the joint on the lateral side will be present on varus stress.

Management

Many isolated injuries heal well with conservative treatment. Treatment is with physiotherapy and bracing for 6 weeks. Minor tears heal well without bracing.

Surgical advancement is sometimes required for chronic unstable injuries.

Prognosis

The knee usually returns to normal after a period of rehabilitation.

Patellar dislocation

Introduction

The patella is prevented from dislocation by anatomical features such as a large lateral femoral condyle and the insertion of the vastus medialis oblique muscle and medial patellar femoral ligament (Fig. 22.6).

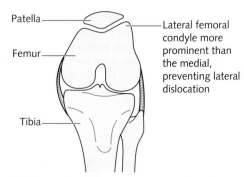

Fig. 22.6 Anatomical features that prevent lateral dislocation of the patella.

Incidence

Patellar dislocation is quite common.

Aetiology and pathology

Patellar dislocation can be habitual or traumatic.

Those suffering habitual dislocation are often young women with ligamentous laxity and a hypoplastic trochlea. This group gets recurrent dislocations after minor injuries, often without trauma, and are difficult to treat.

Traumatic dislocations occur during sports, usually with the knee slightly flexed with side impact. The dislocation occurs laterally and damage may occur to the joint surface as an osteochondral fracture. Structures along the medial border of the patella are torn.

Clinical features

A first-time dislocation is extremely painful and the patient arrives in casualty with a history of dislocated knee. The patella might have spontaneously reduced if the knee was extended to allow transport. If not, it will be laterally placed.

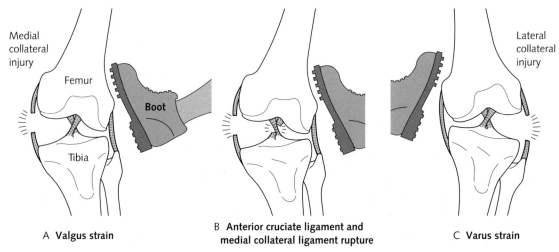

Fig. 22.5 Mechanism of injury in collateral ligament tears. (A) Valgus strain; (B) anterior cruciate ligament and medial collateral ligament rupture; (C) varus strain.

166

There is often tenderness over the medial side of the knee and an effusion.

Later, when the acute injury has settled, the patient may have patellar apprehension and a J-sign. Patients who suffer habitual dislocation may show evidence of generalized laxity in other joints such as fingers, thumbs, elbows and knees (hypermobility syndrome). Both groups may have wasted or deficient vastus medialis.

Diagnosis and investigation

X-ray examinations should be made after reduction, including a tunnel and skyline view looking for any osteochondral defects.

Management

Conservative

Initial reduction is required, usually under sedation in the accident and emergency (A&E) department. A short period on crutches may be helpful but long periods of immobilization are not helpful. Physiotherapy is the mainstay of treatment once pain and swelling allow, improving range of movement and quadriceps strength specifically to try to stabilize the patella.

Surgical

Osteochondral fractures should be repaired or removed arthroscopically.

Recurrent dislocations may require surgical realignment. Repair or reconstruction of the medial patellofemoral ligament is carried out where physiotherapy has failed and persistent dislocation is causing symptoms.

SHOULDER DISLOCATION

Incidence

The shoulder is the most commonly dislocated large joint in the body.

Aetiology and pathology

The shoulder is at risk of dislocation because the joint has very little inherent bony stability, with reliance instead on capsule, labrum and rotator cuff muscles. The joint has sacrificed stability for movement.

The dislocation can be anterior or posterior. Anterior dislocation (Fig. 22.7) accounts for 95% and usually occurs when the arm is forced back in a ball-throwing position of external rotation and abduction. In anterior dislocation, the labrum can be damaged anteroinferiorly, leaving a so-called Bankart lesion predisposing to further dislocations. Recurrent dislocations cause a Hill-Sachs lesion due to impaction of the glenoid on the posterior part of the humeral head.

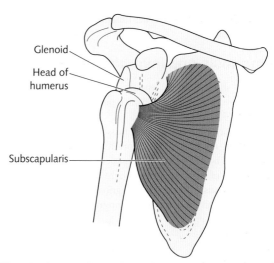

Fig. 22.7 Anterior dislocation of the humerus.

In older patients, the rotator cuff is torn rather than a Bankart lesion developing.

Posterior dislocations are far less common, occurring in fewer than 5% of cases. Posterior dislocations occur with high-energy trauma, epileptic seizures and electrocutions.

Clinical features

The patient is often a sports player—typically rugby—and has an acute injury to the shoulder, as described above. The injury is intensely painful and the shoulder is held supported by the other arm (Fig. 22.8).

Examination findings include:

- loss of normal contour
- palpable glenoid
- complete loss of movement

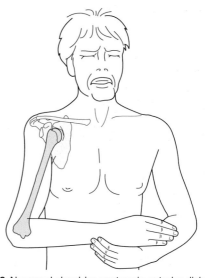

Fig. 22.8 Abnormal shoulder contour in anterior dislocation of the humerus.

Check that the axillary nerve is functioning before and after any intervention.

Diagnosis and investigation

Anterior dislocation is usually obvious and confirmed with X-ray examinations (always performed to exclude a fracture).

Posterior dislocation is often missed as the initial anteroposterior X-ray image looks normal to the untrained eye. This should be suspected in any patient who has fixed internal rotation of the shoulder. The light bulb sign (Fig. 22.9A) should raise suspicion, but the diagnosis is made on axillary view (Fig. 22.9B) or computed tomography scan.

Treatment

Conservative

The dislocation needs to be promptly reduced in the A&E department under sedation.

Posterior dislocation often requires a general anaesthetic and may need open reduction.

Once the dislocation is reduced, the joint is rested in a collar and cuff and once the pain has settled, supervised early rehabilitation with a physiotherapist can commence.

Surgical

Surgery is reserved for recurrent dislocations to repair bone or labral defects.

Prognosis

Men have a higher rate of recurrence than females. The younger the patient at the time of first dislocation, the higher the recurrence rate (as high as 80% in teenage men).

In the more elderly population, shoulder stiffness is more of a problem than recurrence.

ANKLE SPRAIN

Incidence

Ankle sprains are very common injuries, lateral more so than medial.

Aetiology and pathology

These injuries are commonly found on the sports field but anyone can sprain an ankle. The mechanism of injury is inversion or eversion with damage to the lateral ligament and medial ligament complexes respectively.

In a lateral ligament sprain, the talus tilts in varus in the ankle mortice and the anterior talofibular and calcaneofibular ligaments are torn (Fig. 22.10). In a medial ligament sprain, the talus tilts in valgus in the ankle mortice and the deltoid ligament complex is torn.

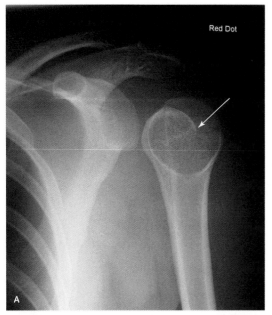
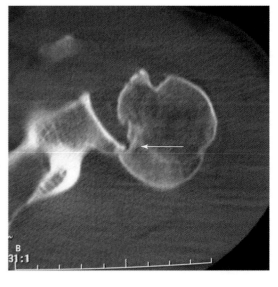

Fig. 22.9 Posterior dislocation of the shoulder. (A) Anteroposterior X-ray showing the light bulb sign (*arrow*); (B) computed tomography scan showing axial view. There is posterior subluxation of the head with impaction of the head from the glenoid rim (*arrow*).

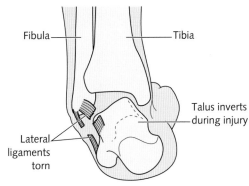

Fibula — — Tibia

Talus inverts during injury

Lateral ligaments torn

Fig. 22.10 Ankle ligament rupture.

Clinical features

The patient experiences pain and may feel something go; swelling occurs rapidly.

Chronic ankle instability leads to the joint giving way.

Clinically, the patient has a variable amount of swelling and tenderness over either the lateral or medial ligament complex.

Patients may have instability of the ankle joint with a positive anterior drawer test and opening of the lateral side.

Diagnosis and investigation

X-ray examinations are performed only if there is bony tenderness or inability to bear weight (Ottawa ankle rules).

Management

Conservative

All sprains are initially treated conservatively with analgesia, RICE and physiotherapy.

Surgical

Arthroscopy of the ankle is sometimes performed for associated osteochondral injuries.

Ligament reconstruction is rarely required for a chronically unstable ankle.

● Chapter Summary

- A locked knee is often caused by a meniscal tear but can also be caused by loose bodies in the joint.
- Meniscal tears are often treated conservatively, but if symptoms are present they can be either repaired or excised by arthroscopic techniques.
- The classic history for a meniscal tear is one of twisting trauma to the knee. A popping sensation is often felt with a rapid onset of effusion.
- Collateral ligaments supply lateral stability to the knee and can be injured with any significant valgus stress.
- The patella does not normally dislocate because strong ligaments hold it in line; however, in those with lax ligaments, such as in connective tissue disorders, patellar dislocations are much more common.
- The shoulder is a ball and socket joint where the majority of stability comes from muscular and ligamentous attachments. It is more prone to dislocation than other joints due to its large rang of motion and shallow depth.
- Shoulder dislocations are most frequently anterior–inferior and should be managed with reduction under sedation as soon as safely possible.
- Surgical treatment in the form of reconstruction for ACL rupture is indicated in high functioning individuals with good rehabilitation potential. It is possible to lead a normal life without an ACL.
- Ankle sprains are frequent and rarely require surgical intervention. However, X-ray examination should be performed to confirm this.

FURTHER READING

Orthobullets website www.orthobullets.com

Solomon, L., Warwick, D., Nayagan, D. (Eds.), 2010. Apley's System of Orthopaedics and Fractures. 9th ed. Hodder Arnold, London.

Soft tissue disorders 23

INTRODUCTION

Soft tissue disorders are common. They are responsible for many days of absence from work and contribute significantly to the workload in primary care, accident and emergency departments, rheumatology and orthopaedic clinics. This chapter will discuss their presentation, diagnosis and management.

TENDON LESIONS

The three main pathologies that affect tendons are:

- tendinopathy
- tenosynovitis
- rupture

Tendinopathy

Definition

Pain arises from strain or injury to tendons and their insertions to bone. The term enthesopathy is used to describe cases with a significant periosteal component, such as lateral or medial epicondylitis.

Aetiopathogenesis

The pathogenesis of tendinopathy is poorly understood. Some cases occur as part of a systemic inflammatory condition and others are related to injury from overuse. However, most cases of tendinopathy are idiopathic.

Clinical features

The most frequent sites of tendinopathy are:

- shoulder
- elbow
- Achilles tendon

Patients complain of pain that is worsened by active movement. Examination findings include:

- Tenderness of the tendon and its insertion.
- An increase in pain when active movement is performed against resistance.
- Soft tissue swelling (not always present).

Examples:

Rotator cuff (shoulder)—Beneath the acromion is the subacromial space. If this space becomes narrowed, irritation of supraspinatus can occur giving rise to tendinopathy.

Tennis elbow

The common extensor origin, at the lateral epicondyle, is tender and pain is exacerbated by resisted wrist extension (Fig. 23.1A).

Golfer's elbow

The common flexor origin, at the medial epicondyle, is tender and pain is exacerbated by resisted wrist flexion (Fig. 23.1B).

Investigation

Tendinopathy can be diagnosed clinically and investigations are often unremarkable. Radiographs may show abnormalities, such as calcification in chronic rotator cuff disease. Ultrasound scan and magnetic resonance imaging may also detect changes in the tendon and surrounding tissue.

Management

The interventions shown below may lead to improvement of symptoms. The strategies at the top of the list should be employed early in the disease process, whilst those at the bottom should be reserved for resistant cases:

- rest or avoidance of precipitating cause
- nonsteroidal antiinflammatory drug therapy
- physiotherapy
- local corticosteroid injection
- surgery

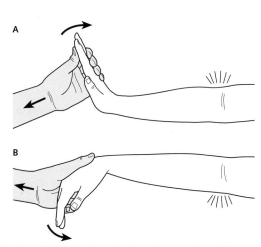

Fig. 23.1 The pain of tennis elbow is exacerbated by resisted wrist extension (A). The pain of golfer's elbow is exacerbated by resisted wrist flexion (B).

Tenosynovitis

Definition

Tenosynovitis is inflammation of the synovial lining of a tendon sheath.

Aetiology

The two main causes are:

- inflammatory arthritis
- trauma

Trauma is usually a result of repetitive or unaccustomed movement.

Clinical features

Patients present with pain in the region of the affected tendon. Common sites of tenosynovitis are the abductor pollicis longus and extensor pollicis brevis tendons (de Quervain tenosynovitis) and finger flexors. On examination, the tendon is swollen and tender and crepitus may be felt on palpation.

A trigger finger or thumb results from tenosynovitis of the flexor tendons. A nodule can develop on the tendon in response to constriction of the tendon sheath. The nodule catches as it enters or leaves the flexor tendon pulleys and a snapping or flicking movement of the digit occurs on flexion or extension. In severe cases, the digit may be held in flexion, requiring the patient to release the triggered digit with the other hand.

Management

Treatment includes rest, splinting and local corticosteroid injection. Surgical decompression of the tendon sheath may be required.

Tendon rupture

Aetiology

Tendon rupture may result from chronic inflammation and degeneration or trauma. For example, rupture of the extensor tendons of the fingers is often seen in rheumatoid arthritis.

Clinical features

The resulting clinical features are loss of movement at the joint to which the tendon provides power, deformity and sometimes swelling. After rupture of the long head of the biceps tendon, a bulge formed by the lateral muscle belly is seen in the upper arm: Popeye sign. Extensor tendon rupture at the distal phalanx can occur after a direct blow to the fingertip, causing aggressive flexion of the distal interphalangeal joint. It results in an inability to extend the flexed distal interphalangeal joint (mallet finger; Fig. 23.2).

Management

Sometimes no intervention is required, such as a long head of biceps tendon rupture, because function is preserved with

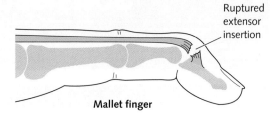

Fig. 23.2 Mallet finger.

other muscles: in that case, short head of biceps, brachialis and supinator. Sometimes splintage is all that is required: a mallet splint in the case of a mallet finger. However, surgery is often required to restore function. This may require direct repair of the tendon or a tendon transfer.

BURSITIS

Bursae are small sacs of fibrous tissue that are lined with synovial membrane and secrete synovial fluid. They reduce friction where ligaments and tendons pass over bone. Inflammation of a bursa (bursitis) can be idiopathic, part of a systemic inflammatory disease or due to injury, infection or gout. Some types are notifiable industrial disorders (e.g., coal miner's 'beat' knee).

Olecranon bursitis, prepatellar bursitis and trochanteric bursitis are common.

Olecranon bursitis

This can be precipitated by excessive friction at the elbow, for example by resting the elbow on a desk. Infection can occur in addition to olecranon bursitis, causing pain on elbow flexion. Idiopathic and traumatic cases are usually only painful when pressure is applied to the bursa; movement of the elbow is not usually uncomfortable or impaired. On examination, the bursa is distended and tender.

Bursal fluid should be aspirated only in cases of sepsis, to guide antibiotic treatment in a sick patient. It should not be routinely aspirated as the patient can develop a chronic sinus, which takes several months to settle. Local corticosteroid injection can help in nonseptic cases, but in most cases antiinflammatory medication and rest are preferable. Infection should be treated with appropriate antibiotics.

COMMUNICATION

Soft tissue lesions are commonly precipitated by injuries caused by overuse. It is therefore important to ask patients about their work and leisure activities.

Prepatellar or infrapatellar bursitis (housemaid's knee)

This type of bursitis is common in people such as carpet fitters who spend a lot of time kneeling. A hot, red swelling develops over the front of the patella (prepatellar bursitis) or patella tendon (infrapatellar bursitis). Active knee extension is usually quite painful. Infection and gout should be excluded by aspirating fluid. Treatment involves rest. Recurrent episodes may require surgical excision of the bursa. Antibiotic therapy should be given for sepsis.

Infected bursitis that fails to settle with antibiotics requires formal incision and drainage.

Trochanteric bursitis

The trochanteric bursa is located lateral to the greater trochanter of the femurs and allows motion of the fascia lata over the trochanter. When this bursa becomes inflamed, the patient will develop pain over the affected trochanter, exacerbated by movement. Patients will often complain of hip pain; however, careful questioning and examination will identify pain localized to the trochanter as opposed to the groin or buttock pain of hip joint pathology. Treatment consists of physiotherapy in the first instance, with steroid injections used in more severe cases. Persistent and debilitating trochanteric bursitis may require surgery.

DUPUYTREN CONTRACTURE

Definition

Dupuytren contracture is a common condition, characterized by fibromatosis of the palmar fascia, resulting in flexion contractures of the metacarpophalangeal and interphalangeal joints of one or more fingers.

Fibromatosis might affect other areas of the body: plantar fascia (Ledderhose disease), penis (Peyronie disease) or knuckle pads (Garrod disease). It is important to ask whether the patient has any symptoms or deformity elsewhere.

Incidence

Before the age of 55 years, the incidence of Dupuytren contracture is much higher in men than in women. After this age, the incidence is equal.

Aetiology

Several factors predispose to Dupuytren contracture. These are shown in the box, Clinical notes:

Factors associated with Dupuytren contracture. Historically, Dupuytren contracture was felt to be a disease of northern Europeans and whilst there is a preponderance, it is also common in those of Mediterranean or Japanese descent.

Clinical features

The ulnar side of the hand is most commonly affected. Patients complain of an inability to extend one or more fingers, usually the ring and little fingers. It is rarely (perhaps never) painful. The fibromatosis may remain stable or progress. Progressive cases can result in marked deformity and loss of function, with the fingers held in a fixed position curled into the palm.

In early cases, nodules may be felt in the palm or on the palmar surface of the finger. In more advanced cases, flexion at the metacarpophalangeal joints is seen (Fig. 23.3) and

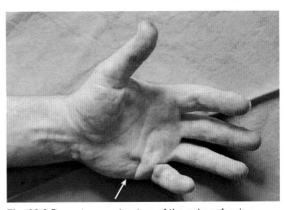

Fig. 23.3 Dupuytren contracture of the palmar fascia (*arrow*). From Hochberg MC, Silman AJ, Smolen JS, et al (eds): Rheumatology, 3rd ed. St Louis, Mosby, 2003.

the palm of the hand cannot be placed flat on a table (positive tabletop test). In severe cases, the proximal and distal interphalangeal joints are involved.

Management

The most effective treatment is surgery. The decision to progress to surgery can either be made when the patient has a positive tabletop test or when the deformity starts to affect the patient's quality of life. Palmar fasciectomy is the most commonly performed procedure. Complete correction of the deformity is more difficult the more advanced the disease. There is a risk of recurrence postoperatively.

Chapter Summary

- Tennis elbow affects the lateral epicondyle at the elbow.
- Golfer's elbow affects the lateral epicondyle at the elbow.
- Tendon rupture can be either traumatic or chronic. In some cases, such as in the Achilles tendon, it can be severely disabling.
- Bursitis is an inflammation of a bursa around a joint. It often settles down with antiinflammatory medication but it can occasionally become infected, requiring antibiotics.
- Dupuytren contracture involves a fibrous change in the palmar fascia causing thickening and fixed flexion of a digit. Multiple joints can be involved.

FURTHER READING

Orthobullets website www.orthobullets.com

Hazleman, B., Riley, G., Speed, C. (Eds.), 2004. Soft Tissue Rheumatology. Oxford University Press, Oxford.

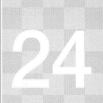
Most doctors will treat orthopaedic patients undergoing surgery during their career. However, the surgical procedure is only a very small part of the overall surgical process. This chapter aims to take you through the patient's journey, starting with the preoperative period, through the basics of orthopaedic surgery to postoperative management.

PREOPERATIVE ASSESSMENT

Patients undergoing elective surgery are seen a few weeks before surgery in the preoperative assessment clinic. It is important that concurrent medical problems are stabilized and new conditions identified, investigated and treated appropriately. Trauma patients are seen prior to surgery in a similar way to optimize their care prior to surgery.

General

The following should be recorded:

- Observations (blood pressure, pulse, temperature): the patient may have undiagnosed atrial fibrillation or hypertension.
- History, including past medical history and drug history: for example, the patient might be on warfarin and will need to stop taking it prior to surgery and might need admission for intravenous heparin if metallic valves are in place.
- Detailed systemic enquiry: the patient may have shortness of breath on exertion and chest pain (angina). After investigation, such patients might eventually have coronary bypass surgery prior to the orthopaedic operation.
- Examination: a detailed cardiorespiratory examination, e.g., the patient may have a heart murmur.
- Blood tests (unnecessary in young, fit patients for simple surgery): full blood count (FBC), glucose, urea and electrolytes (U&E), liver function tests and clotting screen. Arterial blood gases might be required if the patient has respiratory disease.
- Blood group should be identified for all major joint surgeries and cross-matched if significant blood loss is expected.
- Urinalysis for urinary tract infection (UTI). If a patient has a UTI, it should be treated prior to any orthopaedic operation that plans to leave metal work in situ.
- Electrocardiogram (EKG) and chest X-ray examination (if indicated).
- Further investigations should be ordered if required, e.g., echocardiogram in cases of aortic stenosis.

COMMUNICATION

Consent should be obtained from all patients and the correct joint or limb marked for theatre. In the case of elective joint surgery, this is a process occurring over the weeks and months prior to the procedure, with a member of the team capable of carrying out the operation. The signing of the consent form should be the culmination of a detailed consent process starting on the first clinic visit. It is no longer adequate for the most junior member of the team to place a form in front of the patient on the morning of surgery.

Local

The patient should be asked whether the limb is still painful because the surgery might be unnecessary.

The limb is examined.

Note skin condition (there might be a rash or skin breakdown over the operation site), pulses and range of movement and look for any distal infection. For example, a knee replacement procedure should not be carried out in a patient with an infected ingrowing toenail.

IMMEDIATE PREOPERATIVE CARE

Additional monitoring such as an arterial line and central venous line can be inserted in the anaesthetic room for patients expected to have a complicated anaesthetic.

A urinary catheter is important to assess fluid balance in patients who may lose significant amounts of blood.

SURGERY

There are several things a surgeon can do for a painful joint.

Joint debridement

A diseased joint can be debrided surgically in an attempt to improve range of movement or to reduce symptoms such as pain and swelling. Osteophytes are often removed in osteoarthritis but debriding a joint does not cure or stop the progression of the disease process, e.g., a cheilectomy of the first metatarsophalangeal (MTP) joint (Fig. 24.1).

Arthroscopy

Keyhole surgery techniques have become routine in recent years.

In the past, arthroscopy was seen as a diagnostic procedure, but now a number of operations are possible by purely arthroscopic means. Examples are stabilization or rotator cuff repair in the shoulder and meniscal repair or anterior cruciate ligament reconstruction in the knee.

It is now commonplace for arthroscopy to be used on many joints, including the knee, shoulder, ankle, hip and wrist.

Joint excision (excision arthroplasty)

This operation has been mostly superseded by joint replacement. It is still occasionally performed for severe arthritis of the first MTP joint (Keller procedure) and also in the hip (Girdlestone procedure) if the patient has had an infected joint (Fig. 24.2).

The operation leaves the joint unstable and it may still be painful.

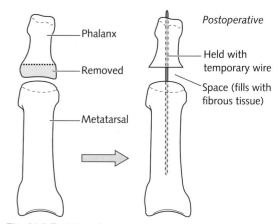

Fig. 24.2 Excision of a joint.

Joint arthrodesis

Arthrodesis or fusion is performed to make the bones heal across a joint. Movement is obviously lost, but if the fusion is sound, the joint will be strong and pain free.

Bones are most commonly fused around the foot and ankle or hand and wrist, usually in patients with rheumatoid arthritis. Examples include ankle fusion, subtalar fusion and wrist fusion.

Fusion can be achieved by different means, such as:

- internal fixation such as screws, staples, plates (Fig. 24.3A)
- intramedullary nail (Fig. 24.3B)
- external fixation (Fig. 24.7)

A bone graft may be used to encourage union.

Joint arthroplasty

Almost any joint can now be replaced. Pain is the primary reason to replace a joint.

The advantage of replacement over fusion is that movement is maintained and therefore function can return to near normality.

Implants are usually made from metal; however, the actual bearing surfaces can be made from a combination of a metal, high-density polyethylene or ceramic. The joint surfaces are highly polished for low friction.

The joint components are either cemented in place or uncemented.

Joint replacements are available for almost any joint, although the most commonly performed are:

- knee (Fig. 24.4)
- hip (Fig. 24.5)
- shoulder

The majority of replacements should last more than 15 years, but this is partly dependent on the patient. A young patient is more likely to wear out a prosthesis due to higher demand.

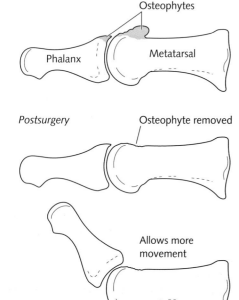

First metatarsophalangeal joint arthritis

Osteophytes

Phalanx   Metatarsal

Postsurgery   Osteophyte removed

Allows more movement

Fig. 24.1 First MTP joint cheilectomy.

A

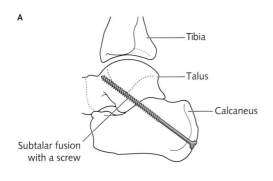

- Tibia
- Talus
- Calcaneus

Subtalar fusion with a screw

B

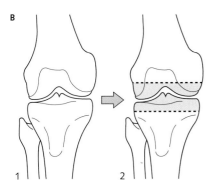

1   2

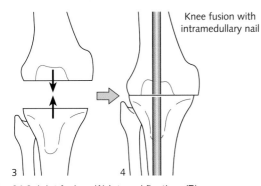

Knee fusion with intramedullary nail

3   4

Fig. 24.3 Joint fusion. (A) Internal fixation. (B) Intramedullary nail.

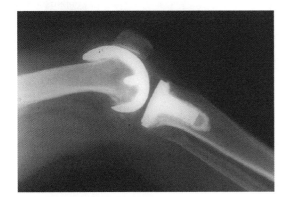

Fig. 24.4 Total knee replacement.

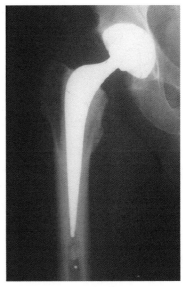

Fig. 24.5 Total hip replacement.

The most common reasons for failure of an implant are loosening, infection and fracture (Fig. 24.6).

HINTS AND TIPS

INFECTED ARTHROPLASTY

Replaced joints are often red in the early postoperative phase and care should be taken before giving antibiotics if infection is suspected. Samples should be taken (preferably in theatre) unless the patient is septic, prior to giving antibiotics, because such medication will make any samples less likely to grow on culture. Ultimately, infection in a joint replacement is unlikely to be cleared by antibiotics alone and often requires two-stage revision.

Osteotomy/deformity correction

An osteotomy is an operation to cut a bone and realign the joint or deformity.

The most common place for this to occur is the first ray of the foot, in the case of hallux valgus. Osteotomies are also performed at the knee to offload arthritic compartments in younger patients, reducing pain and postponing the need for arthroplasty.

Deformity can occur for other reasons such as malunion of fractures (tibia and femur) and congenital deformity (e.g., clubfoot) and correction of such deformity is an important part of orthopaedic surgery.

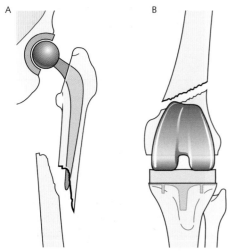

Fig. 24.6 Periprosthetic fracture of the femur: (A) at the hip; (B) at the knee.

It is also possible to lengthen bones gradually with external fixation, usually in the form of circular frames with a variety of hinges and movable rods (Fig. 24.7).

Synovectomy

In the case of inflammatory arthritides, a synovectomy may be performed. The aim of this operation is to remove the synovial lining of the diseased joint or the tenosynovium around tendons. The procedure needs to be performed early and has three possible beneficial effects:

- reduction of swelling
- slowing of disease progression
- prevention of tendon rupture

Unfortunately, it is impossible to remove the whole synovium with synovectomy and symptoms often return. This procedure is usually performed around the wrist.

POSTOPERATIVE CARE

General

Patients are taken to recovery until fully awake, then they are transferred to the ward. High-risk patients might need to be transferred to a high-dependency unit or intensive therapy unit.

Regular recordings are made of blood pressure, pulse and oxygen saturation.

Adequate pain relief is very important.

After major surgery requiring an inpatient stay, patients will need:

- FBC and U&E checked the day after surgery.
- X-ray examination of the operated joint.

Once patients are well, every effort is made to mobilize them and encourage early safe discharge. Deep vein thrombosis (DVT) prophylaxis is continued until patients are fully mobile.

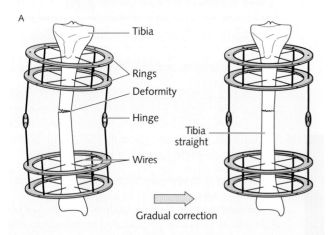
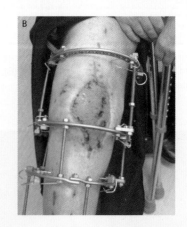

Fig. 24.7 Deformity correction with frames. (A) The use of an external fixator frame to achieve gradual correction of a deformity over several weeks. Note that the frame is also bent but straightens out as the bone is corrected. (B) Ilizarov frame on a fractured tibia. (With permission from Sala F, Catagni M, Pili D, Capitani P, Elbow arthrodesis for post-traumatic sequelae: surgical tactics using the Ilizarov frame; J Shoulder Elbow Surg, 2015 24(11):1757–1763).

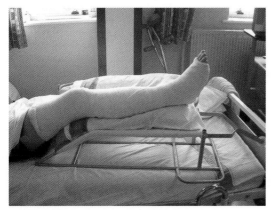

Fig. 24.8 Braun frame used to elevate a lower limb.

A multidisciplinary approach is needed to achieve this with input from physiotherapy, occupational therapy, social workers, nursing staff and sometimes physicians.

Home modifications might be required for patients after joint arthroplasty, but they generally return to having very good function.

Local

Elevation in a Bradford sling (for an arm) or on a Braun frame (Fig. 24.8) is very important to reduce swelling.

Distal neurovascular observations are performed to check the perfusion and function of the limb distal to the operation.

Physiotherapy is encouraged as soon as possible to mobilize the limb.

COMPLICATIONS

Any surgical procedure has risks and complications and knowledge of these helps minimize and prevent them.

Patients need to be made aware of these important complications before informed consent is obtained.

Complications are divided into:

- local (specific to that operation)
- general (common to any operation)

We further subdivide complication on the basis of the time that has elapsed after surgery into:

- immediate (within 24 hours)
- early (days/weeks)
- late (months/years)

General respiratory

Chest infections

Complications affecting the respiratory system are very common postoperatively.

A chest infection typically presents early with fever and shortness of breath. Elderly patients may be confused.

There may be signs of consolidation on examination and a low PO_2.

Treatment is with physiotherapy, nebulizers and antibiotics.

Venous thromboembolism

Immobile orthopaedic patients with traumatized limbs are very susceptible to DVT. Risk is reduced by mechanical aids (foot pumps, graduated compression stockings) and chemical agents (heparin, Clexane, aspirin, warfarin) and early mobilization.

If the clot propagates and then breaks off, it travels to the lungs (a pulmonary embolus), which can be fatal. The patient becomes acutely short of breath and has pleuritic chest pain with signs of tachycardia, tachypnoea and a low PO_2. An EKG might show a sinus tachycardia, arrhythmias or the classic, but rare, S1Q3T3.

Treatment should be started immediately in the form of low-molecular-weight subcutaneous heparin if suspected and diagnosis is proven with a computed tomographic pulmonary angiogram (CTPA).

Cardiac

Myocardial infarction

Myocardial infarction (MI) is a relatively common postoperative complication, particularly in the elderly or those with preexisting heart disease. Patients do not always have typical central crushing chest pain radiating to the left arm associated with sweating and nausea and the cardiac event might be silent or occur during anaesthesia. This should be suspected in any patient with unexplained hypotension.

Diagnosis is made based on EKGs and elevated troponin cardiac enzymes.

Treatment includes oxygen and aspirin. Further agents can be used based on advice from the physicians (it is usually impossible to give thrombolytic drugs to postoperative patients owing to the risk of bleeding).

Left ventricular failure

This can result from a cardiac event or from aggressive fluid management over the perioperative period. It is important not to give too much fluid, particularly to elderly patients with little physiological reserve.

These patients present with shortness of breath and signs include a raised jugular venous pressure and bibasilar crackles. Simple measures such as sitting the patient up and giving oxygen can dramatically improve the patient's condition. Further treatment includes diuretics, morphine/diamorphine and nitrates.

Blood loss and blood transfusion

Most patients do not require a blood transfusion postoperatively, even after a total hip or knee replacement. Blood transfusions are expensive (£400 per unit) and are associated with transfusion reactions, transmission of infections (hepatitis, human immunodeficiency virus (HIV), variant Creutzfeldt-Jakob disease) and immunosuppression. Blood should therefore be prescribed sparingly. Most patients can tolerate haemoglobin of 80 g/L, although higher values are often aimed for in those with known ischaemia.

Gastrointestinal

Bleeding

The most important complication of the gastrointestinal (GI) system is bleeding and the most common reason for this on orthopaedic wards is nonsteroidal antiinflammatory drug (NSAID) therapy.

Patients with haematemesis or melaena have a suspected upper GI bleed until proven otherwise. Diagnosis is confirmed with upper GI endoscopies performed as soon as possible. Supportive measures including starting a proton pump inhibitor, cross-matching blood, fluid resuscitation, careful observations and oxygen if required.

Referral to a gastroenterologist or surgeon is needed.

Paralytic ileus

This is a less serious complication presenting with abdominal distension and nausea. Operations or trauma to the spine predispose to ileus, which usually spontaneously corrects after a few days on intravenous fluids and a nasogastric tube.

Renal

Renal failure

Preexisting renal impairment is common in orthopaedic patients and the additional burden of a fracture or surgery with the associated blood loss can tip the balance, causing renal failure.

Factors influencing the development of renal failure include drugs (diuretics, NSAIDs, antibiotics) and hypovolaemia. It is very important to keep patients well hydrated with enough fluid to prevent prerenal failure.

Careful monitoring of fluid input with hourly urine output and daily U&E measurement is important when assessing such a patient.

HINTS AND TIPS

FLUID

Low urinary output postoperatively is almost always due to hypovolaemia and patients require fluid. It is very important to assess fluid balance carefully, so that diuretics are not given to such patients just to increase the output. This may precipitate renal failure!

Urinary tract infection

Postoperative UTIs are very common. Diagnosis is made on urinalysis and a midstream urine sample is sent to microbiology. Generic antibiotics are started after samples have been taken and refined once sensitivity results are known.

Local

Table 24.1 lists local complications, their timing, causes, signs and symptoms and management.

INFECTION

Infection is the major concern in elective orthopaedic surgery. Deep infection in joint replacement surgery is disastrous when it occurs as simple measures such as antibiotics and abscess drainage will not eradicate the infection. The patient may be worse off than before surgery and might require lengthy hospital stays with extensive further surgery and significant risks.

The risk of infection is minimized by the following preoperative, perioperative and postoperative factors.

Preoperative factors

- cleaning the skin
- avoidance of concurrent infection (e.g., UTI)
- preoperative antibiotics on induction of anaesthesia
- a healthy, well-nourished patient

Perioperative factors

- clean laminar airflow theatre (air is specially filtered)
- adequate skin preparation and impervious exclusion drapes
- sterile instruments and prostheses
- careful surgical technique (including haemostasis)
- the use of antibiotic-loaded cement in joint arthroplasty

Postoperative factors

- wound dressing
- prophylactic antibiotics for possible bacteraemia (e.g., during catheterization)
- postoperative antibiotics

SHOCK

Shock is defined as an inability to maintain adequate tissue perfusion and oxygenation.

Every doctor should be able to recognize shock.

On the orthopaedic wards, the most likely causes are hypovolaemic, septic and cardiogenic shock, although neurogenic shock can occur when setting major trauma. Anaphylactic shock is less common, but possible if patients are allergic to drugs or latex.

Table 24.1 Local complications of orthopaedic surgery

Postoperative timing	Complication	Cause	Signs/symptoms	Management
Immediate up to first 24 hours	Tight cast	Swelling Dressing/cast too tight	Pain, tingling in toes/fingers Poor distal perfusion Numbness Ischaemia of limb	Elevation Split cast
	Compartment syndrome	Swelling in a closed fascial compartment (usually postfracture)	Pain: pain on passive stretch, tense compartments Altered sensation	Fasciotomy
	Primary haemorrhage	Technical problem at surgical site, e.g., bleeding vessel Other risk factors include: major surgery, e.g., total hip replacement; drugs, e.g., warfarin; obesity	Haemodynamic instability Anxiety Slow capillary refill Tachycardia Hypotension Low urine output Confusion	Replace losses: fluids ± blood Reverse cause, e.g., warfarin Pressure dressing Clamp drains If heavy bleeding, reexamine wound
	Nerve injury	Usually retractor, e.g., sciatic nerve in hip replacement	Pain, weakness, paraesthesia	Wait and see Usually recovers
Early up to first 4 weeks	Secondary haemorrhage	Occurs at 5–10 days, usually secondary to infection	Bleeding with signs of infection	Treat infection Wound debridement and washout
	Infection (see Chapter 20)	Infection at time of surgery Can occur later with haematogenous seeding	Early: red, hot, swollen, discharging, temperature Late: persistent pain, loosening of prosthesis	Early: debridement and washout Late: removal of implant and debridement Reimplantation at second stage once infection treated
	Wound dehiscence (breakdown)	Within first week: usually due to poor surgical technique Later: invariably infection and poor healing	Wound gapes open Other features in keeping with infection may be present	Early: clean wounds are taken back to theatre for primary closure Later: treat infection as above
Late (in theory these can occur at any time)	Dislocation of total hip replacement	Patient: inappropriate patient activity, poor stem or cup position Excessive wear Infection	Severe pain, shortening External rotation (anterior) Internal rotation (posterior)	Reduce hip Abduction brace for 6 weeks if early Revision surgery if there is a problem with position of implant
	Periprosthetic fracture	Intraoperative: if a prosthesis is too big for the bone when inserted Late: loosening of the prosthesis, infection or trauma	Increased pain, deformity, unable to bear weight	Intraoperative: fixation of fracture Late: revision of prosthesis
	Heterotopic ossification	Abnormal bone formation in soft tissues: more common in head-injured patients and with hip surgery or trauma	Stiffness	Surgical excision and immediate nonsteroidal antiinflammatory drugs or radiotherapy postoperatively
	Aseptic loosening	Loosening of prosthesis occurs because particle wear of the implant triggers macrophages. These cause osteolysis around the prosthesis	Pain, instability	Revision of the prosthesis

Hypovolaemic

Haemorrhage is the most likely cause of hypovolaemic shock, which is due to inadequate circulatory volume. These patients require intravenous fluids and sometimes blood to restore blood pressure. Postoperative patients may also be behind with their fluid balance and those who have undergone spinal anaesthesia may be hypovolaemic due to venous pooling caused by the spinal anaesthetic.

Cardiogenic

The heart is unable to maintain adequate cardiac output, usually because of infarction. Intravenous fluids may further overload the heart and positive inotropes such as noradrenaline (norepinephrine) may be required.

Neurogenic

This is due to peripheral vasodilatation secondary to injury to the central nervous system.

It is important not to overload such a patient with fluid in an attempt to raise the blood pressure (the blood pressure remains low because of loss of peripheral resistance). A systolic blood pressure of 100 mmHg is normally acceptable in these patients.

Septic

Peripheral vasodilatation is due to bacterial endotoxins in severe infection. Patients require intravenous antibiotics, whilst receiving haemodynamic support.

Anaphylactic shock

This occurs in patients already sensitized to an allergen. There is an aggressive immune response resulting in massive histamine release from basophils. The patient may rapidly deteriorate and develop generalized urticaria, with stridor (upper-airway narrowing), wheeze and shortness of breath. There is massive vasodilatation and tachycardia associated with hypotension. Treatment should be rapid, including emergency airway procedures, oxygen, nebulizers, intravenous hydrocortisone, antihistamines (chlorphenamine) and intramuscular or intravenous adrenaline (epinephrine) and fluid resuscitation.

Treatment

Basic treatment for shock should be instituted immediately and includes oxygen therapy and fluid resuscitation, with catheterization to monitor urine output and regular observation. Admission to a high-dependency unit should be considered if the patient is unstable or requires intensive input.

● Chapter Summary

- A preoperative assessment is vital prior to performing surgery because this is the stage at which potential perioperative problems can be identified and managed. A poor preassessment often causes delays or cancellations on an operating list.
- Arthroplasty for osteoarthritis and rheumatoid arthritis has been around for many years and is considered to be highly successful. If a hip replacement patient is fortunate enough to avoid complications, they are usually very happy with their outcome.
- Basic postoperative care involves regular observation and careful fluid management. Some patients may require a higher level of care. Postoperative blood tests are frequently done and most orthopaedic operations will require a postoperative X-ray examination.
- Complications of surgery are listed in detail in Table 24.1. These are a very common exam question and extra attention should be paid to them.
- Complications of orthopaedic surgery are reduced where possible. DVT prophylaxis is now standard, patients are mobilized quickly after surgery, blocks are given preoperatively to reduce pain postoperatively and to speed up recovery, transfusions are given to keep blood counts above 8 g/dL and many other changes are made to mitigate surgical risks.
- Infection is a devastating complication in arthroplasty and necessitates the removal of all components and a staged revision.

FURTHER READING

Canale, S.T., 2006. Campbell's Operative Orthopaedics, 11th ed, 1–4. Mosby, St Louis

Sweetland, H., Conway, K., 2004. Crash Course in Surgery. Mosby, Edinburgh. www.orthobullets.com

SELF-ASSESSMENT

Single best answer (SBA) questions

Chapter 1 Taking a history

1. A 55-year-old woman develops tingling and umbness in the radial 3.5 fingers of her right hand. Which is the most relevant part of her medical history to be considered in the diagnosis?
   A. A family history of hypertension.
   B. A drug history including nonsteroidal use.
   C. A medical history of underactive thyroid.
   D. A social history of working as an accountant.
   E. A systemic enquiry revealing marked fatigue.

2. A 55-year-old woman presents with a fragility fracture. She undergoes a dual-energy X-ray absorptiometry (DEXA) scan revealing osteoporosis. Which of the following is the most important in terms of her medical history?
   A. A family history of traumatic hip fracture.
   B. Prednisolone 10 mg daily for several years for poorly controlled asthma.
   C. Menopause aged 53 years.
   D. Living in South America for several years.
   E. A personal history of type 2 diabetes mellitus.

3. A 64-year-old man presents with severe pain in his fingertips and skin colour changes (see image). What in his history would help differentiate between primary and secondary Raynaud disease?
   A. A recent history of difficulty in swallowing.
   B. A social history of alcohol misuse.
   C. A family history of osteoarthritis.
   D. A drug history of nifedipine use.
   E. A medical history of chronic obstructive pulmonary disease (COPD).

4. A 44-year-old normally fit and well woman presents with bilateral swollen ankles and knee joints, which occurred a few weeks after a chest infection. The joints are warm and stiff for 2 hours upon waking. She has not been experiencing fever. She feels tired but is otherwise well. Her family history includes a brother with ankylosing spondylitis. What is the likely diagnosis based on the history?
   A. Gout.
   B. Rheumatoid arthritis.
   C. Ankylosing spondylitis.
   D. Reactive arthritis.
   E. Septic arthritis.

Chapter 2 Examining joints

1. A 38-year-old electrician presents with a painful swollen right knee. His knee has become progressively more painful and swollen over a week. On examination, there is a large erythematous swelling anterior to the patella, which is tender to palpate. The skin appears thickened. There is no effusion in the knee joint. He is able to flex his knee to 45 degrees before he is limited by a combination of pain and tightness.
   What is the likely diagnosis?
   A. Osteoarthritis.
   B. Septic arthritis.
   C. Baker cyst.
   D. Patellar fracture.
   E. Prepatellar bursitis.

2. What causes a locked knee?
   A. Anterior cruciate ligament tear.
   B. Radial medical tear.
   C. Medial collateral ligament tear.
   D. Bucket-handle meniscal tear.
   E. Tibial plateau fracture.

3. A patient with an acquired foot drop will most likely present with which type of gait?
   A. Trendelenburg.
   B. Antalgic.
   C. Circumduction.
   D. Waddling.
   E. High-stepping

4. A young man experiences a wrist fracture while skiing. Afterwards, he is unable to lift his thumb off a table when the hand is placed flat. The tendon of which muscle has likely been damaged?
   A. Adductor pollicis.
   B. Extensor pollicis longus (EPL).
   C. Abductor pollicis brevis.
   D. Opponens pollicis.
   E. Extensor digitorum.

5. A patient with a severe burning sensation in her hands presents with bilateral thenar and hypothenar wasting. The pain occurs over her thumb, index finger and middle finger. She has a history of hypothyroidism. What is the most likely cause of her symptoms and signs?

A. Carpal tunnel syndrome.
B. Hypothyroid-related peripheral neuropathy.
C. Peripheral vascular disease.
D. C8 radiculopathy.
E. Golfer's elbow.

Chapter 3 Investigations

1. A 33-year-old Asian woman presents to her physician complaining of fatigue, myalgia and weight loss. She finds it more painful to bear weight compared with 6 months ago. She is losing her hair and there is a non-itchy rash over her nose and cheeks.
    Which test is most likely to confirm the diagnosis?
    A. Anti-double stranded DNA antibodies.
    B. Eerythrocyte sedimentation rate (ESR).
    C. Skin biopsy of the rash.
    D. Thyroid function tests.
    E. MRI of her hips.

2. A 68-year-old woman presents to her GP with fatigue. She has a history of rheumatoid arthritis and has recently had several flares requiring her medication to be increased. The GP performs some blood tests:

Liver function:

Alkaline phosphatase	78 (range 44–147)
Aspartate aminotransferase (AST)	138 (range 10–40)
Alanine aminotransferase (ALT)	179 (range 10–56)
γ-glutamyl transpeptidase (GGT)	36 (range 3–48)
Bilirubin	17 (range 0–22)

   What is the likely cause of the above results?
    A. Primary biliary cirrhosis.
    B. Methotrexate hepatotoxicity.
    C. Acute viral hepatitis due to immunocompromised state.
    D. Gallstones.
    E. Alcohol.

3. A 28-year-old woman presents with Raynaud phenomenon, which ulcerated last winter, progressive tightness in her hands and small red dots on her chest that branch out like spiders.
    Which antibody is she likely to have?
    A. Jo-1.
    B. Anti-dsDNA.
    C. Anti-SCL-70.
    D. p-ANCA.
    E. Histone.

4. A 45-year-old man is getting out of a car when he twists his leg and feels a pop in his knee. He is immediately unable to bear his weight and the joint proceeds to swell.

Which investigation will be most helpful in arriving at a diagnosis?
    A. Joint aspiration.
    B. X-ray knee.
    C. Ultrasound scan (USS).
    D. MRI.
    E. Erythrocyte sedimentation rate (ESR).

Chapter 4 Regional pain

1. A 68-year-old woman presents with a history of lower back pain and fatigue.
    Which of the following additional findings with regard to back pain would warrant urgent investigations?
    A. A history of urinary incontinence.
    B. A raised erythrocyte sedimentation rate (ESR).
    C. A family history of psoriasis.
    D. Abnormal thyroid function tests (TFTs).
    E. A positive antinuclear antibody (ANA; 1:40).

2. A young woman presents to A&E after playing sports. She twisted and felt a pop in her knee and now the joint is swollen, tense and tender.
    Joint aspiration is undertaken: the fluid is bloodied with white/yellow globules mixed in.
    What does the aspirate imply?
    A. A rheumatoid knee.
    B. Ruptured anterior cruciate ligament (ACL).
    C. Septic arthritis.
    D. Patellar dislocation.
    E. Pseudo gout.

3. A 61-year-old retired bricklayer presents with chronic back pain. His pain is exacerbated by walking, particularly downhill, and radiates into his buttocks, thighs and calves bilaterally. Examination shows a stooped gait with reduced motion in the lumbar spine. His symptoms are worsened by extension of the spine.
    What is the diagnosis?
    A. Prolapsed intervertebral disc.
    B. Mechanical back pain.
    C. Spinal stenosis.
    D. Spondylolisthesis.
    E. Spinal malignancy.

4. A 77-year-old man has bilateral shoulder pain, which is aching in nature, stiffness and difficulty in dressing. He is also fatigued, more so over the past 3 months.
    Which test is the most useful in establishing the diagnosis?
    A. Nerve conducting studies.
    B. Bilateral shoulder X-ray image.
    C. Urinary Bence Jones protein.
    D. Erythrocyte sedimentation rate (ESR).
    E. MRI of the neck.

5. Following a stroke, a patient develops severe hand pain, with skin changes, hypersensitivity and arm swelling.
   What is the diagnosis?
   A. Arterial insufficiency.
   B. Upper limb deep vein thrombosis (DVT).
   C. Factitious pain.
   D. Phantom-limb pain.
   E. Complex regional pain syndrome.

Chapter 5 Widespread musculoskeletal pain

1. A 68-year-old woman presents with bilateral hip and shoulder pain. She has an elevated erythrocyte sedimentation rate (ESR; 68). She is prescribed steroids and a provisional diagnosis of polymyalgia rheumatic (PMR) is reached.
   Two months later she is seen in clinic and despite the steroids she is still symptomatic, has developed synovitis and has lost 2 stone in weight.
   What is the next investigation to consider?
   A. CT thorax, abdomen and pelvis.
   B. Vitamin D.
   C. Muscle biopsy.
   D. Check rheumatoid factor.
   E. Skeletal survey.

2. A 35-year-old Asian woman presents with widespread pain, fatigue, dry eyes and a rash over her nose and cheeks.
   Which is the best test to confirm the diagnosis?
   A. Erythrocyte sedimentation rate (ESR).
   B. Anti-dsDNA antibodies.
   C. Schirmer test.
   D. Rheumatoid factor.
   E. Urine dip.

3. A 38-year-old woman presents with pain throughout the shoulders, arms and hip girdle. She has intermittent loose stools/constipation, low mood and severe fatigue.
   Investigations show the following:

Erythrocyte sedimentation rate	9 mm/h (normal 0–29 mm/h)
Calcium	2.27 mmol/L (normal 2.20–2.70 mmol/L)
Vitamin D	78 nmol/L (normal 70–100 nmol/L)

Which of the following drugs would you consider using in treating her condition?
   A. Naproxen.
   B. Adalimumab.
   C. Pregabalin.

D. Methotrexate.
E. Oxycodone.

4. A 42-year-old woman is unable to walk. She has focal neurological findings indicative of a specific neurological lesion but is tender over her greater trochanters, lower back and quadriceps. She is tearful and discloses a history of insomnia and intermittent paraesthesia. She has pain in 14/18 trigger points.
   Her initial blood tests are normal. Her chest X-ray and EKG are similarly unremarkable.
   What is the next best step?
   A. MRI of the spine.
   B. Autoimmune profile.
   C. Electromyography.
   D. Reassurance.
   E. Intravenous immunoglobulins.

5. Which of the following are not typical features of fibromyalgia?
   A. Altered sleeping pattern.
   B. Pain in multiple tender points.
   C. Altered bowel habit.
   D. Headache.
   E. Foot drop.

Chapter 6 An acute hot swollen joint

1. A 62-year-old diabetic woman presents with an acutely hot swollen right knee. She has recently been treated for a foot ulcer. She is febrile.
   Her bloods show a white cell count of 15.5 and a C-reactive protein of 113.
   What will her joint aspirate most likely show?
   A. Gram-positive cocci.
   B. Gram-negative bacilli.
   C. Needle-shaped negatively birefringent crystals.
   D. Rod-shaped positively birefringent crystals.
   E. Blood.

2. A 25-year-old man presents with acute monoarthritis of the left knee. He has a history of an itchy, flaky rash affecting the knees and his lower back. He has had painful distal finger joints in the past.
   How would you start to treat his condition?
   A. Antibiotics.
   B. Disease-modifying antirheumatic drugs (DMARDs).
   C. Paracetamol.
   D. High dose steroids.
   E. Topical emollients.

3. A 48-year-old man presents with acute arthritis of the right ankle. The joint is red and inflamed and he has difficulty bearing weight on it.

Which of the following features would favour gout rather than septic arthritis?

A. A low-grade fever.
B. A high C-reactive protein (CRP).
C. A previous history of right ankle swelling and pain.
D. A history of immunosuppression.
E. A family history of rheumatoid arthritis.

Chapter 7 A child with a limp

1. Which of the following is not a risk factor in the development of Perthes disease?
   A. Delayed bone age.
   B. Hypothyroidism.
   C. Low socioeconomic group.
   D. Low-birthweight children.
   E. Family history.

2. A 13-year-old overweight boy presents with severe right hip pain, with a background of 2 weeks of groin pain. There is no history of trauma and he is otherwise well. He is unable to bear his weight, holds his hip in external rotation and flexion and has a decreased range of motion in all axes because of pain. Inflammatory markers are normal. What is the likely diagnosis?
   A. Perthes disease.
   B. Septic arthritis.
   C. Neck of femur fracture.
   D. Osteoarthritis.
   E. Slipped upper femoral epiphysis.

3. A 3-year-old girl is brought to A&E by her mother with a 24-hour history of a left leg limp. Her mother states there is no history of trauma. The child localizes the pain to her groin. The patient has an unremarkable medical history, although her mother notes she had a cold last week. On examination, the child is apyrexial and is systemically well. She is refusing to bear her weight fully and has a decreased range of motion in all axes secondary to pain. X-ray examination shows no abnormality and her blood tests are normal.
   What is the likely diagnosis?
   A. Transient synovitis.
   B. Septic arthritis.
   C. Slipped upper femoral epiphysis.
   D. Perthes disease.
   E. Malignancy.

4. A 7-year-old boy is brought to A&E by his father having been in pain for 6 hours and with reduced range of motion in his hip. He was recently admitted with pneumonia. He appears unwell and is febrile. His pulse is elevated and he is clammy to the touch.
   What is the most appropriate next step?

A. Aspiration of the painful joint.
B. Await blood tests and await culture results to direct treatment.
C. Ultrasound scan hip.
D. Immediate resuscitation and IV antibiotics.
E. X-ray examination of both hips.

Chapter 8 A limb swelling

1. A normally fit and well 45-year-old woman presents to her GP with a lump on her wrist. She describes a 1-year history of a marble-sized lump on the volar aspect of her wrist. She states the lump comes and goes and is not painful. On examination, there is a 1 × 1 cm fluctuant lesion on the volar aspect of her left wrist. It is fixed to underlying tissues.
   What is the most likely diagnosis?
   A. Soft-tissue sarcoma.
   B. Lipoma.
   C. Ganglion.
   D. Osteophyte.
   E. Rheumatoid nodule.

2. A 73-year-old lady reports symptoms of pain and a large lump in her thigh. She is kept awake at night by this and has been struggling to bear her weight. She reports weight loss and informs you she was diagnosed with Paget disease several years ago. What is the most likely diagnosis?
   A. Osteosarcoma.
   B. Lipoma.
   C. Osteophyte.
   D. Ewing sarcoma.
   E. Deep vein thrombosis.

3. A 44-year-old lady presents with a complaint of a lump on the back of her leg behind the knee. She reports it is painless and has been there for several months not changing in size. She is walking normally and does not report night pain. On examination, it is soft, immobile and transilluminates.
   What is the most likely diagnosis?
   A. Popliteal aneurysm.
   B. Osteochondroma.
   C. Lipoma.
   D. Baker cyst.
   E. Sebaceous cyst.

Chapter 9 Back pain

1. In the case of a prolapsed vertebral disc, pain is caused when the nerve root is compressed by:
   A. Annulus fibrosis.
   B. Posterior longitudinal ligament.
   C. Ligamentum flavum.
   D. Nucleus pulposus.
   E. Interspinous ligament.

2. Which of the following is a sign of impending cauda equina syndrome?
   A. Severe unilateral sciatic-type pain.
   B. Bilateral sciatic-type pain.
   C. Prolonged duration of symptoms.
   D. Leg pain and altered sensation.
   E. Muscle weakness.

3. Which is the most important investigation in diagnosing impending cauda equina syndrome?
   A. Blood test including urea and electrolytes, C-reactive protein and white cell count.
   B. MRI scan.
   C. CT scan.
   D. X-ray examination.
   E. White cell count scan.

4. A 61-year-old retired bricklayer presents with chronic back pain. He describes his pain as exacerbated by walking, particularly downhill, and radiating into his buttocks, thighs and calves bilaterally. Examination reveals a stooped gait and a reduced range of motion in the lumbar spine. His symptoms are exacerbated by extension of the spine.
   What is the diagnosis?
   A. Prolapsed intervertebral disc.
   B. Mechanical back pain.
   C. Spinal stenosis.
   D. Spondylolisthesis.
   E. Spinal malignancy.

5. A 72-year-old male presents with back pain and mild weakness in both legs. An X-ray examination is performed and shows a sclerotic lesion in the L5 vertebrae. What is the most likely underlying diagnosis causing this man's problem?
   A. Multiple myeloma.
   B. Malignant sarcoma.
   C. Metastatic prostate cancer.
   D. Metastatic lung cancer.
   E. Paget disease.

Chapter 10 Altered sensation and weakness

1. A distal radius fracture with significant dorsal angulation is most likely to cause altered sensation in the distribution of which nerve:
   A. Ulnar nerve.
   B. Superficial radial nerve.
   C. Medial cutaneous nerve of the forearm.
   D. Median nerve.
   E. Axillary nerve.

2. A 56-year-old woman with rheumatoid arthritis presents to her GP with a 6-month history of altered sensation and pain in both her hands, the right worse than the left. She describes pins and needle in her index, middle and ring fingers and pain at night, which frequently wakens her from sleep. She also describes decreased grip strength. On examination, there is wasting of the thenar eminences and percussion at the wrist crease exacerbates her symptoms.
   What is the diagnosis?
   A. Cervical radiculopathy.
   B. Cubital tunnel syndrome.
   C. Peripheral neuropathy.
   D. Carpal tunnel syndrome.
   E. Transient ischaemic attacks.

3. A patient presents with numbness in the hand, worse at night, in the radial three digits. It passes off rapidly, but she has begun to notice loss of fine movements in the hand. Which of these tests will be most helpful in confirming the diagnosis?
   A. Blood tests including urea and electrolytes, C-reactive protein and full blood count.
   B. MRI cervical spine.
   C. Nerve conduction studies.
   D. X-ray examination of the wrist.
   E. CT of the brain.

4. A 67-year-old lady with a previous history of myocardial infarction presents with numbness and tingling in her left arm of only 6 hours' duration. She is mildly confused and has 60% power in the left arm with numbness throughout. What is the likely diagnosis?
   A. Transient ischaemic attack (TIA).
   B. Carpal tunnel syndrome.
   C. Brachial plexus injury.
   D. Prolapsed cervical disc.
   E. Ulnar nerve entrapment.

Chapter 11 Osteoarthritis

1. Which of the following is not a typical finding from an X-ray examination in osteoarthritis?
   A. Lytic bone lesions.
   B. Joint space narrowing.
   C. Sclerosis.
   D. Cyst formation.
   E. Osteophytes.

2. A 77-year-old man sees his GP for left knee pain, gradually worsening over a month. He is now struggling to bear weight on it and the joint appears slightly swollen. The pain is achy and is affecting his ability to walk. He has now started to experience pain at night.
   What would an X-ray examination reveal?
   A. Erosions.
   B. Osteophytes.

C. Hairline fracture.
D. Osteopenia.
E. Soft tissue swelling.

3. An 80-year-old woman complains of worsening stiffness in her hands for 6 months. She finds it difficult to button up her clothes and her hands ache after gardening and doing household chores.
What might you expect to find on clinical examination?
A. Ulnar deviation.
B. Boutonniere deformity.
C. Heberden nodes.
D. Dupuytren contracture.
E. Metacarpophalangeal (MCP) swelling.

4. A 65-year-old former factory worker presents to his physician with pain in his hips. He has trouble sitting and standing. The pain increases after walking and radiates to his knees. Resting makes it better.
What is the next most appropriate step in his management?
A. Glucosamine.
B. Joint replacement.
C. Trial of steroids.
D. Physiotherapy.
E. Joint injection.

Chapter 12 Rheumatoid arthritis

1. A 65-year-old woman with stable rheumatoid arthritis (RA) notices loss of sensation in the lateral 3.5 fingers, palmar aspect.
Which is the most appropriate therapy for this more recent condition?
A. Splinting.
B. Oral steroids.
C. Methotrexate.
D. Physiotherapy.
E. Intramuscular gold injections.

2. An 80-year-old man presents to his GP with pain in his fingers and joints for 6–12 months. He is struggling to work in his garden and is finding dressing himself difficult. He has flattened knuckles, swan-neck deformity of his fingers and z-thumb deformity of the thumbs. There is slight ulnar deviation.
Which might you not expect to see on an X-ray image of his hands?
A. Juxtaarticular erosions.
B. Joint effusion.
C. Narrowed joint space.
D. Osteopenia.
E. Soft tissue swelling.

3. A 48-year-old woman presents with 8-week onset of bilateral stiffness and intermittent swelling of the metacarpophalangeal joints. She is otherwise fit and well. On further questioning, she admits to similar episodes over the previous 2 years.
She is anti-CCP and rheumatoid factor positive, with high erythrocyte sedimentation rate and C-reactive protein. X-ray images show erosive arthropathy.
What is the next most appropriate management step?
A. Physiotherapy.
B. MRI of the hands.
C. Start disease-modifying antirheumatic drugs (DMARDs).
D. Hydrotherapy.
E. Start nonsteroidal antiinflammatory drugs (NSAIDs).

4. An 86-year-old woman goes to her GP with pain in her fingers and toes for 6 months. It is intermittent and her fingers feel stiff and tender. Stiffness is greatest when she wakes and eases as the day goes by. She has also noticed firm subcutaneous lumps forming on the extensor side of her elbow. Her medical history states she has had bleeding from a duodenal ulcer.
Which of the following would be best avoided in this woman?
A. Hydroxychloroquine.
B. Methotrexate.
C. Paracetamol.
D. Naproxen.
E. Sulfasalazine.

5. A 58-year-old woman with longstanding rheumatoid arthritis and secondary osteoporosis presents with progressive worsening breathlessness. She has been on methotrexate and sulfasalazine for many years and has had considerably long courses of steroids.
Which is the least likely cause for her breathlessness?
A. Rheumatoid lung disease.
B. Anaemia.
C. Methotrexate-induced lung fibrosis.
D. Acquired kyphosis.
E. Constrictive pericarditis.

Chapter 13 Spondyloarthropathies

1. A 22-year-old man develops an acute swelling of his left knee and ankle with painful heels. There was no trauma.
A week previously he had conjunctivitis and a fever. Blood and urine samples are taken for culture.
Which of the following is NOT the likely pathogen?
A. *Haemophilus influenzae*.
B. *Chlamydia trachomatis*.
C. *Salmonella typhi*.
D. *Neisseria gonorrhoeae*.
E. *Escherichia coli*.

2. A 53-year-old woman complains of bloody diarrhoea and abdominal pain. She experiences low-grade fever, nausea and weight loss. A colonoscopy is conducted, which shows ulcerative lesions in her rectum.

   During this period her shoulders becomes progressively stiffer and she develops pain and swelling in her right knee. The intensity of the pain has worsened with her bowel symptoms.

   What is the most appropriate immediate management for this woman?
   A. Nonsteroidal antiinflammatory drugs (NSAIDs).
   B. Corticosteroids.
   C. Panproctocolectomy.
   D. Biologic therapy.
   E. Sulfasalazine.

3. A 45-year-old man presents to his GP with joint pain and stiffness in both wrists, knuckles and distal interphalangeal joints. There is a slight degree of swelling in the right and left middle fingers, giving them a sausage-like appearance. The GP notices dry skin around his hairline and back of his ears.

   Which of the following nail changes is he most likely to have?
   A. Keratoderma blennorrhagica.
   B. Koilonychia.
   C. Subungal hyperkeratosis.
   D. Leuconychia.
   E. Paronychia.

4. Which of the following is not associated with ankylosing spondylitis?
   A. Amyloidosis.
   B. Apical lung fibrosis.
   C. Aortic incompetence.
   D. Anticardiolipin antibody.
   E. Acute anterior uveitis.

5. Which of the following types of spondyloarthropathy is most closely associated with HLA B27 positivity?
   A. Psoriatic arthritis.
   B. Enteropathic arthritis.
   C. Reactive arthritis.
   D. Undifferentiated spondyloarthritis.
   E. Ankylosing spondylitis.

Chapter 14 Connective tissue diseases

1. A 63-year-old man presents with a headache for 3 days. It is severe and unilateral, only affecting the left side of his head. It radiates to his scalp.

   He has no visual disturbance or pain in his jaw on eating, but feels sore when he brushes his hair. The pain is constant, with only temporary relief from analgesia.

What investigation is most useful in confirming the diagnosis?
   A. Temporal artery biopsy.
   B. Erythrocyte sedimentation rate (ESR).
   C. Antineutrophil cytoplasmic antibody (ANCA) screening.
   D. Lumbar puncture.
   E. MRI of the aortic arch.

2. A 58-year-old man presents to the respiratory clinic with breathlessness. He is found to have a raised pulmonary artery pressure. High-resolution CT of the chest shows pulmonary fibrosis.

   He also complains of painful discolouration of his fingers when outdoors, has evidence of skin thickening in the fingers and hands with hard deposits under the skin, and small red spider-like lesions on the chest and face.

   What is the most likely explanation for the findings.
   A. Systemic lupus erythematosus (SLE).
   B. Systemic sclerosis.
   C. Linear scleroderma.
   D. Paraneoplastic syndrome.
   E. Multiple sclerosis.

3. A 48-year-old woman complains of dry eyes, dry mouth and lethargy. There is evidence of oral candidiasis and dental caries. She also complains of pains in multiple joints. Her GP questions what her diagnosis may be.

   Which is the most likely test to confirm the diagnosis?
   A. HIV test.
   B. Schober test.
   C. Schirmer test.
   D. Transoesophageal echocardiogram.
   E. Trendelenburg test.

4. A 60-year-old woman comes to the GP with stiffness, fatigue and muscle pains affecting her shoulder and hips. The onset was over several days. On examination, she is slow to rise from a chair, has difficulty in raising her arms and cannot undo her bra-strap. She also complains of a right sided headache, which isn't made better by simple analgesia and which is progressively worsening.

   What should you do immediately?
   A. Check erythrocyte sedimentation rate (ESR).
   B. Refer for temporal artery biopsy.
   C. Refer for muscle biopsy.
   D. Administer prednisolone.
   E. Administer a nonsteroidal antiinflammatory drug.

5. A 67-year old man presents to the GP complaining of difficulty in rising from a chair. He has also noticed the development of erythematous plaques over his

knuckles and a lilac discolouration of his eyelids. The GP decides to order some tests to confirm the diagnosis.
Which test has the highest diagnostic yield?
A. Erythrocyte sedimentation rate (ESR).
B. Antinuclear antibodies.
C. Chest X-ray.
D. X-ray of the affected joints.
E. Serum creatine kinase levels.

6. A 35-year-old woman is admitted as an emergency to A&E with breathlessness, haemoptysis, chest pain and signs of shock. She receives thrombolysis and is seen to improve. Contrast CT of the pulmonary arteries confirms bilateral pulmonary emboli.
She gives a history of stillbirth in the past and a retinal vein occlusion.
What is the most appropriate next investigation for this woman?
A. Antiphospholipid antibody.
B. Anti-double-stranded DNA antibody.
C. Antineutrophil cytoplasmic antibody (ANCA).
D. Prothrombin time.
E. Syphilis serology.

Chapter 15 Metabolic bone disease

1. An 85-year-old presents to his GP with lower back pain for 2 days. Over the previous 3 years he has noticed his shirts seem to be getting longer but not looser. He had a rib fracture a year ago after slipping off a chair.
Blood tests are performed, which show the following:
Calcium: 2.38 mmol/L (normal 2.12–2.65 mmol/L)
Phosphate: 1.1 mmol/L (normal 0.8–1.4 mmol/L)
Alkaline phosphatase: 98 U/L (normal 30–150 U/L)
What is the most likely diagnosis?
A. Osteoporosis.
B. Myeloma.
C. Osteomalacia.
D. Paget disease.
E. Potts disease (spinal tuberculosis).

2. A 58-year-old woman presents to her GP with hip pain for 3 weeks. On examination, she has bowing of her tibias. She seems to be having difficulty hearing and the doctor has to keep repeating himself. Her father had a similar issue with bowing of the tibias.
What would be the next most appropriate step in diagnosis?
A. Coeliac serology.
B. Bone biochemistry.
C. Dual-energy X-ray absorptiometry (DEXA) scan.
D. MRI of the tibias.
E. Test for rheumatoid factor.

3. An 80-year-old man who has chronic renal failure starts developing bony tenderness and muscle weakness. He even finds walking with a zimmer frame difficult due to pain. Blood tests are performed:
Calcium: 1.56 mmol/L (normal 2.12–2.65 mmol/L)
Phosphate: 0.62 mmol/L (normal 0.8–1.4 mmol/L)
Alkaline phosphatase: 198 U/L (normal 30–150 U/L)
What is not a possible consequence of his condition?
A. Skeletal deformity.
B. Tetany.
C. Polydipsia.
D. Convulsions.
E. Arrhythmias.

4. A 56-year-old woman presents to her physician with pain shooting down her right leg from her back and also with sore knees. They feel warm to touch. She also has pain when walking. Bone biochemistry is checked and the results are as follows:
Calcium: 2.38 mmol/L (normal 2.1–2.65 mmol/L)
Phosphate: 1.1 mmol/L (normal 0.8–1.4 mmol/L)
Alkaline phosphatase (ALP): 220 U/L (normal 30–150 U/L)
What is the likely diagnosis?
A. Osteoarthritis.
B. Prolapsed vertebral disc.
C. Septic arthritis.
D. Paget disease.
E. Gout.

5. A 68-year-old woman presents to her GP feeling tired, with myalgia and bone pain. The GP does a broad battery of blood tests and these are her results:
Calcium: 1.87 mmol/L (normal 2.12–2.65 mmol/L)
Phosphate: 0.58 mmol/L (normal 0.8–1.4 mmol/L)
Alkaline phosphatase: 202 U/L (normal 30–150 U/L)
Haemoglobin: 10.3 g/dL (normal 11.5–16.0 g/dL)
Mean cell volume: 101 fL (normal 76–96 fL)
Iron: 9 μmol/L (normal 11–30 μmol/L)
Folate: 1.9 μg/L (normal 2.1 μg/L)
Which investigation would be most useful to confirm the diagnosis?
A. Anti-double-stranded DNA antibody.
B. Antiphospholipid antibody.
C. Anti-smooth muscle antibody.
D. Anti-vitamin D3 antibody.
E. Anti-tissue transglutaminase antibody.

Chapter 16 Gout and pseudogout

1. A 75-year-old man develops pain in his right wrist and right third metacarpophalangeal joint. The joints are red, warm, swollen and tender. He cannot do his usual activities due to pain. Aspiration of his wrist shows rhomboid calcium pyrophosphate crystals. An X-ray examination of the joint reveals

chondrocalcinosis, subchondral sclerosis and osteophytes. He is given co-codamol for pain relief. What is the next most effective step in his management?

A. Antibiotics.
B. Disease-modifying antirheumatic drugs.
C. Joint replacement.
D. Physiotherapy.
E. Splinting.

2. A 59-year-old obese man presents to his physician with acute onset of pain and swelling in his left first metatarsophalangeal joint. It is red, swollen, tender and warm. He is unable to bear weight on it. The physician also finds unusual white lumps on his fingers. The joint is aspirated.
What will the fluid microscopy probably show?

A. Gram-positive bacteria.
B. Calcium pyrophosphate.
C. Pus.
D. Monosodium urate crystals.
E. Clear synovial fluid.

3. A 55-year-old woman comes to her doctor with an excruciatingly painful right first metatarsophalangeal joint for 24 hours. The overlying skin is warm, shiny and the joint is swollen and immobile. She has a history of chronic kidney disease. Last year she had a similar short-lived episode that resolved and left her symptomless.
What is the most likely explanation for her condition?

A. This is an autoimmune condition where T-lymphocytes attack the synovial lining of joints, eventually causing erosion of the cartilage and underlying bone.
B. There is an ongoing chronic infection in the joint.
C. Chronic hyperuricemia leading to the formation of sodium urate crystals that get deposited in the synovium, causing inflammation.
D. Calcium pyrophosphate crystals have deposited in the joint space.
E. Degeneration of the weight-bearing cartilage and subsequent eburnation of subchondral bone.

4. A 72-year-old man presents with a 24-hour history of a painful swollen knee. There is no history of trauma. He is otherwise well. He is apyrexial. His knee is mildly erythematous and is tender on palpation with decreased range of motion. An X-ray examination is performed (see image). Erythrocyte sedimentation rate and C-reactive protein are mildly elevated, but the white cell count is normal.
What is the most likely diagnosis?

A. Gout.
B. Pseudogout.
C. Septic arthritis.
D. Rheumatoid arthritis.
E. Haemarthrosis.

5. A 65-year-old man presents with a warm, hot, swollen and tender right ankle. He has a history of gout and has had recurrent flares of his disease. He currently takes 200 mg of allopurinol daily. His GP treats acutely with colchicine and his symptoms settle. Sometime later, his uric acid level is checked and is found to be 460 μg/mL. His other blood tests are normal, including renal function.
What is the next appropriate step in managing this man's gout?

A. Increase allopurinol to 300 mg daily.
B. Add febuxostat 120 mg daily.
C. Start long-term prednisolone 10 mg daily.
D. Add colchicine 500 μg twice daily.
E. Start ibuprofen 400 mg three times daily.

Chapter 17 Paediatric joint disease

1. The majority of the blood supply to the femoral head in adults arises from:

A. Artery of ligamentum teres.
B. Lateral femoral circumflex artery.
C. Obturator artery.
D. Medial femoral circumflex artery.
E. Profunda femoris artery.

2. A 12-year-old boy attends the hospital with a new onset of pain in his left hip. He is overweight and has not started puberty. He is unable to bear weight on this leg and on examination all movements are generally painful. An X-ray examination reveals that he has an abnormality of the femoral neck in keeping with a SUFE. In what position is his leg most likely to lie?

A. Internal rotation.
B. External rotation.
C. Flexion.
D. Abduction.
E. Adduction.

3. A baby is assessed in the birthing room after delivery at term. An abnormality is noted involving an inward pointing foot and calf wasting. The father tells you he had the same thing as a child. What is the most likely diagnosis?

A. Talipes equinovarus.
B. Normal variant.
C. Cerebral palsy.
D. Pes planus.
E. Spina bifida.

4. A 6-year-old boy attends the fracture clinic with a fracture of his wrist, which has been treated in a cast

and seems to be healing. His mother tells you he also recently broke his other wrist and had a supra-condylar fracture 1 year ago, all with low-energy trauma. He seems happy and well-dressed but is small in stature and on examination has a subtle scoliosis. What is the most likely underlying diagnosis here?
A. Marfan syndrome.
B. Idiopathic scoliosis.
C. Nonaccidental injury.
D. Osteoporosis.
E. Osteogenesis imperfecta.

5. A patient is admitted to an orthopaedic ward with a proximal tibia fracture whilst awaiting surgery. During the night the patient experiences a severe increase in pain. This is initially settled with opiate analgesia but rapidly returns and eventually opiate analgesia is no longer effective.
What are you primarily concerned about?
A. Further displacement of the fracture.
B. Deep vein thrombosis.
C. Compartment syndrome.
D. Embolic arterial occlusion.
E. Nerve injury following the fracture.

6. A 68-year-old woman is seen 3 days after a total hip replacement. Initially progressing well, she suddenly develops sharp left-sided chest pain and shortness of breath. On examination, she has slight pyrexia (37.5°C) and is hypoxic on room air (SpO2 91%) and tachycardic (heart rate 110 bpm).
What is the cause of her symptoms?
A. Pulmonary thromboembolism.
B. Myocardial infarction.
C. Basal atelectasis.
D. Fat embolism.
E. Pneumothorax.

7. What is the main principle when choosing internal fixation over casting of fractures?
A. Lower complication rate.
B. Cheaper.
C. Early mobilization.
D. Ensure union of fracture.
E. Less pain.

8. A young man is involved in an road traffic accident and is brought into A&E with a collar in situ. He has a Glasgow Coma Scale of 15, but after completing an ABCDE survey he is found to be unstable due to a suspected unstable pelvic fracture. What is the first step to take in dealing with this?
A. Place an external fixator while in A&E.
B. Urgent angiogram.
C. Place a pelvic binder.

D. Laparotomy and pelvic packing.
E. Anteroposterior X-ray examination of the pelvis.

9. A 92-year-old lady who is normally fit and well presents to A&E with a painful hip and not able to bear weight. She is normally mobile in the home but has chronic obstructive pulmonary disorder and a poor maximum walking distance. She is examined and her hip is found to be in external rotation and shortened. She is seen to have an intracapsular neck of femur fracture on X-ray examination. What is the best treatment for her?
A. Hemiarthroplasty.
B. Dynamic hip screw (DHS).
C. Total hip replacement.
D. Girdlestone procedure.
E. Conservative management.

Chapter 19 Trauma

1. A man arrives in A&E following a car accident, with a suspected pelvic fracture. He is unresponsive, hypotensive and tachycardic. Which is the first step in the management of this patient?
A. Obtain intravenous access and commence fluid resuscitation.
B. Apply a pelvic binder.
C. Get an anteroposterior pelvis X-ray examination.
D. Crossmatch the patient for type-matched blood.
E. Assess the airway whilst stabilizing the cervical spine.

2. A 20-year-old patient is involved in a road traffic accident, fracturing their femur. They are brought into the A&E and assessed using an ABCDE approach. Their blood pressure is noted to be 100/60 and their pulse is 110. What is their likely percentage blood loss?
A. 0%–15%
B. 15%–30%
C. 30%–40%
D. >40%

3. An 80-year-old patient trips in her bathroom and hits her head on a toilet seat. She is admitted to A&E D and undergoes evaluation using an ABCDE approach. She is found to have a bruise on the back of her head and complains of neck pain. She has a GCS of 14 and no neurological abnormalities. She is on warfarin with an INR of 3. Which is the next best investigation?
A. MRI head and C-spine.
B. X-ray examination of C-spine.
C. CT angiogram.
D. CT head and C-spine.
E. Bone scan.

Chapter 20   Infection of bones and joints

1. Which is the most common pathogen in septic arthritis in adults?
   A. *Streptococcus sp.*
   B. *Mycobacterium tuberculosis.*
   C. *Staphylococcus aureus.*
   D. *Haemophilus influenzae.*
   E. *Enterobacter sp.*

2. A 64-year-old man with a background of diabetes presents with a 24-hour history of progressive atraumatic left knee pain. He is unable to bend his knee and unable to bear weight. On examination, he is pyrexial and his left knee is hot and erythematous. He has a large effusion, virtually no range of movement and global tenderness around the knee. What is the most important step in this man's management?
   A. Anteroposterior and lateral X-ray examination of the knee.
   B. Commence intravenous antibiotics.
   C. Aspiration of the knee.
   D. Bloods for inflammatory markers.
   E. Ultrasound scan of the knee.

3. A 38-year-old electrician presents with a painful swollen right knee. He states that over the past week his knee has become increasing swollen and red and he now has a decreased range of motion. On examination, there is a large erythematous swelling anterior to the patella, which is tender to palpate. There is thickened skin over the anterior of the knee. There is no effusion in the knee. He is able to flex his knee to 45 degrees before he is limited by a combination of pain and tightness in the knee. What is the likely diagnosis?
   A. Osteoarthritis.
   B. Septic arthritis.
   C. Baker cyst.
   D. Patellar fracture.
   E. Prepatellar bursitis.

4. In the case of septic arthritis in intravenous drug abusers, which of the following pathogens is most likely?
   A. *Staphylococcus aureus.*
   B. *Pseudomonas.*
   C. Fungal infections.
   D. *Streptococcus sp.*
   E. All of the above.

Chapter 21   Malignancy

1. A 30-year-old man presents with an intensely painful right proximal tibia with no history of trauma. He experiences pain during the day and night. Of note, he states that aspirin relieves his pain significantly. On examination, there is significant tenderness over the proximal tibial metaphysis. X-ray examination shows a small lucent area in the tibial metaphysis with dense sclerosis surrounding it.
   What is the most likely diagnosis?
   A. Enchondroma.
   B. Osteoid osteoma.
   C. Chondrosarcoma.
   D. Osteochondroma.
   E. Lymphoma.

2. A 24-year-old, normally fit and healthy woman presents with a 4-month history of gradually increasing pain in her left knee. There was no history of trauma. She is now having difficulty bearing weight and is frequently woken at night with pain. She also notes weight loss in the same timeframe. X-ray examination of her knee demonstrates an expansile and lytic lesion in her distal femur, with cortical destruction and significant periosteal reaction.
   What is the most likely diagnosis?
   A. Tuberculosis.
   B. Osteosarcoma.
   C. Enchondroma.
   D. Osteomyelitis.
   E. Stress fracture.

3. An 89-year-old man presents with a painful lumbar spine and difficulty mobilizing. He tells you this has only been present for 6 weeks but that he has noticed some weight loss and feels generally unwell. He undergoes an X-ray examination of the spine, which shows sclerotic change through L5 and S1.
   What is the most likely underlying diagnosis?
   A. Prostate cancer.
   B. Renal cancer.
   C. Lung cancer.
   D. Thyroid cancer.
   E. Bowel cancer.

4. Which of these common bony structures visible on X-ray images might be an indication of malignancy?
   A. Looser zones.
   B. Periarticular erosions.
   C. Osteophytes.
   D. Periosteal reaction.
   E. Vertebral trabecular thickening.

Chapter 22   Sports injuries

1. What causes a locked knee?
   A. Anterior cruciate ligament tear.
   B. Radial meniscal tear.
   C. Medial collateral ligament tear.
   D. Bucket handle meniscal tear.
   E. Tibial plateau fracture.

2. An 18-year-old football player presents to A&E with a knee injury. He describes turning quickly and twisting his right knee, precipitating immediate pain. He states his knee was grossly swollen before he left the pitch. On examination, there is a tense effusion, no joint line tenderness and a poor range of motion. Lachman test is positive, but otherwise the knee is stable. What is the diagnosis?
   A. Medial meniscal tear.
   B. Posterior cruciate ligament tear.
   C. Medial collateral ligament tear.
   D. Patellar dislocation.
   E. Anterior cruciate ligament tear.

3. A 23-year-old man walks into A&E reporting pain in his left shoulder. He has an obvious deformity and is unable to move the shoulder. A dislocation is diagnosed. What is the most likely position for the humerus to lie, in relation to the glenoid?
   A. Anterior, medial.
   B. Posterior.
   C. Anterior superior.
   D. Anterior inferior.
   E. Superior.

4. Which of the following conditions make a patellar dislocation more likely?
   A. Patella fracture.
   B. Cerebral palsy.
   C. Anterior cruciate ligament injury.
   D. Hypoplastic trochlea.
   E. Osteoarthritis.

Chapter 23 Soft tissue disorders

1. De Quervain tenosynovitis involves inflammation of which tendon sheath?
   A. Extensor pollicis longus.
   B. Abductor pollicis longus.
   C. Extensor indicis.
   D. Flexor pollicis longus.
   E. Extensor carpi radialis longus.

2. A 55-year-old man presents with pain and swelling over his left elbow. He has an obvious swelling but not much redness at the olecranon and a normal range of motion. His C-reactive protein is 6 and his white cells 7.3. What is the first line treatment for this condition?
   A. Nonsteroidal antiinflammatory drugs (NSAIDs) and rest.
   B. Aspiration and culture.
   C. Intravenous antibiotics.
   D. Open washout.
   E. Bursectomy.

3. Which tissue is primarily involved in the development of Dupuytren contracture?
   A. Flexor tendons.
   B. Palmar fascia.
   C. Metacarpophalangeal joint capsule.
   D. Flexor tendon sheaths.
   E. Skin.

Chapter 24 Principles of orthopaedic surgery

1. An 82-year-old female undergoes hemiarthroplasty after fracture of her left hip. Six hours after the operation, her pulse is 70 bpm and her blood pressure is 80/40. She is not confused but is not producing any urine. Which is the most likely cause for her condition?
   A. Cardiogenic shock.
   B. Hypovolaemia.
   C. Anaphylaxis.
   D. Sepsis.
   E. Neurogenic shock.

2. A 79-year-old male presents to A&E with pain in his right hip. He is unable to move and reports that he simply bent over to do up his shoe lace and felt a severe pain in his hip. Of note in his history, he had a total hip replacement on the right side 9 years previously but had been functioning well. What is the most likely cause for his pain?
   A. Hip dislocation.
   B. Periprosthetic fracture.
   C. Implant loosening.
   D. Deep infection.
   E. Implant failure and breakage.

3. A 55-year-old female had a total hip replacement carried out 6 months previously. She has constantly struggled with pain and has leakage through the wound. She has a C-reactive protein of 110 and white cell count 12.0. She has attended the A&E today but remains haemodynamically stable. What is the best treatment?
   A. Immediate intravenous antibiotics and admission.
   B. Admission, observation and aspiration in theatre.
   C. Single stage revision total hip replacement.
   D. Admission and bone scan.
   E. Discharge and review in clinic.

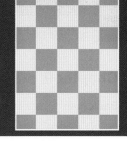

Each answer can be used once, more than once or not at all.

Chapter 7 A child with a limp

Paediatric hip disorders

A. Perthes disease
B. Juvenile idiopathic arthritis
C. Developmental dysplasia of the hip
D. Congenital talipes equinovarus
E. Slipped upper femoral epiphysis
F. Septic arthritis
G. Osteomyelitis
H. Reactive arthritis
I. Ewing tumour
J. Osgood-Schlatter disease.

Read the clinical details of each patient below and decide which is the most appropriate diagnosis from the list above.

1. A 13-month-old baby presents with a limp as the child begins to walk. The left leg looks shorter than the right. The child has a waddling gait but is not in obvious discomfort.
2. A 13-year-old boy presents with a 1-week history of left leg pain radiating from the groin down the thigh and into the knee. The pain is worse on activity and partially relieved by rest. Clinically, he has an externally rotated left leg with pain on all movements. The anteroposterior X-ray image of the hip shows a smaller epiphysis than on the right. The frog lateral view clinches the diagnosis.
3. A 12-year-old boy has been unwell for a few months with pain and swelling in his right knee. He has also been more tired than usual and not himself. On further questioning, it becomes clear that other joints are involved. The right knee is swollen with a small effusion. At presentation, he is noted to have decreased visual acuity in his right eye.
4. A 14-year-old boy is a keen footballer and presents with bilateral knee pain that is worse on movement and very tender if touched. On examination, he is well and has tenderness over the tibial tubercle just beneath the patellar ligament.
5. A 7-year-old boy presents with a 1-year history of right knee pain, gradually increasing. He has a pronounced limp and has been off school for 1 month. On examination the right knee is normal but the hip is irritable and abduction is markedly decreased. X-ray images show sclerosis of the femoral head.
6. An 8-week-old baby girl is very ill on the paediatric intensive care unit. She has features of sepsis, including a raised temperature and WCC and blood cultures have grown *Staphylococcus aureus*. There is no obvious focus of infection. An ultrasound scan of both hips is normal.

Chapter 8 A limb swelling

Orthopaedic investigations

A. MRI
B. X-ray examination
C. CT scan
D. Ultrasound scan
E. MRI arthrogram
F. Dual-energy X-ray absorptiometry (DEXA) scanning
G. Isotope bone scanning

For each scenario choose the most appropriate imaging modality from the list above.

1. A 70-year-old lady returns to the clinic 6 weeks after bilateral distal radius fractures. She is comfortable out of cast. She has also recently broken her hip.
2. A 44-year-old man presents to the emergency department with a swelling over his 3rd metatarsal on his left foot. He reports a gradual onset of pain and difficulty in bearing weight. The lump is fixed and hard and is not changing in size.
3. A 70-year-old male attends with a pain in his hip. He has also noticed recent deafness and X-ray imaging shows markedly thickened cortices to his femur and skull.
4. An 80-year-old presents with gross swelling of the leg and a lump taking up the majority of her thigh. She reports pain for a number of years in the leg and no other systemic symptoms.
5. A 25-year-old man presents with a lump over his left groin. He is an IV drug user and has recently injected. The lump is red and extremely painful with some discharge.
6. A 14-year-old boy presents with insidious onset of pain and a lump above his left knee. An X-ray examination shows a lytic lesion with a periosteal reaction and he has a new onset of jaundice.

Chapter 9 Back pain

Back pain

A. Spondylolisthesis
B. Spinal stenosis
C. Prolapsed intervertebral disc
D. Discitis
E. Chronic musculoskeletal back pain
F. Spinal metastases
G. Acute low back pain
H. Ankylosing spondylitis
I. Abdominal aortic aneurysm
J. Cauda equina syndrome

Read the clinical details of each patient below and decide which is the most appropriate diagnosis from the list above.

1. A 60-year-old man presents with low back pain and aching in both legs. The pain is worse on walking and relieved by rest. The leg pain radiates down the leg and into both calves. Examination shows reduced movements of the spine and pain on extension. Sciatic stretch testing is normal. X-ray images show osteoarthritis of the spine.
2. A 60-year-old woman has unrelenting low back pain which is not mechanical in nature. Night pain is severe and not relieved by simple analgesia. On examination she is pale and thin. Her abdominal system reveals a palpable liver edge. X-ray examination of her lumbar spine shows loss of a pedicle (winking-owl sign).
3. A 56-year-old diabetic patient with chronic renal failure is admitted for dialysis. He also complains of new back pain. The patient becomes unwell with a raised temperature, a white cell count of $22.5 \times 10^9/L$, C-reactive protein 125 mg/L and erythrocyte sedimentation rate 79 mm/h. The renal physicians treat him for line sepsis but he fails to respond. One week later, an X-ray examination of the lumbar spine shows loss of disc space between L3 and L4 with bony destruction of the end plates.
4. A 32-year-old GP presents with a short history of back pain after straining in the garden. He has bilateral leg symptoms with pain radiating down both legs into his feet. He says the saddle area of his bottom feels odd when sitting down and he has difficulty passing urine. When he arrives in A&E he is in acute urinary retention and the crossover sign is positive.
5. A 30-year-old man complains of low back pain after digging at work. The pain does not radiate and is worse on movement. He feels well and examination shows muscle spasm, reduced movements and some tenderness across the lower lumbar spine.

6. A 15-year-old boy presents with increasing low back pain for 1 year. He is a county-level fast bowler and big things are expected of him. The pain does not radiate and is worse after prolonged activity. Examination shows a well boy with well-maintained spinal movements and normal neurology. Pain is significant on extension. Oblique X-ray images of the lumbar spine show a typical Scottie dog appearance with a pars defect at L5–S1.

Chapter 10 Altered sensation and weakness

Causes of peripheral upper limb symptoms

A. Ulnar nerve compression
B. Cervical rib
C. Pancoast tumour
D. Carpal tunnel syndrome
E. Axillary nerve palsy
F. Radial nerve palsy
G. C6–C7 cervical disc prolapse
H. Peripheral neuropathy

Read the clinical details of each patient below and decide which is the most likely diagnosis from the list above.

1. A 21-year-old man complains of numbness in his little and ring fingers and over the medial aspect of his forearm with weakness in his hand. This only seems to occur in certain positions, especially when his arm is raised above his head. His hand also turns white on occasions. There is wasting of the small muscles of the hand.
2. A 65-year-old heavy smoker complains of weakness in his left hand. He has had a persistent cough for the last 3 months and has lost 13 kg in weight. On examination he has wasting of the small muscles of the hand. The doctor also notes that he has a constricted pupil on the left side with drooping of the eyelid and dry skin over the left side of his forehead.
3. A 26-year-old man crashes his motorbike at 40 mph. He sustains a spiral fracture to the mid-shaft of his right humerus. He has altered sensation over the first dorsal web space of his right hand and has weakness of extension of his wrist, fingers and thumb.
4. A 40-year-old woman develops a sudden onset of severe neck pain after turning suddenly. This is associated with pain in her middle finger and weakness straightening her arm. She has no significant past medical history.
5. A 40-year-old man is tackled heavily during a rugby game and lands awkwardly on his left shoulder. His shoulder has lost its normal contour and he finds all movements painful. He notices some tingling over the outer aspect of his upper arm.

Chapter 16 Gout and Pseudogout

Gout and pseudogout

A. Gout
B. Pseudogout
C. Haemarthrosis
D. Psoriatic arthritis
E. Reactive arthritis
F. Septic arthritis

Read the presenting signs and clinical details of each patient below and decide which is the best diagnosis for them based on the information.

1. A man who presents with a tense, acutely swollen knee after twisting getting out his car. His past medical history is of atrial fibrillation and high blood pressure.
2. An elderly man who was recently treated for a chest infection presents with an acutely hot and painful right wrist. His past medical history includes osteoarthritis, blepharitis and asthma.
3. A young man presents with a swollen knee and ankle, and burning on micturition. He has had recurrent anterior uveitis in the past.
4. A woman with episodic severe foot pain, redness and swelling, which has recently started to affect her ankle.
5. A young woman who has developed a hot swollen knee. She also complains of problems with her nails and swollen, sausage-like toes.
6. A middle-aged man presenting with a hot tender shoulder. He feels faint, is sweaty and looks unwell. He is a type 1 diabetic.

Chapter 17 Paediatric joint disease

Paediatric joint disorders

A. Nonaccidental injury
B. Cerebral palsy
C. Talipes equina varus
D. Osgood-Schlatter disease
E. Fracture tibial shaft
F. Perthes disease
G. SUFE
H. Developmental dysplasia of the hip
I. Normal variant
J. Osteogenesis imperfecta
K. Rickets
L. Septic arthritis hip

Read the clinical details of each patient below and decide which is the most appropriate diagnosis from the list above.

1. An 8-year-old girl presents with her mother who is concerned by the appearance of her knees. She walks comfortably without pain but has noticed a knock-kneed appearance with her knees in a valgus position. Both knees are symmetrical.
2. A 7-year-old boy presents to the fracture clinic for the third time in a year. He has an isolated fracture of his ulnar shaft on his right arm and previously had a fracture of his left arm. He is shy and not very clear about how he got these injuries. However, his father says he fell off his bike.
3. A 5-year-old boy presents to the clinic with pain in his left knee. He mobilized well up until 4 weeks ago but has gradually started to struggle. An X-ray examination shows a normal knee but an abnormality to the femoral head including loss of epiphyseal height and subchondral fracture with partial collapse. His inflammatory markers are normal.
4. A 15-year-old boy presents to the clinic with anterior knee pain. This has been present for 2 weeks. He is specifically tender over the tibial tuberosity and can walk normally but is in severe pain when running.
5. A 1-year-old girl is sent to the clinic with an abnormality to her right lower leg. She is struggling to crawl and has not yet learned to walk. She has an equinus deformity that her mum reports as present since birth. When she is examined, she is found to have spasticity in all muscles of the right leg with a contracture at the Achilles tendon.

Chapter 18 Fractures

Fractures

A. Salter-Harris fracture
B. Simple fracture
C. Pathological fracture
D. Open fracture
E. Complex regional pain syndrome
F. Compartment syndrome
G. Nonaccidental injury

Read the clinical details of each patient below and decide which is the most appropriate diagnosis from the list above.

1. A 10-year-old boy falls out of a tree and lands on his left wrist. He cries immediately and his mother brings him to A&E because his wrist is deformed. When the doctor takes an X-ray image, he explains that the child has a fracture.
2. A 50-year-old man suddenly feels pain in his right thigh and falls to the ground. He is alarmed to find that his leg is badly angulated and X-ray examination in the Casualty Department confirms a fracture. He explains that he has had pain in this leg for some time and over the last few months has lost weight. He also mentions that he has been coughing up blood and worries that his lifelong smoking habit is the cause.

3. A 30-year-old footballer is kicked hard in his shin during a game. He does not feel too uncomfortable initially and can bear weight, but over the next 3 hours his pain becomes severe. The team doctor examines his leg and finds that his leg is swollen and tense. He has altered sensation over the dorsum of his foot and passive movement of his toes is extremely painful. Foot pulses are normal.

4. An 18-month-old girl is brought to A&E by her mother following a fall from the settee at home. She has a painful swollen forearm. Radiographs show a transverse fracture of the forearm with callus formation. The grandmother says that the arm hurt a few days ago.

5. A 46-year-old secretary falls from a ladder on to her forearm. Her arm is badly angulated and there is a tiny wound over the middle part of the forearm. The junior doctor straightens her arm and places it in a cast and brings her back to clinic 2 days later. His consultant reviews the case and is very angry.

Postoperative complications

A. Hypovolaemia
B. Sepsis
C. Anaphylaxis
D. Neurogenic shock
E. Cardiogenic shock
F. Drugs
G. Epidural anaesthesia

Read the clinical details of each patient below and decide which is the most appropriate diagnosis from the list above.

1. A fit 65-year-old woman returns to the ward 2 hours after a total hip replacement. The nurse is worried because her blood pressure is only 90/60 mmHg. Her pulse rate is 74 bpm and she has a good urine output. She feels well and capillary refill is 2 seconds. Her legs feel numb but sensation is slowly returning.

2. A 60-year-old man presents with a very painful right hip and feeling unwell. He has a history of type 2 diabetes mellitus and chronic obstructive airway disease for which he takes oral steroids. Recently he has had a bad chest, for which the GP prescribed antibiotics. On examination, his hip is held in fixed flexion and he will not move it. His temperature is 38°C. Pulse is 120 bpm and blood pressure is 80/40 mmHg. His veins are distended and he has warm peripheries.

3. A 25-year-old kitchen fitter is ejected from his van at high speed when he crashes on a motorway. He has lower back pain but is alarmed because he can no longer feel his legs. When he arrives in the emergency department he is fully examined by the doctor, including a log roll and per rectum

examination. This is normal apart from a boggy swelling at the level of L1 and loss of sensation and power in his legs. Pulse rate is 60 bpm and blood pressure is 100/50 mmHg.

4. The night doctor is called urgently to review an 80-year-old woman on the ward 4 days after a hemiarthroplasty for a fractured neck of femur. She looks very unwell. On examination, she has a pulse of 110 bpm, shallow and rapid breathing with crepitations at the bases, a raised jugular venous pulse and is sweaty and clammy. Blood pressure is only 84/40 mmHg. The electrocardiogram (EKG) shows ST elevation in the lateral leads, which is new compared with the preoperative EKG.

5. A 40-year-old man is being nursed in the recovery room in theatre after having a complex total hip replacement. His blood pressure is 90/50 mmHg despite 2 litres of intravenous fluids. His pulse rate is 120 bpm. His urine output is poor and he looks pale, sweaty and anxious. Capillary refill time is 5 seconds and his peripheries are cool.

Chapter 19 Trauma

Trauma

A. Tension pneumothorax
B. Pelvic fracture
C. Lumbar spine fracture/dislocation
D. Wedge fracture lumbar spine
E. Haemothorax
F. Fracture of the seventh cervical vertebra
G. Neck sprain
H. Hip dislocation
I. Osteomyelitis

Read the clinical details of each patient below and decide which is the most appropriate diagnosis from the list above.

1. A 30-year-old man falls 6 metres from some scaffolding. On admission to A&E he complains of shortness of breath and chest pain. On examination he is cyanosed and unable to complete sentences. His trachea is deviated to the right and he has absent breath sounds on the left side. Blood pressure is low, pulse rate is 120 bpm and oxygen levels are only 80% on high-flow oxygen.

2. A heavy steel girder falls directly on to a 45-year-old man on a construction site, crushing his lower abdomen. He is rushed to the Emergency Room and is noted to have bruising around his lower abdomen and groin. His airway and breathing are stable, but his blood pressure is low and he has tachycardia. Intravenous fluids are started, which correct the hypotension. On secondary survey, a doctor finds blood at the urethral meatus and notes that the man has not passed urine.

3. A 23-year-old woman loses control of her car at high speed and crashes. Unfortunately, she is not wearing her seat belt and is ejected from the vehicle. When the paramedic arrives, she complains of severe lower back pain and says that she cannot feel her legs. When the paramedic examines her lower back, he can feel a step in her lumbar spine. Later in hospital she is unable to pass urine, so a catheter is inserted, which drains 1000 mL of clear urine.

4. An 80-year-old man loses balance and falls on to his bottom on the pavement. He complains of lower back pain but is just about able to walk. His legs feel normal and he has normal bladder and bowel function. After 1 week, the pain has not gone so he consults his doctor and is sent for an X-ray examination.

5. A 32-year-old mountain biker goes over his handlebars and lands head first on the ground. He feels immediate neck pain but is otherwise normal. He rides home, but the pain is severe so his wife brings him to A&E. He tells the doctor that he remembers hitting his chin against his chest quite hard. Examination reveals tenderness at the level of C7. Neurological examination is normal. A lateral X-ray examination of the man's neck shows from C1 to C6 is normal. The doctor therefore reassures the man and discharges him. On the way home, the man develops tingling in his right little finger.

6. A 40-year-old lawyer is stationary in his car at the traffic lights. He is wearing his seatbelt. Suddenly he feels a shunt from behind as a van crashes into him at moderate speed. He gets out of his car. The back bumper has been damaged but otherwise the car is untouched. After 10 minutes, the man notices that his neck feels stiff. He goes home, but during the night his neck becomes very painful and he develops a headache.

Chapter 20   Infection of bones and joints

Infection

A. *Staphylococcus aureus*
B. Anaerobic bacteria
C. *Mycobacterium tuberculosis*
D. Methicillin-resistant *Staphylococcus aureus*
E. *Haemophilus influenzae*
F. *Neisseria gonorrhoeae*
G. *Escherichia coli*

Read the clinical details of each patient below and decide which is the most appropriate diagnosis from the list above.

1. A 2-year-old child is admitted with a hot, painful swollen left knee associated with a high fever. She will not move the knee because of pain. On further questioning, it is revealed that the child has never had any vaccinations because her mother has read in the newspapers that vaccinations are dangerous.

2. A 60-year-old woman with known osteoarthritis of her left hip is admitted feeling unwell with a high temperature. Her hip is now very painful and she will not allow the doctor to move it. She says she has been unwell recently with a 'water infection'.

3. A 51-year-old Caucasian woman presents with back pain. She has not been well for the last 3 months. Recently, she has lost weight and had night sweats. She mentions that she lived in India for 10 years when she was 20. On examination, she has a gibbus in the middle region of the thoracic spine and has tenderness on palpation.

4. A 10-year-old girl is admitted with pain in her left tibia and a fever. There is no history of recent illness. X-ray examination shows osteomyelitis in the proximal tibia.

5. A farmer falls 3 metres from a ladder in his cattle yard. He sustains an open fracture of his tibia, which is heavily contaminated.

Chapter 21   Malignancy

Joint and bone pain

A. Paget disease
B. Osteomalacia
C. Rickets
D. Osteoporosis
E. Myeloma
F. Leukaemia
G. Lymphoma
H. Osteogenesis imperfecta
I. Osteoid osteoma
J. Hypercalcaemia

Read the clinical details of each patient below and decide which is the most appropriate diagnosis from the list above.

1. A 70-year-old man presents with pain in both hips and thighs. The history is gradual but night pain is now a feature. Examination shows a normal gait but some restriction of hip movements, particularly hip internal rotation. An X-ray examination shows some early osteoarthritis of the hip but also areas of abnormal bone architecture in the pelvis and left femur. His alkaline phosphatase is 250 U/L.

2. A 12-year-old boy of Asian origin presents with joint aches and pains, particularly of the wrists. He a small and has some diffuse swelling over the wrists with tenderness. X-ray examination shows widened epiphyses with cupping of the physis.

3. A 72-year-old woman presents with back pain and an obvious kyphosis. She had a fall several months ago, which made matters worse. She has no history of previous fractures. X-ray examination shows loss

of height in several thoracic vertebral bodies but the pedicles are intact. All blood tests are normal.

4. A 7-year-old boy presents with severe right hip pain. He has been unwell for several weeks with weight loss and various aches and pains, but the hip pain has come on over the last 24 hours. Clinically, the child looks unwell and any movement of the hip is extremely painful. He is apyrexial and his white cell count (WCC) is abnormal at 1.2×10^9/L. The orthopaedic registrar is worried about septic arthritis and takes the patient to theatre for a washout of the right hip. The culture from theatre is negative.

5. A 10-month-old baby is brought to the casualty department for the fourth time, unsettled and in pain. The pain appears to be located in the right arm. The mother is sure she has not dropped the baby and has supervised the baby well. The A&E senior house officer thinks she might have a case of nonaccidental injury and refers the baby to the paediatric doctors who admit the child. A full skeletal X-ray examination shows several rib fractures and a humeral fracture with a thin cortex and osteopenia.

6. A 14-year-old boy presents with severe right lower leg pain that has been getting worse over 2 months. The pain is present at rest and night pain is a feature. The pain is relieved by ibuprofen, prescribed by the GP. X-ray images show a thickened cortex of the distal shaft of the tibia. A computed tomography scan shows a nidus within a cortical lesion.

Malignancy

A. Prostate metastasis
B. Lung metastasis
C. Myeloma
D. Kidney metastasis
E. Bowel metastasis
F. Breast metastasis
G. Osteosarcoma
H. Thyroid metastasis
I. Osteochondroma

Read the clinical details of each patient below and decide which is the most appropriate diagnosis from the list above.

1. An 80-year-old man presents with pain in the hip. An X-ray shows a sclerotic lesion in the proximal femur with a poorly defined zone of transition. He has a history of hesitancy and weak urine stream.

2. A 10-year-old boy presents with a short history of severe pain around the knee. Examination reveals a tender mass just below the joint in the proximal tibia. An X-ray examination shows cortical destruction and periosteal elevation.

3. A 55-year-old man presents with a pathological fracture of his left clavicle after lifting a suitcase. On

the X-ray image, there is a diffuse area of abnormal bone. The skull shows numerous lytic lesions and his erythrocyte sedimentation rate (ESR) is 130 mm/h.

4. A 15-year-old girl presents with a gradual swelling around the knee. It occasionally gives some discomfort. Examination reveals a hard mass over the distal femur. X-ray examination shows a pedunculated well-defined lesion in continuity with the cortex of the bone.

5. A 60-year-old woman presents with a complete flaccid paralysis of the legs. Prior to this, she had 3 weeks of severe back pain. X-ray images show complete collapse of T12 vertebra. Chest X-ray examination, abdominal and thyroid ultrasound scans are normal. The ESR is 30 mm/h and serum electrophoresis is normal.

6. A 66-year-old man who has been a lifelong smoker has pain in his right arm. X-ray images reveal a lesion in the proximal humerus on and his chest X-ray examination is abnormal.

Chapter 23 Sports injuries

Knee injuries

A. Anterior cruciate ligament rupture
B. Medial meniscal tear
C. Osteoarthritis
D. Pseudogout.
E. Medial collateral ligament sprain
F. Osteochondritis dissecans
G. Patella dislocation
H. Tibial fracture
I. Posterior cruciate ligament injury
J. Patellar tendon rupture

Read the clinical details of each patient below and decide which is the most appropriate diagnosis from the list above.

1. A 30-year-old patient presents after a road traffic accident. The only injury is to the left knee, which hit the dashboard of the car on impact. The knee is generally tender and has a large effusion and a posterior sag. X-ray examination shows no obvious fractures.

2. A 25-year-old woman is playing netball and twists her knee with the foot on the ground. The 'knee went in'. She hobbled off the court but was able to bear weight. Examination shows no effusion but there is tenderness medially above the joint line. Lachman test is negative.

3. A 55-year-old man presents with gradually increasing left knee pain over 6 months. He played football as a young man and has always had 'dodgy knees'. He remembers a few injuries but simply bandaged his knee and played again the following week. He stands

with a varus deformity and has a mild effusion with reduced range of movement and crepitus.

4. A 30-year-old woman has an accident on her first skiing holiday when her ski is caught in the snow at slow speed. The boot stayed in the ski and her right knee was twisted. She felt something go and the knee immediately became swollen. Clinical examination is difficult due to pain, but she does have an effusion.

5. A 35-year-old man presents with knee pain after a relatively minor injury at work several months ago. The knee was bent and twisted when carrying something down the stairs. The knee was very sore initially but settled to some extent. He still has the feeling of something catching and does not fully trust the knee. Examination is normal apart from medial joint line tenderness and a small effusion.

6. A 36-year-old man suffers an injury playing rugby. He is not sure what happened exactly but was tackled and felt severe pain in his right knee. Examination shows swelling and tenderness below the patella. He is unable to raise his leg straight.

Painful joint

A. Osteoarthritis
B. Rheumatoid arthritis
C. Reiter syndrome
D. Septic arthritis
E. Gout
F. Avascular necrosis
G. Ankylosing spondylitis
H. Enteropathic arthritis.
I. Psoriatic arthropathy

Read the clinical details of each patient below and decide which is the most appropriate diagnosis from the list above.

1. A 65-year-old woman presents with a gradual history of pain in the first metatarsophalangeal (MTP) joint. The pain is worse on walking, particularly when she pushes off from that foot. She is only able to wear certain shoes and finds her walking boots surprisingly comfortable. Examination shoes a bony lump over the dorsum of the metatarsal and diminished movements of the joint with crepitus. She has no other joint problems.

2. A 25-year-old soldier comes home on leave after being on duty for 3 months. She has been complaining of knee pain and swelling for several weeks. She has also recently been diagnosed by her GP as having conjunctivitis. Examination reveals a diffusely swollen knee with a large effusion and bilateral eye redness. She has recently also had dysuria.

3. A 40-year-old man presents with pain and swelling of his right hand with multiple swollen joints, particularly the metacarpophalangeal (MCP) joints. He has had a rash over the extensor part of the arm, which has slightly itched but has never really troubled him.

4. An 80-year-old woman, a resident of a nursing home, is normally pleasantly confused and mobile around the home. Over the last few days, she has been unwell and has not used her right arm. She has become drowsy and listless and it is very difficult to obtain a history from her. There is swelling of her right shoulder, which she holds close to her body. Her temperature is 38.6°C and her white cell count (WCC) is 19×10^9/L.

5. A 40-year-old man presents with an acutely inflamed left first MTP joint. He is a heavy drinker and works as a sales representative, entertaining clients a lot in the evenings. He is apyrexial and an X-ray examination is normal. His serum uric acid is normal.

6. A 28-year-old man presents with back pain over several months. He was a keen cricketer but is now unable to play the sports he enjoys because of pain and stiffness. The stiffness is worse in the morning. Clinically, he has diminished movement of the lumbar spine, as demonstrated by Schober test. The sacroiliac joints are also tender. X-ray examination reveals calcification between vertebral bodies.

Lower leg pain

A. Physiotherapy
B. Antiinflammatory tablets
C. Unicompartmental knee replacement
D. Total knee replacement
E. X-ray of the hip
F. X-ray of the spine
G. Realignment surgery
H. Arthroscopy

Read the clinical details of each patient below and decide which is the most appropriate action from the list above.

1. A 40-year-old heavy manual worker presents with a 2-year history of painful right knee. He says the pain is always on the inside of his knee and is worse after activity. He also experiences stiffness and finds that the pain is starting to affect his ability to work. Examination reveals severe varus deformity of the knee. X-ray images show arthritis in the medial compartment with a normal lateral compartment.

2. A 35-year-old plumber presents to clinic with pain in his right knee. This occurred after he stood up from a squatting position. His knee swelled over 24 hours. The pain is on the medial aspect of his knee and he cannot fully straighten his knee. On examination, he has a moderate effusion and has lost 20 degrees of extension.

3. A 67-year-old farmer presents with constant pain on the inside of his left knee. He still works as a farmer, but the pain is making it difficult. The pain is worse

after walking and despite painkillers he gets night pain, which affects his sleep. On examination, he has a swollen left knee, tenderness over the medial joint line and mild varus deformity with a good range of movement. Radiographs show osteoarthritis confined to the medial compartment.

4. A 55-year-old patient has been referred by her GP for a total hip replacement. She complains of left hip pain but also complains of numbness in her buttock that radiates down into her foot. Pain is relatively constant, but she does not find that hip movements worsen her symptoms. She has a good range of hip movement on examination. X-ray examination of her hip shows mild osteoarthritis.

5. A 78-year-old retired miner presents with right knee pain. This is all over his knee and is associated with swelling and clicking. He has not slept properly because of the pain for the last 6 months and he can no longer cope with his symptoms. He has mild chronic obstructive airway disease but is relatively fit otherwise. He lives alone, his property has stairs and he normally walks with a stick. Examination reveals a fixed flexion deformity of 10 degrees and a Baker cyst in the popliteal fossa. X-ray images reveal loss of joint space, subchondral sclerosis and cyst, with large osteophytes. He would like an operation to help his pain.

Chapter 23 Soft tissue disorders

Imaging

A. CT scan
B. MRI
C. Plain X-ray image
D. Bone scan
E. Nerve conduction study
F. Ultrasound scan
G. Venous Doppler scan

Read the clinical details of each patient below and decide which is the most appropriate investigation according to what you think the most likely diagnosis is.

1. A 56-year-old housewife says she gets pins and needles and pain, especially at night in her index, middle and half her ring fingers. This is relieved by hanging her hand over the end of the bed. She has a history of type 2 diabetes.

2. A 40-year-old woman reports a 6-month history of shooting pains from her left buttock, radiating down the back of her leg into her foot. She has altered sensation over the lateral aspect of her lower leg and the sole of her foot.

3. A 68-year-old man attends A&E with a swollen, tender left leg. He had a left total knee replacement 6 weeks previously. Movements of his ankle are quite painful.

4. A 30-year-old man presents with a lump on the palmar aspect of his left wrist. He has had this for many years, but recently it has slightly increased in size and can be painful as it catches on his watch. On examination, it is mobile to the skin and underlying muscle and soft and has smooth round borders. It is not pulsatile.

5. A 56-year-old man has renal cell carcinoma. He complains of pain in his right forearm.

Chapter 24 Principles of orthopaedic surgery

Orthopaedic gait assessment

A. Ataxic
B. Trendelenburg
C. Waddling
D. Antalgic
E. Foot drop
F. High-stepping
G. Shuffling
H. Spastic

Read the clinical details of each patient below and decide which is the most likely gait pattern from the list above.

1. A 62-year-old man presents with pain in his left hip, which he has suffered with for many years. X-ray images show osteoarthritis. When asked to stand on his left leg, his pelvis drops. When standing on his right leg, his pelvis tilts up.

2. A 35-year-old football hooligan is seen in clinic saying that he cannot walk properly. He was involved in a fight 6 weeks previously and says the policeman hit him very hard just below his right knee with a truncheon. He has some numbness over the dorsum of his foot but has no pain. When he walks, he brings his right knee much higher than the left.

3. A 10-year-old boy is seen in the orthopaedic clinic for review. When walking, he displays muscular incoordination and has his feet quite wide apart. His old notes state that he had meningitis as an infant.

4. A 30-year-old woman is seen in clinic with a painful ankle after she twisted it falling down a kerb. When walking, she hobbles and has a reduced-stance phase on the affected side.

5. An 8-year-old boy is seen in clinic with his mother. His lower-limb function has worsened over the last few years. He has flexed and adducted hips and walks with a stiff gait. His feet are in equinus.

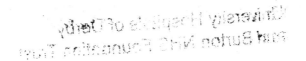

SBA answers

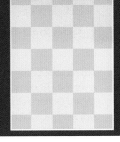

Chapter 1 Taking a history

1. C. A medical history of an under-active thyroid. This is commonly associated with carpal tunnel syndrome. A family history of hypertension is important but does not clarify the diagnosis. Many patients try multiple analgesics to relieve the pain from this condition. Her social history might reveal exacerbating factors such as typing at a keyboard but does not narrow the diagnosis. Marked fatigue often occurs with hypothyroidism but is not directly associated with carpal tunnel syndrome.

2. B. Prednisolone 10 mg daily for several years. Corticosteroids are a well-recognized risk factor in developing osteoporosis. Corticosteroid use of 7.5 mg prednisolone (or equivalent) daily for more than 3 months is considered to be sufficiently high to warrant bone protection. A family history of traumatic hip fracture is unlikely to present significant increased risk of osteoporosis, as is the case of menopause at the age of 53 years, which would be considered normal. Living abroad might confer a protective effect against osteoporosis as increased sunlight exposure improves vitamin D metabolism. A personal history of type 2 diabetes does not increase your risk of osteoporosis.

3. A. A recent history of swallowing trouble. These are features of CREST syndrome (systemic sclerosis), an important cause of secondary Raynaud disease. Primary Raynaud disease does not typically ulcerate, nor is it associated with other connective tissue diseases. Alcohol misuse is not a recognized risk factor for secondary Raynaud disease, nor is a family history of osteoarthritis. Nifedipine and other calcium channel blockers are commonly used to help all forms of Raynaud phenomenon. COPD is not associated with secondary Raynaud disease.

4. D. Reactive arthritis. This inflammatory joint condition can occur after bacterial infections (such as mycoplasma pneumoniae in lower respiratory tract infections) and favours the larger joints of the lower limbs. Acute polyarticular gout is unlikely in someone as a first presentation. Rheumatoid arthritis is a symmetrical inflammatory arthritis typically affecting the hands and feet. Ankylosing spondylitis is an axial spondyloarthropathy affecting the back, although it is commonly associated with the HLA-B27 antigen, as is reactive arthritis. Polyarticular septic arthritis is rare and usually presents as life-threatening sepsis.

Chapter 2 Examining joints

1. E. Prepatellar bursitis. This is common in patients who work a lot on their knees; the patient's signs and symptoms are suggestive of this. Osteoarthritis tends to occur slowly over many months and years and in older patients. Septic arthritis is often associated with an acute illness where the patient is septic or systemically unwell. A Baker cyst typically presents with pain at the back of the knee. A patellar fracture is unlikely as there is no history of trauma.

2. D. Bucket-handle meniscal tear. The handle segment flips over and becomes trapped in the joint resulting in the knee locking. The patient is unable to extend the knee fully.

3. E. High-stepping gait. This is because the leg must be lifted higher to clear the ground in patients with a foot-drop. Trendelenburg gait is seen in patients with abnormal hip abductor function. An antalgic gait is a painful gait often seen in osteoarthritis or any painful condition. A circumduction gait occurs in hemiplegia. Waddling gait is seen in patients with congenital hip dislocations, amongst other conditions.

4. B. Extensor pollicis longus. The tendon of EPL runs over the radial side of the wrist joint and is commonly affected by displaced wrist fractures. It controls thumb extension and can be tested by asking the patient to straighten the distal joint of the thumb or lift the thumb off a flattened surface with the palm face-down. Adductor pollicis controls thumb adduction, abductor pollicis brevis controls abduction and opponens pollicis controls thumb opposition. Extensor digitorum is responsible for extension of the metacarpophalangeal, proximal interphalangeal and distal interphalangeal of the digits.

5. A. Carpal tunnel syndrome. Her hypothyroidism is a risk factor for the condition. The classic presentation is of pain occurring in the thumb, index and middle finger and the thumb side of the ring finger. Systemic causes of peripheral neuropathy most commonly cause a glove-and-stocking distribution of pain or anaesthesia. Peripheral vascular disease causes intermittent claudication, typically found in the legs.

C8 radiculopathy would result in altered sensation over the C8 dermatome, which covers the 4th and 5th digits. Golfer's elbow is an acute swelling of the medial epicondyle, which would typically affect the ulnar nerve if any.

Chapter 3 Investigations

1. A. Anti-double stranded DNA antibodies. These are highly specific for systemic lupus erythematosus (SLE). ESR would be elevated, but it is nonspecific. Skin biopsy can be useful for cutaneous lupus but in a classic photosensitive malar rash it would be unlikely to help confirm the diagnosis. Thyroid disease is important to consider but would not confirm the diagnosis of SLE.

2. B. Methotrexate hepatotoxicity. It is important that a patient's blood is closely monitored when increasing doses of methotrexate. Signs of toxicity include flu-like symptoms, nausea, diarrhoea, fatigue and recurrent mouth ulcers. Blood shows a hepatitic pattern of derangement. Primary biliary cirrhosis is associated with rheumatoid arthritis but presents insidiously with itching and cholestatic blood. Acute viral hepatitis is unlikely and typically the derangement would be far more severe. Gallstones cause painful jaundice with elevated alkaline phosphatase, GGT and bilirubin. Alcohol abuse is a possibility, but there is nothing in her history to suggest overuse.

3. C. Anti-SCL-70. This woman has systemic sclerosis with secondary Raynaud phenomenon, sclerodactyly and telangiectasia. Jo-1 is associated with antisynthetase syndrome. Anti-dsDNA is very specific for SLE. p-ANCA is associated with vasculitis. Histone antibodies are seen in drug-induced lupus.

4. D. MRI. The twisting mechanism with a popping sensation suggests a meniscal tear for which MRI is the best investigative procedure. Joint aspiration, in the context of trauma, is likely to show haemarthrosis but will not facilitate the diagnosis. X-ray examination is limited to diagnosing bony issues. Ultrasound is useful for looking at soft tissue, but it is technically difficult to get deep views of the knee. ESR will be nonspecifically elevated in the context of injury and inflammation.

Chapter 4 Regional pain

1. A. A history of urinary incontinence. This is a red flag feature of back pain and an urgent MRI should be carried out to exclude cord compression. An elevated ESR is nonspecific for inflammation but does not imply an urgent cause for concern. A family history of psoriasis may predispose the patient to psoriatic arthritis with sacroiliitis, but it does not require an urgent MRI. Abnormal TFTs may explain fatigue but are not usually implicated in back pain. A positive ANA is a common nonspecific finding in the general population, particularly at low titres.

2. B. A ruptured ACL. The fluid description of blood with fat globules suggests lipohaemarthrosis, which usually indicates a fracture or ruptured ACL. An inflated rheumatoid joint aspirate would be slightly cloudy yellow. Septic arthritis gives frank pus on aspirate. A patellar dislocation is extremely painful but does not usually present with effusion as its main sign. Pseudogout is a crystal arthropathy seen in the elderly, where the fluid can be cloudy or slightly pus-like.

3. C. Spinal stenosis. The pain is bilateral, radiates and is relieved by flexing the spine (hence the patient's stooped gait). Extension aggravates his symptoms. Prolapsed intervertebral discs give pain in response to an acute injury, which is usually unilateral. Mechanical back pain does not usually give radiating neurological symptoms. Spondylolisthesis pain usually improves on lying flat. The patient does not have red flag features suggesting malignancy.

4. D. ESR. This gentleman has polymyalgia rheumatica, a common cause of bilateral shoulder pain, fatigue and stiffness in the elderly. Treatment is with steroids. Nerve conduction studies are unlikely to yield useful results, nor will X-ray images as his history does not suggest a bony cause for his symptoms. The history is not typical of multiple myeloma, the test for which is a urinary Bence Jones protein. MRI of the neck is helpful in neuropathic disorders to exclude nerve root compression but would not be helpful here.

5. E. Complex regional pain syndrome is characterized by severe pain after an injury, skin changes, hypersensitivity and occasional swelling. Arterial insufficiency causes claudication and ulceration. Upper limb DVT would not normally cause hypersensitivity. Factitious pain is rare and we should be wary of labelling patients with this. Phantom-limb pain is seen postamputation.

Chapter 5 Widespread musculoskeletal pain

1. A. CT thorax, abdomen and pelvis. This woman has an atypical presentation of PMR with overlapping inflammatory joint disease; the possibility of a paraneoplastic rheumatic syndrome must be considered. A CT scan of the thorax, abdomen and pelvis is the first-line test when considering an occult malignancy. Abnormal vitamin D levels would

not explain the synovitis or elevated ESR. Muscle biopsy is usually only undertaken for the diagnosis of myositis. Rheumatoid factor is nonspecific and steroids would normally improve standard rheumatoid arthritis. Skeletal survey is a test for multiple myeloma; it may be undertaken later but would not be a first-line test.

2. B. Anti-dsDNA antibodies. These are highly specific for systemic lupus erythematosus. ESR is nonspecifically elevated in a variety of inflammatory conditions. Schirmer test is useful in confirming reduced lacrimation but is nonspecific. Rheumatoid factor would not be useful in this situation. A urine dip may show blood and protein in lupus nephritis, but this is again nonspecific.

3. C. Pregabalin. This woman has fibromyalgia. A multitherapy approach to treatment is required involving physiotherapy/graded exercise, addressing trigger stressors and analgesia (anticonvulsants are often used). Naproxen is a nonsteroidal antiinflammatory drug and therefore useful. Adalimumab is a monoclonal antibody used in severe inflammatory arthritis. Methotrexate is similarly reserved for inflammatory arthritis. Opiates such as oxycodone are generally avoided in the management of fibromyalgia.

4. D. Reassurance. This woman has fibromyalgia. Her initial tests are normal and she has no neurological deficits. She needs reassurance and referred to services such as physiotherapy, cognitive behavioural therapy and occupational therapy. In the absence of neurological features, MRI is unlikely to have any diagnostic use. Immunology is normal in fibromyalgia. Electromyography is reserved predominantly for disorders affecting the neuromuscular junction. IV immunoglobulins are used in a variety of severe autoimmune conditions but have no role here.

5. E. Foot drop. This usually indicates an L5/S1 nerve root lesion. Altered sleep pattern, pain in multiple tender points, alternating bowel habits and headache are all common features of fibromyalgia.

Chapter 6 An acute hot swollen joint

1. A. Gram-positive cocci. This woman has septic arthritis and the most common organism is *Staphylococcus aureus*, a common skin bacterium. Gram-negative bacilli tend to inhabit the GI tract. Crystal arthropathy is unlikely because she is clinically exhibiting signs of infection. Blood would indicate a haemarthrosis, but she is not known to be on anticoagulants or to have suffered trauma.

2. B. DMARDs. This man has psoriatic arthritis, a common cause of acute inflammatory monoarthritis in young men. His rash is characteristic of the skin symptoms caused by psoriatic arthritis. Methotrexate or leflunomide are usually first-line DMARDs. Antibiotics will not help. Paracetamol may help his pain but not the underlying condition. Systemic steroids often worsen skin symptoms of psoriasis. Topical emollients will help treat the skin symptoms but not the arthritis.

3. C. A previous history of right ankle swelling and pain. This suggests recurrence of a gout flare. Septic arthritis does not typically happen episodically. A low-grade fever can be a feature of either condition as can a high CRP level. A history of immunosuppression favours the diagnosis of septic arthritis. A family history of rheumatoid arthritis is not particularly relevant to either condition.

Chapter 7 A child with a limp

1. B. Hypothyroidism. Hypothyroidism conveys no risk to developing Perthes disease. Hypothyroidism and other hormonal conditions are risk factors in slipped upper femoral epiphysis. Delayed bone age, low socioeconomic group, low birth weight and a family history are all risk factors of developing Perthes disease.

2. E. Slipped upper femoral epiphysis. This condition occurs in adolescents aged 11–14 years and is more common in boys than girls. A background of chronic pain prior to the slip of the

3. A. Transient synovitis. With the history of a recent viral illness and normal radiology and inflammatory markers, transient synovitis is most likely.

4. D. Immediate resuscitation. Whilst the other steps may be important in the management of the patient, they should not delay resuscitation and should be part of an ongoing process of reassessment.

Chapter 8 A limb swelling

1. C. Ganglion. The history of a small fluctuant lesion surrounding a joint with an intermittent history is that of a ganglion.

2. A. Osteosarcoma is rare but most commonly occurs in adolescents and elderly patients with Paget bone disease. It is a highly malignant tumour and requires urgent investigation. An X-ray examination will identify the problem and MRI scanning will better define it.

3. D. Baker cyst. This is a common benign mass on the back of the knee; it is thought to be a sack of joint fluid pushed posterior in the knee. It should be carefully felt for pulsatility to rule out an aneurysm.

Chapter 9 Back pain

1. D. Nucleus pulposus. A disc prolapse occurs when part of the nucleus pulposus herniates through the annulus fibrosus and presses on a spinal nerve root.

2. D. Bilateral sciatic-type pain. Bilateral leg symptoms are suggestive of impending cauda equina syndrome.

3. B. MRI scan. In order to assess for compression of the nerve roots at the cauda equina, MRI is the best investigative procedure. This must be done urgently if clinical suspicion is high. A CT scan can be useful and with modern scanners can give lots of information; however, MRI is gold standard.

4. C. Spinal stenosis. This man has spinal stenosis. The pain in his buttocks, thighs and calves is spinal claudication. Patients walk with a stooped gait to flex the lumbar spine and alleviate their symptoms.

5. C. Metastatic prostate cancer. This is the most likely cause: the spread of tumour into the spine is thought to made more likely by back flow through the venous complex. It has the classic sclerotic appearance on X-ray images.

Chapter 10 Altered sensation and weakness

1. D. Median nerve. A dorsally angulated distal radius fracture can cause compression of the median nerve, giving symptoms of carpal tunnel syndrome.

2. D. Carpal tunnel syndrome. This woman has carpal tunnel syndrome. Her symptoms and their distribution are typical of carpal tunnel syndrome. Percussion at the wrist crease is Tinel sign.

3. C. Nerve conduction studies. These studies can be useful when planning surgery for carpal tunnel disease and will give a grading from 1 to 4 as to how severe it is. Ultimately, the decision to decompress is still made clinically.

4. A. Transient ischaemic attack. This story is much more acute and concerning than that of a simple nerve entrapment and should be investigated for stroke or TIA with a central cause far more likely then a peripheral cause.

Chapter 11 Osteoarthritis

1. A. Lytic bone lesions. This suggests malignant infiltration of the bone. The other four findings are all classic signs of osteoarthritis.

2. B. Osteophytes. This gentleman is suffering from osteoarthritis. Erosions are a feature of inflammatory arthritis. A hairline fracture would have a quicker scale of onset. Osteopenia is usually incidental and not usually a primary cause of pain. Soft tissue swelling is clinically discernible on examination; X-ray examination is primarily an investigation of bony structures.

3. C. Heberden nodes. The patient's clinical history and age are suggestive of osteoarthritis. Ulnar deviation and boutonniere deformity are suggestive of rheumatoid arthritis. A Dupuytren contracture is common with advancing age, but it is not typically painful. MCP swelling is suggestive of inflammatory arthritis.

4. D. Physiotherapy. This man has osteoarthritis (OA). The evidence for glucosamine is poor. Joint replacement may be warranted but most patients explore nonsurgical options first. Systemic steroids to not have a role to play in managing OA, although joint injection can help with pain; however, the hip joint is a challenging joint to inject and must be done under ultrasound or X-ray guidance.

Chapter 12 Rheumatoid arthritis

1. A. Splinting. The patient is developing carpal tunnel syndrome, a recognized complication of RA. Steroids, methotrexate and gold have no place in the treatment of this: they are disease-modifying antiinflammatory drugs. Physiotherapy tends not to be helpful. Surgery may be a late consideration if conservative measures fail.

2. B. Joint effusion. Hand joints are very small and therefore detecting an effusion on X-ray images is particularly challenging. Erosions and joint space narrowing may be seen in rheumatoid arthritis (RA). Osteopenia may be seen in a number of conditions but is typically described as periarticular in RA. Soft-tissue swelling may be noted; however, this is a clinical finding!

3. C. Start DMARDs. In the absence of other issues, methotrexate would be the drug of choice. Physiotherapy has a role to play in the management of rheumatoid arthritis but will not quickly alleviate the synovitis. MRI of the hands is unnecessary

and will delay treatment. Hydrotherapy again may have a role to play, but the focus on early disease is inducing remission. NSAIDs are good for treating symptoms.

4. D. Naproxen. This is an nonsteroidal antiinflammatory drug with an associated risk of gastrointestinal bleeding. Hydroxychloroquine, methotrexate and sulfasalazine are disease-modifying antirheumatic drugs used to treat rheumatoid arthritis, whilst paracetamol is an analgesic used for pain relief. In the context of nodulosis, the patient should be warned that methotrexate might make it worse, but it would not be considered a contraindication to taking it.

5. E. Constrictive pericarditis. This is a very rare complication of longstanding pericardial inflammation, which is no longer seen as common in rheumatoid arthritis (RA) due to improvements in treatment. Rheumatoid lung disease and methotrexate-induced fibrosis still occur though the incidence is relatively low. Anaemia is common in RA for a number of reasons. An acquired kyphosis is common in osteoporosis, commonly seen in patients who have had significant corticosteroid treatment.

Chapter 13 Spondyloarthropathies

1. A. Haemophilus. This is a respiratory pathogen. The man has Reiter syndrome, which is associated with gut infections and sexually transmitted infections.

2. B. Corticosteroids. These will act fast to settle both the bowel and joint symptoms. They can be given systemically or via rectal foam in the first instance. NSAIDs often aggravate gastrointestinal symptoms. Panproctocolectomy is the surgery of last-choice in patients with IBD who fail with medical management. Biological specimens are useful but are not indicated first-line in the absence of severe disease; they are very useful in axial disease involvement. Sulfasalazine is commonly used as maintenance therapy in inflammatory bowel disease and enteropathic arthritis, but steroids are more appropriate acutely to induce remission.

3. C. Subungal hyperkeratosis. This occurs in psoriatic arthritis. Keratoderma blennorrhagica is associated with reactive arthritis. Koilonychia (spoon-shaped nails) is associated with iron-deficiency anaemia. Leuconychia is a generally benign condition of white marks on the nail due to trauma or injury to the growing nail. Paronychia is an infection of the skin adjacent to the nail.

4. D. Anticardiolipin antibody. This is associated with connective tissue disease and antiphospholipid syndrome. AS is a seronegative spondyloarthropathy. The other four are the four As associated with ankylosing spondylitis.

5. E. Ankylosing spondylitis. 90% of patients are HLA B27 positive. Around 60%–80% of patients with psoriatic and reactive arthritis are positive. 60% for enteropathic arthritis and 25% for undifferentiated spondyloarthritis.

Chapter 14 Connective tissue diseases

1. A. Temporal artery biopsy. This is the gold standard test for giant cell arteritis. ESR should be elevated but this is nonspecific. ANCA screening is likely to be negative. Lumbar puncture is used to test for headaches caused by meningitis, encephalitis and elevated intracranial pressure. MRI of the aortic arch is a sensitive test for aortic vasculitis, but there is no guarantee that any lesions would be visible.

2. B. Systemic sclerosis. This patient has evidence of widespread multisystem sclerosis and fibrosis with pulmonary hypertension, pulmonary fibrosis, Raynaud phenomenon, scleroderma and calcinosis in the hands and telangiectasia. Linear scleroderma is a limited cutaneous pattern of the disease. SLE presents differently and would not give calcinosis. Paraneoplastic syndrome is generally associated with few signs and would not give pulmonary fibrosis. Multiple sclerosis is a neurological disorder characterized by progressive weakness and spasticity.

3. C. Schirmer test. This test is used in the diagnosis of Sjögren syndrome. An HIV test is a reasonable second-line test if no cause is found for these symptoms. Schober test measures lumbar spine mobility. Transoesophageal echography is used to exclude valvular lesions such as endocarditis. Trendelenburg test is used to assess hip muscle weakness.

4. D. Administer prednisolone. This woman has polymyalgia rheumatica with features of giant cell arteritis. It requires urgent treatment to preserve vision and reduce the risk of stroke. Checking ESR is an important part of diagnosis, as is arranging a temporal artery biopsy, but it should not obstruct treatment. Muscle biopsy is not required in this scenario. Nonsteroidal antiinflammatory drugs are good for treating the symptoms of inflammation but will not alter the disease process.

5. E. Serum creatine kinase levels. Dermatomyositis will produce inflamed muscles, which leak enzymes due to oedema in the cells. Elevated creatine kinase levels are seen, usually several orders of magnitude compared with normal. ESR may be elevated but is nonspecific and positive antinuclear antibodies are seen in many connective tissue diseases. Chest X-ray examination should be performed to exclude malignancy but is not diagnostic of dermatomyositis and X-ray examination of the affected joints does not normally reveal erosions.

6. A. Antiphospholipid antibody. A stillbirth and two vascular events suggest antiphospholipid syndrome, which is also associated with levido, migraines, low platelets and systemic lupus erythematosus. Other antibodies should be checked given the association, but the primary antiphospholipid syndrome must be confirmed. A prothrombin time may be checked after thrombolysis to monitor coagulation but is nondiagnostic. Syphilis serology is occasionally checked in unusual cases of thrombosis and arteritis but is a very unlikely cause.

Chapter 15 Metabolic bone disease

1. A. Osteoporosis. Vertebral height loss, back pain from a probable vertebral fracture and previous history of low-energy fracture all suggest osteoporosis. Myeloma would cause back pain for weeks or months, hypercalcaemia and weight loss. Osteomalacia is a disorder of low vitamin D levels. It results in low calcium levels/low phosphate and raised alkaline phosphatase. Paget disease would cause an elevated alkaline phosphatase level and is not associated with vertebral height loss. Potts disease is very rare and is associated with systemic upsets including weight loss, night sweats and unexplained persistent pyrexia.

2. B. Bone biochemistry. The patient has Paget disease of bone and this simple blood test will show an elevated alkaline phosphatase level. Coeliac serology should be tested if vitamin D deficiency is thought to be the cause. DEXA is used for diagnosing osteoporosis. MRI would give the diagnosis but is costly and will take time to organize. Isotope bone scanning is therefore the imaging modality of choice. Rheumatoid factor will not help in this diagnosis.

3. C. Polydipsia. The patient has renal osteomalacia where vitamin D fails to be metabolized into the active form by chronically failing kidneys. Polydipsia is a commonly seen symptom in hypercalcaemia but is not associated with low calcium or low phosphate levels. The other features are all possible.

4. D. Paget disease. Back pain, knee pain with increased blood flow and high levels of alkaline phosphatase suggest this. Osteoarthritis should not cause an increase in ALP. A prolapsed disc may explain her back pain but not the biochemical changes of the knee warmth. Septic arthritis rarely involves so many joints in a patient who seems otherwise well. Gout would again not explain the biochemistry picture.

5. E. Anti-tissue transglutaminase antibody. Coeliac disease is a common malabsorptive cause of osteomalacia causing low levels of iron, folate, vitamin D and other essential vitamins and minerals. Anti-dsDNA is found in lupus. Antiphospholipid antibodies are seen in patients with recurrent venous and arterial thrombus. Anti-smooth muscle antibody is found in lupus and autoimmune liver disease. Anti-vitamin D3 antibodies is not a readily available test, but the picture remains more complex than straightforward osteomalacia due to isolated vitamin D deficiency.

Chapter 16 Gout and pseudogout

1. E. Splinting. This will allow the joint time to rest and pain relief to be given. Aspiration has not grown organisms and antibiotics are therefore not required. DMARDs are not indicated in pseudogout. Joint replacement is not performed in an acute setting such as this. Physiotherapy is likely to be required, but only once the inflammation has settled.

2. D. Monosodium urate crystals. These are found in acute gout. The white lumps are tophi. Bacteria need to be excluded from an acute hot joint but the presence of tophi make septic arthritis less likely. Calcium pyrophosphate crystals occur in pseudogout, mainly seen in the elderly in knees and wrists. Pus is possible, but white tophus is more likely given the finger deposits. Clear synovial fluid is unlikely; fluid tends to be slightly cloudy when inflammation is present.

3. C. Chronic hyperuricemia. This leads to the formation of sodium urate crystals that are deposited in the synovium, causing inflammation. This is the underlying process in gout. Chronic kidney disease often leads to asymptomatic hyperuricemia and gout develops when these crystals are deposited in tissue. The patient's history is not suggestive of rheumatoid arthritis, chronic septic arthritis, pseudogout or osteoarthritis.

4. B. Pseudogout. Both gout and pseudogout would occur without trauma, but given the finding of chondrocalcinosis from the X-ray examination, the joint involved and age, pseudogout is most likely. Septic arthritis is unlikely if the patient is well, with

normal temperate and white-cell count. Rheumatoid arthritis is unlikely and there is no trauma or anticoagulant use as a risk for haemarthrosis.

5. A. Increase allopurinol to 300 mg daily. The patient's blood should be rechecked within 12 weeks and the dose increased as required to maintain serum uric acid below 360 μg/ml. There is no indication for changing to febuxostat at this time. Steroids can be useful in the acute setting but are avoided long term. Colchicine and nonsteroidal drugs such as ibuprofen are typically used for acute flares but are sometimes continued in the medium term in difficult-to-manage cases.

Chapter 17 Paediatric joint disease

1. D. Medial femoral circumflex artery. The majority of the blood supply to the femoral head in adults arises from the medial femoral circumflex artery. There is a lesser contribution from the lateral femoral circumflex artery. The artery of the ligamentum teres supplies a negligible blood supply in adults.

2. B. External rotation. The classic position for a leg to lie after SUFE is in external rotation and on flexion this will persist due to the impingement of the displaced anterior-lateral femoral metaphysis (Drehmann sign). The hip will be painful on all movements and it is likely to have lost internal rotation, flexion and abduction.

3. A. Talipes equinovarus. This baby has a deformity that is commonly called a clubfoot. The initial treatment is a cast and then further assessment should be made if this is unsuccessful. It is likely that the foot will always appear abnormal but this often does not affect the quality of life.

4. E. Osteogenesis imperfecta. There is a chance that this child is the victim of NAI and this should be explored. However, given the scoliosis, short stature and multiple low-energy fractures, a diagnosis of osteogenesis imperfecta should be considered and investigated.

5. C. Compartment syndrome. The principal symptom of compartment syndrome is pain. Any patient who has a severe increase in pain following a fracture should be assessed for compartment syndrome. Proximal tibial fractures are at increased risk of developing compartment syndrome.

6. A. Pulmonary thromboembolism. Although rare, pulmonary thromboembolism is a recognized complication of arthroplasty surgery. The onset and nature of the patient's symptoms are highly suggestive of this condition.

7. C. Early mobilization. The main principle of internal fixation is to allow early mobilization.

8. C. Apply a pelvic binder. Whilst the others are sensible options, a pelvic binder can be quickly and simply applied by anybody and should be the FIRST step taken if it has not already been done. Blood samples should also be taken.

9. A. Hemiarthroplasty. Fixation with DHS is not an option because the blood supply to the femoral head will be compromised. The patient is not fit enough for total hip replacement. Girdlestone is a complete disarticulation of the hip and is a last resort if all other options have failed. Conservative treatment in a previously mobile patient would be a poor option, committing her to several months of pain and immobility.

Chapter 19 Trauma

1. E. Assess the airway whilst stabilizing the cervical spine. In the assessment of any trauma patients, follow the ABCDE pathway and assess systems in order of importance. Do not become distracted by the perceived main issue. All patients should be assumed to have a cervical spine injury until proven otherwise.

2. B. They are likely to have lost 15%–30% of blood volume. Their blood pressure has fallen in response to volume depletion and their pulse rate has gone up in order to attempt to maintain perfusion of end organs.

3. D. A CT scan should be obtained of the head and C-spine. It is likely this patient also has an intracranial abnormality. If the patient already needs to undergo a CT scan and has symptoms, C-spine X-ray examination will be an extra, unhelpful step. Whilst an MRI is informative, it is difficult to obtain in an emergency situation, unlike a CT scan.

Chapter 20 Infection of bones and joints

1. C. *Staphylococcus aureus*. *S. aureus* is the most common pathogen in septic arthritis in adults, followed by *Streptococcus* and *Enterobacter*. *S. aureus* is the most common pathogen in all ages.

2. C. Aspiration of the knee. This man has septic arthritis until proven otherwise. It is important that this is confirmed via joint aspiration as soon as possible. X-ray examination and blood tests can be performed first, but joint aspiration is the most important investigation. When possible, antibiotics should be withheld until after joint aspiration has been performed.

3. E. Prepatellar bursitis. Prepatellar bursitis is common in patients who kneel when working (e.g., electricians, plumbers). This patient's signs and symptoms suggest an obvious bursitis and do not highlight an intraarticular pathology.

4. E. All of the above. Intravenous drug abusers inject themselves with potentially contaminated drugs through a dirty needle. They are also frequently immunosuppressed and undernourished; consequently, they are at risk of a wide range of infections. As a result, they will require a broad range of antibiotics to cover potential pathogens.

Chapter 21 Malignancy

1. B. Osteoid osteoma. Osteoid osteoma presents insidiously, giving rise to intense pain and tenderness over the affected area, sometimes with a history of night pain. A central lucent nidus surrounded by a dense area of reactive bone will be seen on X-ray image. Salicylates greatly reduce the pain.

2. B. Osteosarcoma. Osteosarcoma is most common between the ages of 10 and 40 years and frequently occurs around the knee. The symptoms of night pain and weight loss are suspicious of malignancy. The X-ray findings are typical of osteosarcoma.

3. A. Prostate cancer. The finding of a sclerotic lesion makes prostate cancer the most likely cause for this metastatic deposit. Prostate cancer often metastasizes to the spine due to the venous drainage connection.

4. D. Periosteal reaction. This is the Codman triangle appearance on an X-ray image whereby, in aggressive lesions, the cortex does not have time to remodel and there is a raised multilayered edge of periosteum. Looser zones are present in osteomalacia, vertebral trabecular thickening is seen in Paget disease and the other changes are in keeping with osteoarthritis.

Chapter 22 Sports injuries

1. A. Bucket handle meniscal tear. The handle part of a bucket handle tear flips over, becoming trapped in the joint and preventing full extension.

2. E. Anterior cruciate ligament tear. An anterior cruciate ligament tear is normally caused by a twisting injury to the knee. Patients will describe immediate pain and rapid swelling. Examination will reveal a large effusion, due to the haemarthrosis, and laxity in the AP axis. Lachman test and anterior drawer test are used for diagnosis.

3. D. The majority of dislocations come out anterior inferior due to the weakness of the muscle cover in this position.

4. D. Hypoplastic trochlea. A shallow trochlea will increase the risk of patellar dislocation, which is particularly common in young women and can be difficult to treat.

Chapter 23 Soft tissue disorders

1. B. Abductor pollicis longus. De Quervain tenosynovitis is inflammation of the tendon sheaths of abductor pollicis longus and extensor pollicis brevis.

2. A. This is olecranon bursitis and should initially be treated with a period of rest and NSAIDs.

3. B. Palmar fascia. Dupuytren contracture is a disease in which palmar fascia undergoes fibrosis and contracture.

Chapter 24 Principles of orthopaedic surgery

1. B. Hypovolaemia. The patient is likely to be still very hypovolaemic postoperatively. This should be corrected but not too aggressively in an older patient.

2. A. Hip dislocation. Given the patient's history, he is most likely to have suffered a dislocation of his hip replacement. This normally happens with a low impact mechanism; a periprosthetic fracture would usually require more force.

3. B. This is a problem frequently encountered on the orthopaedic ward. If the patient is well, antibiotics should be withheld until samples have been taken. Immediate single stage revision would be unwise in the presence of likely infection. A bone scan would add little as infection is extremely likely with this history. This patient clearly requires investigation and should not be discharged.

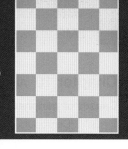

Chapter 7 A child with a limp

Paediatric hip disorders

1. C. Developmental dysplasia of the hip. Late-presenting developmental dysplasia of the hip presents with a painless limp and leg-length discrepancy. All the other conditions on the list will present with pain.

2. E. Slipped upper femoral epiphysis. The patient is the correct age and the history of pain is typical. The femoral head in slipped upper femoral epiphysis rotates posteriorly and leaves an externally rotated leg. The frog lateral X-ray image shows the slip more obviously than the AP X-ray image.

3. B. Juvenile idiopathic arthritis. Presentation with monoarthritis is common, with other joints involved later. Generalized symptoms suggest a systemic disorder. The presence of eye symptoms is worrying as blindness can result.

4. J. Osgood-Schlatter disease. The disease is often bilateral and occurs during the adolescent years. Tender swollen tibial tuberosities are present bilaterally.

5. A. Perthes disease. The boy is the right age to have Perthes and the history of knee pain is typical. The loss of abduction is worrying as it could mean impending joint subluxation. The sclerosis of the femoral head is due to avascular necrosis.

6. G. Osteomyelitis. Diagnosis is difficult in the very young child. In this case, the child clearly has an infection. In the absence of an obviously swollen joint and with a normal hip ultrasound scan, the most likely cause is osteomyelitis.

Chapter 8 A limb swelling

Orthopaedic investigations

1. F. DEXA scan: for osteoporosis. The best method to quantify bone density is DEXA. In any patient suffering fragility fractures, this should be considered.

2. B. X-ray examination: march fracture. A stress fracture of one of the metatarsals at the distal third. Caused by repetitive stress on foot. Often causes a lump but usually self-limiting.

3. G. Isotope bone scanning: Paget disease. Although an X-ray examination will demonstrate disorganized patterns of affected bone, a bone scan is much more sensitive for identifying pagetic lesions.

4. A. MRI: lipoma. This patient has a very large lipoma that has been growing for some time. When a benign lesion grows large enough, it will cause venous congestion and the whole limb can become swollen. MRI scanning will help to define it properly and to plan surgery.

5. D. Ultrasound scan: abscess/aneurysm. This patient requires imaging of this lump prior to incision to ensure no involvement of the major vessels. It is common to find a large aneurysm in the groin of people who inject intravenous drugs regularly.

6. C. CT scan: Ewing sarcoma. This boy has a very worrying presentation and the jaundice implies metastatic spread. He should undergo a staging CT scan urgently.

Chapter 9 Back pain

Back pain

1. B. Spinal stenosis. The history is typical and pain is often worse on extension. The X-ray image often only shows osteoarthritis and a CT or MRI scan will confirm the presence of spinal stenosis.

2. F. Spinal metastases. The history sounds sinister, with unrelenting pain. The X-ray image showing loss of the pedicle (winking-owl sign) means bony destruction by tumour.

3. D. Discitis. This condition often presents late after the patient has had a number of normal investigations. This patient is at risk of sepsis, having diabetes and chronic renal failure. The X-ray image shows the typical features of long-standing discitis.

4. J. Cauda equina syndrome. This is a typical history. Bilateral symptoms are suspicious. Any patient with sciatica and new urinary or bowel disturbance should be investigated urgently.

5. G. Acute low back pain. Very common and usually resolves. Note the absence of leg pain.

6. A. Spondylolisthesis. Fast bowlers in cricket are at increased risk. The features seen on the X-ray image in this case are diagnostic.

Chapter 10 Altered sensation and weakness

Causes of peripheral upper limb symptoms

1. B. Cervical rib. Occurs in 1 in 200 people and may be bilateral. An extra rib from C7 (may just be a fibrous band) articulates with the first rib or may be free distally. This may cause vascular (subclavian artery) disturbance such as Raynaud phenomenon or neurological symptoms, normally in the distribution of C8/T1 dermatomes. The T1 myotome supplies the small muscles of the hand.

2. C. Pancoast tumour. An apical lung tumour has resulted in compression of the sympathetic nerves that arise from T1 and run up to supply the eye and forehead. This results in Horner syndrome (ipsilateral meiosis, ptosis and facial anhidrosis) on the affected side. The tumour is also compressing the T1 myotome.

3. F. Radial nerve palsy. The radial nerve runs in the spiral groove on the posterior aspect of the midshaft of the humerus. It is in direct contact with the bone at this point, which makes it prone to injury.

4. G. C6/C7 cervical disc prolapse. A disc at this level would compress the C7 nerve root, causing numbness and/or pain in the middle finger. C7 supplies the triceps and flexor carpi radialis and there is resultant weakness of elbow extension and flexion of the wrist.

5. E. Axillary nerve palsy. This man has sustained an anterior dislocation of his shoulder. The axillary nerve leaves the brachial plexus and winds around the surgical neck of the humerus to supply sensation to the army badge area over the upper lateral aspect of the upper arm, and motor function to the deltoid. This injury is normally a result of neuropraxia.

Chapter 16 Gout and Pseudogout

Gout and pseudogout

1. C. Haemarthrosis. This is a tense swelling that occurs after bleeding into the joint. The patient's history of atrial fibrillation suggests probable anticoagulation. These painful effusions often occur after seemingly trivial injuries.

2. B. Pseudogout. Intercurrent infections are a recognized trigger of attacks of pseudogout, which commonly affect the wrist joint. Osteoarthritis is another risk factor, as is the gentleman's elderly age. The blepharitis and asthma are not clinically relevant.

3. E. Reactive arthritis. Pain on micturition in a young man should prompt sexual health screening, because true urinary tract infections are rare in this age group. The larger joints of the lower limbs are often affected in reactive arthritis. Recurrent anterior uveitis suggests this gentleman may be human leucocyte antigen B27 positive.

4. A. Gout. The episodic nature of the pain, with redness and swelling suggests recurrent gout. First metatarsophalangeal joint involvement is the classic presentation of gout, but any joint can be affected. Ankles, knees and wrists often become affected as time proceeds if left untreated.

5. D. Psoriatic arthritis. Nail changes, swollen toes (dactylitis) and knee monoarthritis are all features of psoriatic arthropathy. Sometimes the joint disease can precede skin symptoms.

6. F. Septic arthritis. Diabetes can predispose to infection. The shoulder is not an uncommon site for septic arthritis: joint aspiration must be undertaken urgently to test for bacteria. Urgent administration of antibiotics is key and other supportive treatment should be given as needed.

Chapter 17 Paediatric joint disease

Paediatric joint disorders

1. I. Normal variant. This girl simply has knock knees, which are likely to improve with time. Concerning features would be asymmetry or pain on mobilizing.

2. A. Nonaccidental injury. Whilst many children sustain fractures falling off bikes and are shy when seen, multiple attendances and an inconsistent story should raise suspicion. The inconsistency here is that ulnar shaft fractures are commonly a 'defence wound' and would be odd to sustain falling from a bike and even less likely to happen twice in a year.

3. F. Perthes disease. This boy has findings consistent with Perthes disease on X-ray examination. This can commonly present with knee pain. Abnormal inflammatory markers would suggest possible septic arthritis.

4. D. Osgood-Schlatter disease. This manifests as severe pain at tibial tuberosity. It usually settles with rest and simple analgesia. Complete resolution is normal.

5. B. Cerebral palsy. Whilst this could fit with a clubfoot, the increased spasticity is not in keeping with this condition and fits more with a missed cerebral palsy.

Chapter 18 Fractures

Fractures

1. A.   Salter-Harris fracture. This is a fracture around the growth plate (physis) and these are common injuries in children.

2. C.   Pathological fracture. This is a fracture of abnormal bone. The history alone is suspicious of this. This poor man has developed lung cancer caused by smoking and now has metastasis to his right femur, which has been painful. This bone is therefore weak and low-energy activities such as walking result in fracture. Other primary malignancies that metastasize to bone are thyroid, kidney, breast and prostate.

3. F.   Compartment syndrome. This is unlikely to be a fracture because he could initially walk. Compartment syndrome can occur with or without fractures and this man needs urgent fasciotomy to the compartments (within 6 hours of onset). Absent foot pulses is a very late sign and usually indicates that the limb needs to be amputated.

4. G.   Nonaccidental injury. The history is not consistent with a healing fracture. Be very suspicious of any fracture in children under 2 years old. Take no chances, admit the child and inform the paediatricians.

5. D.   Open fracture. Any wound, no matter how small, on the same limb as a fracture should be assumed to be open until proven otherwise. This woman has a puncture wound from when the bone burst through the skin when it was severely angulated. This woman needs urgent debridement of the wound, stabilization of the fracture and antibiotics to help prevent chronic osteomyelitis.

8. Postoperative complications

1. G.   Epidural anaesthesia. The effect of this can last several hours (numb legs) and peripheral vasodilation causes pooling of fluid in the legs, which results in hypotension. Other causes must be sought before assuming that the cause of hypotension is the epidural, but all other parameters are normal in this case.

2. B.   Sepsis. This man is in septic shock and requires an emergency hip washout to treat his septic hip. He has risk factors for infection, including type 2 diabetes mellitus and steroid treatment (immunosuppression).

3. D.   Neurogenic shock. This man appears to have an isolated spinal injury based on his initial examination. This has resulted in loss of sympathetic tone to his legs and therefore hypotension. There is no evidence that he has any other injuries and therefore hypovolaemia secondary to blood loss is unlikely. In patients with spinal cord injury, this blood pressure reading is acceptable and intravenous fluids should be given cautiously to avoid fluid overload.

4. E.   Cardiogenic shock. This poor woman is having a myocardial infarction, confirmed on the EKG. This has caused left ventricular failure and therefore pulmonary oedema and hypotension. Thrombolysis is contraindicated as she is only 4 days postsurgery.

5. A.   Hypovolaemia. Intraoperative haemorrhage has resulted in hypovolaemic shock and this man's blood pressure has not responded to fluids. He requires an urgent blood transfusion in order to prevent further deterioration. Hypotension within the first 48 hours of surgery is usually secondary to hypovolaemia.

Chapter 19 Trauma

Trauma

1. A.   Tension pneumothorax. This occurs after trauma, creating a one-way valve in the lung or chest wall. This means that air flows into the chest cavity, but not out again, which collapses the lung, causing hypoxia. The mediastinum is displaced to one side, which reduces venous return to the heart and therefore cardiac output. This causes hypotension. This is life-threatening and requires immediate decompression with a large-bore needle (before chest X-ray examination is sought!), followed by insertion of a chest drain.

2. B.   Pelvic fracture. The mechanism here suggests that this poor man has had a heavy crush injury to his pelvis. Venous bleeding can be massive with pelvic fractures and can even be fatal. The man's hypotension and tachycardia are signs of hypovolaemic shock. Associated bladder and urethral injuries are not uncommon and this man may have either a ruptured bladder or a urethral tear, which would explain the blood at his urethral meatus and his inability to pass urine. He should have a retrograde urethrogram before attempted catheterization.

3. C.   Lumbar spine fracture/dislocation. This is a high-energy injury and the lumbar spine fracture dislocation is associated in this case with transection of the spinal cord. Therefore, there is no function below the level of the injury, including nerves to the legs and sacral nerves to the bladder and bowel. The prognosis in this case is very poor.

4. D. Wedge fracture lumbar spine. This is likely to be an osteoporotic wedge fracture. This is a low-energy fracture. It is also important to consider other pathological causes such as myeloma or bone metastasis from a primary malignancy.

5. F. Fracture of the seventh cervical vertebra. Unfortunately, the doctor has missed the diagnosis of a C7 fracture. This is because the X-ray images did not show the whole of the cervical spine. Adequate trauma X-ray examinations for neck injuries are anteroposterior and lateral showing C1 to the top of the first thoracic vertebrae and an odontoid peg view. This patient has a potentially unstable fracture from a significant hyperflexion injury and there is now compression of the right eighth cervical nerve root (learn dermatomes!).

6. G. Neck sprain. This is a classic case of a neck sprain. The damage to the car suggests that this is a low-speed crash and the delayed onset of pain is crucial in making the diagnosis. Patients with significant neck injuries (fractures or ligament tears) develop immediate pain. A neck sprain requires simple analgesia and neck exercises to prevent more stiffness from developing.

Chapter 20 Infection of bones and joints

Infection

1. E. *Haemophilus influenzae*. This used to be the most common cause of septic arthritis in infants but is now rare because of a successful vaccination programme. This unfortunate child's vaccinations are not up-to-date, however.

2. G. *Escherichia coli*. This woman has developed septic arthritis of her hip. This has resulted from haematogenous spread of bacteria to the hip from her urinary tract infection (UTI) and *E. coli* is a common cause of UTIs. Always look for a source when diagnosing septic arthritis.

3. C. *Mycobacterium tuberculosis*. Travel to India may have exposed this woman to tuberculosis, which has remained dormant for many years. This has now become activated, however, and caused collapse of one of her thoracic vertebral bodies, resulting in a gibbus (sharp angulated kyphosis). She will need an MRI scan and then biopsy of the lesion to confirm the diagnosis.

4. A. *Staphylococcus aureus*. This is the most common cause of septic arthritis and osteomyelitis. This girl seems to have developed spontaneous osteomyelitis, which will require antibiotics for 6 weeks and surgical debridement of the bone if indicated.

5. B. Anaerobic bacteria. This man has an open fracture that is potentially contaminated by cattle manure, amongst other things. Anaerobic bacterial and *Clostridium perfringens* (gas gangrene) infections are important to consider here based on the history. The fracture site should be irrigated and debrided urgently in theatre. Heavily soiled wounds should be covered with high-dose antibiotics, including an intravenous cephalosporin, penicillin and metronidazole. Tetanus prophylaxis should be given if vaccinations are not up-to-date.

Chapter 21 Malignancy

Joint and bone pain

1. A. Paget disease. The abnormal bony architecture and high alkaline phosphatase give the diagnosis.

2. C. Rickets. The history is typical for rickets, as are the clinical features and X-ray image findings.

3. D. Osteoporosis, presenting with vertebral fractures. The history with deformity and X-ray image findings point to osteoporotic vertebral fractures. The normal blood tests exclude pathological causes of fractures.

4. F. Leukaemia. The history of prolonged illness with aches and pains suggests a generalized disorder. The low WCC is also suggestive of a haematological disorder and a sterile hip washout makes septic arthritis very unlikely. Leukaemia occasionally presents with musculoskeletal symptoms.

5. H. Osteogenesis imperfecta. The history of spontaneous or low-violence fractures is typical. These cases are often initially diagnosed as nonaccidental injury but here the X-ray examination shows abnormal bone.

6. I. Osteoid osteoma. The history is typical, with intense pain relieved by nonsteroidal antiinflammatory drugs. The findings on X-ray examination and CT scans are typical.

Malignancy

1. A. Prostate metastasis. The history of urinary dysfunction suggests prostate. Metastases from prostate cancer are sclerotic (the others being lytic).

2. G. Osteosarcoma. Although rare, primary malignant tumours do occur in children and metastases are unheard of in this age group. The level of pain is suspicious but it is the X-ray image features that provide the diagnosis.

3. C.   Myeloma. The fracture under normal loads should raise suspicion. The X-ray features are typical of myeloma, as are the high ESR and skull lesions.

4. I.   Osteochondroma. The history is benign, of mild discomfort over long periods, and the X-ray appearance is typical of a benign lesion, in this case an osteochondroma.

5. F.   Breast metastasis. You were not told that she had a breast lump. She has a malignant spinal lesion causing spinal cord compression. The normal investigations exclude all the other potential sources of primary malignancy (except bowel carcinoma, but this rarely metastasizes to the spine), leaving breast carcinoma as the most likely.

6. B.   Lung metastasis. The history of smoking and an abnormal chest X-ray examination indicate the diagnosis.

Chapter 23 Sports injuries

Knee injuries

1. I.   Posterior cruciate ligament rupture. The history is typical, with a backwardly directed force on the tibia. The posterior sag is pathognomonic for posterior cruciate ligament rupture.

2. E.   Medial collateral ligament sprain. The history suggests medial ligament sprain and the fact that she could bear weight afterwards suggests a less serious injury. Tenderness at the joint line would indicate the meniscus but above is more likely to be medial collateral. The absence of an effusion excludes an anterior cruciate ligament rupture.

3. C.   Osteoarthritis. The history is typical for osteoarthritis with gradually increasing pain, a varus deformity and crepitus.

4. A.   Anterior cruciate ligament rupture. The history of a skiing injury and the patient hearing a pop or feeling something go are typical. The presence of an effusion makes it more likely. Often knees such as these are difficult to examine initially but later will have positive Lachman and pivot shift tests.

5. B.   Medial meniscal tear. The history of twisting injury, things settling but persistent niggling symptoms is typical. Joint line tenderness and an effusion also suggest meniscal injury.

6. J.   Patellar tendon rupture. In this case, the history is not helpful but examination findings of being unable to raise the leg straight with swelling and tenderness below the patella provide the diagnosis.

Painful joint

1. A.   Osteoarthritis of the first MTP joint (hallux rigidus). The pain in the toe-off stage is typical as the patient has lost extension. Walking boots can relieve the pain by minimizing this movement. Clinical features are typical of osteoarthritis anywhere, with osteophytes (dorsal bump) and crepitus.

2. C.   Reiter syndrome. A syndrome of arthritis, conjunctivitis and urethritis. It is more common in men but does occur in women.

3. I.   Psoriatic arthropathy. Commonly affects the hands, which can be significantly deformed.

4. D.   Septic arthritis. Can be a difficult diagnosis to make in the elderly. Her raised WCC and temperature point to an infective cause.

5. E.   Gout. Typical history and the usual joint. The serum uric acid is often normal during an acute episode.

6. G.   Ankylosing spondylitis. The condition tends to present in early adult life and the spine is commonly affected and stiffens, eventually ankylosing. The sacroiliac joints are commonly involved.

Lower leg pain

1. G.   Realignment surgery. This man is developing medial compartment osteoarthritis in his knee because of his varus deformity. This results in increased load through the medial part of the knee joint and therefore earlier wear. He is too young for a joint replacement but realignment surgery will correct his deformity so that there is less wear on the medial side. This will hopefully slow down the progression of his osteoarthritis, but he may require a joint replacement when he reaches a suitable age.

2. H.   Arthroscopy. This man has a locked knee secondary to a medial meniscal tear. The meniscus can get trapped in the joint and tears as the knee extends. The meniscus is not very vascular and therefore the bleeding is slow and swelling occurs over 24 hours. An arthroscopy will identify the tear and it can then either be repaired or excised.

3. C.   Unicompartmental knee replacement. This man has developed medial joint line osteoarthritis but his knee is otherwise well preserved. A unicompartmental knee replacement is designed to treat just the affected area of the knee. Its advantage over a total knee replacement is that it is a smaller operation and has a shorter recovery time.

4. F.   X-ray examination of the spine. The doctor has not properly examined this woman. The

changes detected on X-ray examination of the hip are very mild and would not explain the severe pain that this woman complains of. Numbness is more typical of neurological pathology and the fact that the hip has a good range of movement rules out major hip arthritis. This is more likely to be referred pain from the spine and a plain X-ray image may show degenerative change. Performing a hip replacement in this woman could be disastrous as it is a big operation and would not treat the pain.

5. D. Total knee replacement. This man has had a physical job for many years resulting in severe osteoarthritis of the knee. He cannot cope with his symptoms and further conservative treatment is not going to help. He should benefit from a total knee replacement.

Imaging

1. E. Nerve conduction study. The distribution of the pain is in keeping with a median nerve lesion. The diagnosis is carpal tunnel syndrome. This is associated with other conditions such as diabetes mellitus and pregnancy. This is usually confirmed with nerve conduction studies, but if the diagnosis is very obvious the surgeon may proceed to do a carpal tunnel decompression without them.

2. B. MRI. This woman has sciatica, most likely from a disc prolapse in her lumbar spine at the level of L5/S1. X-ray examination might show an obvious cause of the pain, such as osteoarthritis, but it is often unhelpful. MRI will provide detailed images of the soft tissues and vertebral discs. This is also a very useful investigation if sinister spinal disease such as malignancy is suspected. CT is very good at showing detailed images of bones, e.g., for assessment of a complex vertebral body fracture.

3. G. Venous Doppler scan. The leg might be swollen as a result of the surgery, but a total knee replacement puts the patient at high risk of deep vein thrombosis.

4. F. Ultrasound scan. This is likely to be a wrist ganglion. These are usually diagnosed clinically and excised if they cause problems, but if the clinician is unsure, an ultrasound scan is a simple, quick noninvasive test to provide more information. Ganglions are fluid-filled and therefore can change size depending on this. In the past, people were encouraged to bash them with a big book to rupture them!

5. C. Plain X-ray image. This man may have metastasis to his ulna or radial shaft and a plain X-ray image would normally show the diagnosis. Other malignancies that commonly metastasize to bone include thyroid, breast, lung and prostate.

Chapter 24 Principles of orthopaedic surgery

Orthopaedic gait assessment

1. B. Trendelenburg. This man has weakness of his left hip abductors and when asked to stand on his left leg, his pelvis tilts. This results in a Trendelenburg gait. Bilateral weakness of the abductors results in a waddling gait when the pelvis drops with each step.

2. E. Foot drop. The policeman has purposefully hit the man over his common peroneal nerve to disable him. This nerve is very superficial and winds around the fibula neck, supplying sensation to the dorsum of the foot and motor supply to the dorsiflexors of the toes and ankle. The patient lifts his foot high to prevent his toes dragging on the ground. Bilateral foot drop results in a high-stepping gait.

3. A. Ataxic. This boy has cerebral palsy secondary to meningitis as an infant. There is a loss of balance that is overcome by a broad-based gait.

4. D. Antalgic. Any painful condition results in an antalgic gait. This is characterized by a reduced-stance phase (less time is spent bearing weight on the affected side) during walking.

5. H. Spastic. This child has cerebral palsy. Children might display varying degrees of spasticity. Hip adductors contract, resulting in scissoring of the legs. The equinus deformity of his feet will also reduce function. He may benefit from complex surgery to correct the deformities.

Note: Page numbers followed by *f* indicate figures, *t* indicate tables, and *b* indicate boxes.